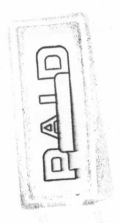

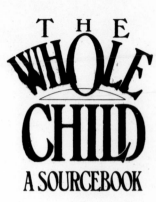

THE
WHOLE
CHILD
A SOURCEBOOK

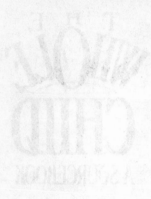

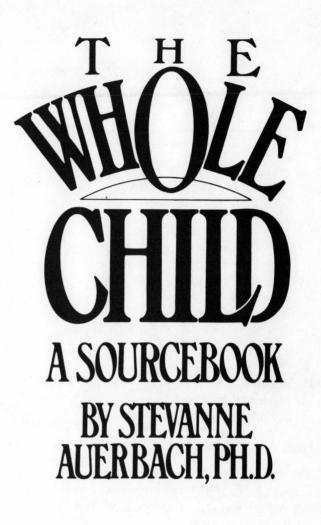

THE WHOLE CHILD

A SOURCEBOOK

BY STEVANNE AUERBACH, PH.D.

A Perigee Book

Dedicated to Amy Beth, with love.

Perigee Books
are published by
G. P. Putnam's Sons
200 Madison Avenue
New York, NY 10016

Library of Congress Cataloging in Publication Data

Auerbach, Stevanne.
  The Whole Child.

  Bibliography: p.
  1. Parenting.   2. Parent and child.
3. Parenting—Information services.
4. Parent and child—Information services.
I. Title.
HQ755.8.A83   1980   649'.1   80-6
ISBN 0-399-50554-7

First Perigee Printing, 1981

Printed in the United States of America

Contents

Special Contributors

Introduction

Having a child is very much like planting a garden. To cultivate a garden, you need good rich soil, sunlight, water and the time it takes to grow each of the plants. Plants, when they are young and tender, need your most loving attention. Recent research shows that plants respond to talk, stimulation and sensitivity. Children are no different. A young baby needs your tender touch, your sensitive voice and your loving responses. Children, as they grow, need understanding, guidance and direction, stimulation and support, and your knowledge about every facet of their lives. In this kind of environment, children will grow, respond and learn to respect others.

We suggest that you share your ideas, work, interests and feelings, and skills with your children. You will reap the rewards of their responses. Knowing that you are doing all you can to create a nurturing atmosphere, your children will thrive and blossom.

The suggestions given in *The Whole Child* are based on research conducted at colleges and universities that are interested in child growth and development. These studies give clues to various aspects of children's behavior: physiological and psychological, social and emotional. These studies are also teaching us much about the ways in which children progress through developmental stages. As adults, we should be aware of these stages and prepare for the different attitudes and responses, both of ourselves and of our children, characteristic of each stage. If we anticipate some of the difficulties children have, for example, when a sibling is born, we are prepared to assist the older child with his or her feelings.

Raising children is not something to be taken for granted or taken lightly. It is a lifetime responsibility. One of the most important decisions of one's life is whether to become a parent. *The Whole Child* has been created to provide you with as many resources as possible to give you assistance and make your role as a parent more enjoyable. Children are a delight (but not always). They can be a manifestation of our highest ideals. They provide us with an opportunity to expand our knowledge, personal understanding and to deepen our emotions. They allow us to create and expand ourselves and our relationships to each other. They also require from us patience, personal skills, and ability to give from our hearts.

Open your mind to new discoveries about children. Open your eyes to new possibilities and activities. Open your ears to new information and to feelings that you have not expressed before. Open your heart to allow the child in you to emerge and be reborn. Having a child can be the rebirth of yourself.

There are no limits when you are a creative parent. Creative parenting means being alert to new possibilities, expressing yourself openly and communicating your deepest feelings in an honest way. As your children go through different stages, try to relax, enjoy and take them in stride. The more relaxed you are, the better parent you will be. But also don't worry when you are feeling tense, tired or upset. Your child will usually understand. Love allows us to be human with each other after all.

Children need your guidance more than ever in today's high-pressure, constantly changing world. They need to know that there are special people who love and care about them. Children are a reflection of the mental health of our country. If our children are well cared for and happy, then family structure as a social entity is safe and secure. What we do affects our children, and what our children do affects us. Respect their need to question and to wonder and don't feel you need to know all the answers. Feel free to talk with your children's teacher or pediatrician, a social worker or another parent. Information and support are available to you if you know where to turn. The organizations listed in the back of the book will be helpful for additional information and referrals.

Most of all, trust your own judgment and feel comfortable with your decisions. You know what is best for your child. *The Whole Child* offers clues and information to assist you. The books that are included can help answer your questions and can help you trust and understand your feelings. If you are interested in reading beyond the books listed which are written for parents, we suggest that you go to your local college or university library and look at books and journals written for professionals.

A Note

The Whole Child will assist you, step by step, in the process of parenting and in preparing yourself, your home, and your environment for the changes that will take place from pregnancy to when your child reaches twelve years of age. We intend to give the help you need in this book, which includes information, resources, organizations, materials, books and many other contributions which we believe will be of value to you as a prospective parent. We have considered and included the needs of single parents, stepparents, parents who adopt children and others who work with families.

This sourcebook is designed to take you through the early stages of planning and into the care and raising of your child. It is a guide to books in child development, psychology, education, health and recreation and many other special books which have been produced over the years. We have found information that will make your job easier, more enjoyable and more productive. Most important, it will result in happier, healthier children.

Raising children is not always easy. We usually do not have adequate training for this most important responsibility. When parents do not know the answers, they need sources to turn to for assistance. Dr. Benjamin Spock's book was a comfort to me very often in my early years as a parent, especially when it was late at night and I hesitated to call the pediatrician. My sources for support and information expanded as my child grew, and so did I. I became aware of the wide diversity of other sources provided by many other specialists in pregnancy, birth, health, nutrition, education, recreation, psychology, television and the arts.

Early in my professional career, I attended many conferences and meetings related to parenting and child development. At such events, which were sponsored by organizations like the National Association for the Education of Young Children, National Education Association, Council for Exceptional Children, and the Association for Childhood Education International, I visited hundreds of exhibits of publishers, manufacturers and programs. I had the opportunity to learn firsthand about the newest materials. I collected information from teachers, manufacturers, and publishers, often wishing for a computer to store all of the data. The development of this book came as a result of gathering the information and finding a practical way to share it with you.

I believe that with accessible information and resources you will enjoy your role as a parent even more, and your child will be the beneficiary.

Being a parent is hard work. It is time-consuming and not always easy. However, it is fulfilling, exciting and rewarding in many ways. Feel good with your child, and your child will feel good with you. The adventure of parenthood is unique, and we hope that you will make it as exciting and rewarding as it can be. If you find our book particularly helpful, we would like to hear what information has been useful to you. You can also send additional information on publications and other resources you feel can help others at any time. This is our book to share and we hope you will share your experiences.

Write: The Institute for Childhood Resources
      1169 Howard Street
      San Francisco, CA 94103

Parents hold the responsibility and future of new life in their hearts and minds and open the doors of the world to their children. As children pass through these doors, we hope they will be prepared for full participation in the society of tomorrow.

We wish the children and their parents Happy Birthday and a safe and fulfilling journey, full of life's promises and love.

—The Editor

Acknowledgments

Compilation of this sourcebook for parents has not been unlike preparing for and having a baby (the first manuscript weighed ten pounds). It has been a long, rewarding and fulfilling process of learning, growing and listening. Many have contributed to the creating of this book—parents, teachers and, most important of all, countless numbers of children. Everyone has expressed his or her own experiences of childhood and parenting. With access to information, we feel parents can make better choices, gain confidence and assist their children in ways that more closely reflect the love they feel.

During the more than three years *The Whole Child* was in the making, many people contributed ideas, reviewed books, researched a specific area, typed and prepared copy. Everyone grew in his or her awareness of children and of the role of parents in the child's natural development. Those who participated came from many areas: education, psychology, journalism, health, social services and the arts. Men and women participated equally. The youngest staff member was twelve years old, the oldest seventy-five. I am grateful that I was privileged to share the creation of this book with these talented, committed and concerned people.

I thank personally all persons listed on the credit page for working as volunteers for whatever time they were able to give to the project. I am grateful to all the contributors who were so generous in their statements. I also thank David Charlsen, one of the great book designers, for his creative talent and full personal commitment. I appreciate the individual support of Marsha Bezan, Becky Bolin, Marlene Cresci-Cohen, Irene Cohn, Georgia Millor, Dena Reiner, Monique Rothschild, Jovana Rudisill, Reva Smilkstein, Carol Tarlen, and Mikki Wening.

I thank photographer Erika Stone, whose work has such enormous range and sensitivity. She has photographed children since her own were infants, and her extensive collection captures every nuance of children's activity. I also thank Suzanne Arms, a talented photographic journalist, for her inspiration and mutual support and for the days of sharing visions while we spent time together with our young daughters, Molly and Amy. I acknowledge Peter Simon, whose photographs I have admired for many years and who so perfectly reflects his love and understanding of children.

I want to express appreciation to all the large and small publishers who responded so generously with contributions of books included in this sourcebook. All the publications, as well as new ones, will continue to be on permanent display for use by parents, professionals and students at the Institute for Childhood Resources in San Francisco, California. The library of the Institute for Childhood Resources is a complete resource center housing books and information to assist parents. We hope with future funding to compile our research and resources on computer.

To Amy Beth, my incredibly special and wonderful daughter, I am grateful for what you have taught me about being a parent and for making all the challenges and learning so full of love. May you and the children of this world inherit a planet with greater vision and caring for its young. I also thank Nancy, Danny and David for the lessons and their love.

The *Sourcebook* was my personal dream. I am appreciative of the opportunity given me by Diane Reverand, editor at G. P. Putnam's Sons, who believed in and allowed me to create this book. I thank Gail Rivers for her inspired assistance.

A note of special tribute to Zvika Greensfield, L. A. Paul, Mark Pierce, Paul Silby, Ted Druch and Mark Zickel for their personal support and unique contributions to the completion of *The Whole Child*. Thanks to Marlene Posner for her editorial and professional contributions.

I also want to thank the many bookstores in San Francisco and New York that I visited and in particular the staffs at I. Gutenberg, Cover to Cover, Solar Light, Books Plus, and B. Dalton Booksellers.

My personal appreciation goes to Charles Flewellen of Bank of America. Lastly, my deepest thanks and respect to my mother, Jeane Sydney Rosen Stockheim, who taught me about parenting and thousands of other new parents as an instructor for The American Red Cross in New York City for so many years. It was she who inspired me to enter the professional field of child development and education.

Photo Credits

Suzanne Arms—pages 9, 15, 25, 29, 34, 37, 38, 64, 89, 168

Peter Simon—pages 3, 6, 17, 71, 90, 111, 123, 142, 148, 161, 165, 171, 180, 188, 224, 232

Erika Stone—pages 11, 13, 16, 21, 26, 39, 40, 48, 53, 57, 60, 63, 73, 77, 81, 86, 100, 115, 120, 128, 137, 156, 185, 195, 199, 202, 213, 219, 229, 238, 245, 249

Special Acknowledgments for Excerpts and/or Other Resources and Contributions

Action for Children's Television
Administration for Children, Youth and Families
American Academy of Pediatrics
Bantam Books
Jesse Bernard, author, *The Future of Marriage*
California Council on Children and Youth
Children's Bureau
Mary Calderone and Sex Information and Education
    Council of the U.S.
Florida Department of Education
Ron Goldman, M.D.
International Childbirth Education Association
La Leche League
March of Dimes Birth Defects Foundation
Mental Health Association
Metropolitan Life Insurance Company
National Association for the Education of Young Children
National Committee for Citizens in Education
National Organization for the Prevention of Blindness
Glen Nimnicht, creator Parent-Toy Lending Library
North American Center on Adoption
Parent's Magazine
Parents Without Partners
Ellen Peck, author *The Baby Trap*
Price/Stern/Sloan Publishers
Single Parent Magazine
State of Utah Office of Child Development
Marda Woodbury, gifted resource center librarian (San
    Mateo, CA)
and to all of the publishers listed in the Appendix who
    contributed books for this project.

If we have omitted anyone from these credits, we apologize. We have attempted to credit all sources and quotes, and acknowledge all participants and contributors throughout the book.

PART I

Planning and Having Your Baby

Parents must be like a tree:
They must have branches
Like open arms that welcome all
    their children.
A bark able to stand rain
Like tears and problems,
Storms and arguments.
Roots making a tree stand on its
    own and nourish itself,
Like the route you need to guide
    your child to independence.
Like leaves, you must explain to
    your child,
The changes he will go about
    during his life.
Parents must be able
To show their child the right path
    to the
Stem of a good life.*

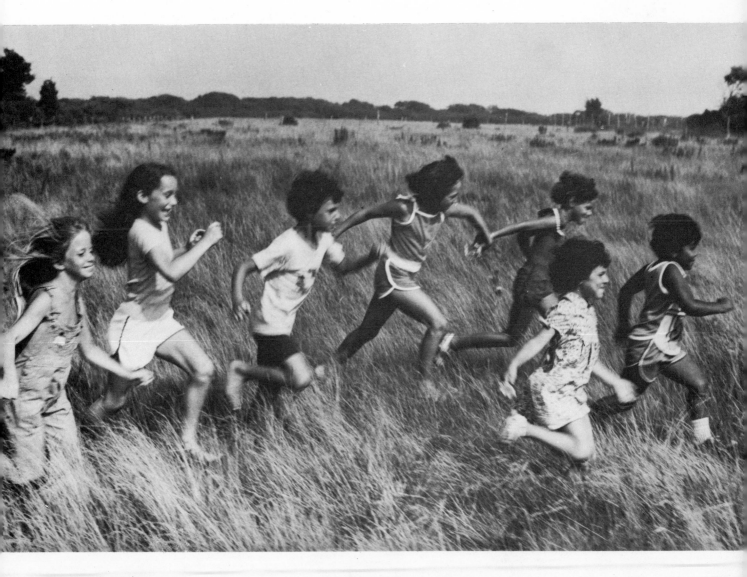

*From *How to Grow a Child: A Child's Advice to Parents*, edited by Bernard Percy, Price/Stern/Sloan Publishers

Preparation for Parenting

In preparing for parenthood, it is important to consider how children will fit into the total structure of your life. Being a parent is one of the most important tasks a person can undertake, not only for one and one's children, but for society in general.

If you are preparing for parenthood, then, you are making a decision that will affect the rest of your life. This is a decision that you must not take lightly. You are wise to think ahead about the responsibilities of having a child; what differences will occur in your life in terms of time and commitment and the planning and arrangements which have to be made. You need to consider your job, economic situation and the many facets of parenthood people often do not think about. It is important to consider these responsibilities seriously before the child is born, so that you have prepared yourself as well as possible. Preparation should take the form of accumulating monetary savings; for women, clarifying your job position with the boss as to maternity leave; being knowledgeable about your mutual wishes as to whether or not both parents should work and for how long before and after the birth. Both parents should be preparing for childbirth through classes, reading and other related activities.

It is preferable that your entire family be happy about and supportive of your pregnancy. Mothers and fathers can be extremely helpful if they feel that the baby is coming at a time when they can also participate in its care. If your parents believe that you should finish school, that you are too young, or this is not a good time (they may be right, but it is, of course, from their own experience that their opinions come), remember: only you and your mate should make the decision.

If you do not have a mate, you have a special set of challenges. You will need to have others in your family or friends who will support you during this period. Whether you are alone or not, it is easy to become blue or discouraged, and you may find yourself crying and sad at times, which is natural. Despite this, your pregnancy can be very exciting and happy. It is important to create supportive resources in your life; that includes family as well as friends.

Mothers-to-be should take a look at themselves. Take the time before pregnancy to explore yourself, your education, your career goals, your work experience and what you want for yourself in the future. If you are very much involved in a career, you may want to stop and think whether having a baby will reduce your chances for advancement and personal growth. If you feel that working part-time will be satisfying to you, then be sure to discuss this with your employer to find out whether part-time opportunities will be available to you, as well as the extent of time allotted for maternity or paternity leave.

In addition, exploring yourself on a personal level is very important. There are a number of courses and opportunities available to you; for example, at colleges and universities, consciousness-expanding groups such as est, transcendental meditation, gestalt therapy, rebirthing and others. The books suggested at the end of this chapter can serve as guides to your own self-development before and during your parenting experience. This is an appropriate time to put yourself on mailing lists for magazines and other materials that will be useful. The names of these publications and additional information you may need for preparation are included in this section. (If you find some information and ideas that assist you during this period which we have not mentioned, we would very much appreciate your writing to us.)

Having a baby is exciting; preparing for its arrival is the first step.

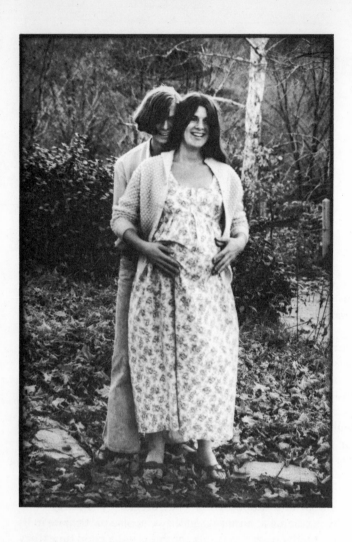

THE ULTIMATE INVESTMENT

The greatest gifts life has to offer are sound health and good relationships—with ourselves, our associates, our environment. Unfortunately both health and relationships are often undermined when we are totally dependent and most vulnerable: that is, during conception, pregnancy, birth and the first five years of life. Consequently, the largest portion of human suffering—illness, loneliness, delinquency, etc. would be greatly diminished if that period were lived in harmony and love. The well-being of the world depends largely on the quality of the relationship between parents or parent substitutes and their children. If they were to live in a loving state of consciousness, the benefit would be universal.

The most effective way to set in motion such an improvement is to initiate it as early as possible in the life of all individuals. A forty-year-old person has an average of thirty years to influence the world. But a new baby has a much longer time to do so. He can touch the lives of hundreds, even thousands of people. And he will touch them in a beneficent way if he is conceived, born and brought up in a welcoming, loving environment.

Laura Huxley
You Are Not the Target
Farrar, Straus & Giroux
1976   paper: $3.00

IDEAL PARENT

Ideal parents are such a rarity that we can practically say they are nonexistent. But a real possibility exists for each of us to be our own ideal parent. This is one of the most effective ways to improve our relationship with ourselves.

We often hear of the distress of parents who, having devoted all they had to the upbringing of their children, feel sadly disappointed by the results. Their vision of what that child could or should have become is shattered by reality. Just as often, the same disappointment occurs in children and adolescents. They too had an image of their ideal parents, an image that was shattered again and again. Mutual disappointment in each other often troubles the relationship between parents and children and consequently the relationship of each person to himself.

At any age the discovery that we can become our own ideal parents is momentous and improves all relationships.

First we must let go of dependence on our parents, whether they are present or absent, loved or unloved, living or dead. We may be unaware of this emotional dependence, which can be buried or on the surface, expressing itself either in rebellion against or in blind conformity to the parents' wishes, opinions and emotions.

Each of us has probably imagined the ideal father or the ideal mother he would like (or would have liked) to have. This father is a paragon of excellence. His qualities include a tremendous interest in and comprehension of ME. How proud *I* am of him! And how delighted with and full of praise for *me* he is! We imagine overhearing our father telling a friend what a wonderful human being his son or daughter is. When the ideal father is severe and even punishing, how justly so! We are even grateful for that just punishment because it is given in a way that relieves our guilt, rather than diminishing or discouraging our self-confidence. His fair punishment makes us feel more secure and ready to go ahead, having learned something very important which might otherwise have taken years and years to learn. This father, although a busy and important man, always has time if we need him, to answer questions, to discuss a viewpoint, to lend a hand in a project.

And our ideal mother? She glows with happy love for the only man who could have given her that very special child—ME! There is a constant unspoken alliance of mother and child to give the father more love, just as there is a constant and unspoken alliance of father and child to cherish and protect this unbelievably lovable woman. It is not necessary to tell her our fears, desires, uncertainties or dreams. She knows—and assuages, reassures and restores our confidence in ourselves and in life. We almost cry when we think of her tenderness. Yes, we cry, overwhelmed by emotion at the thought of our ideal parents. It is marvelous to have such a mother and father, and we are completely aware of our good luck.

It is a rare occurrence to have ideal parents. If you did, you don't need this recipe. I assume you belong to the great majority whose parents did the best they could, yet were not the ideal, the perfect parents. Even if they were endowed with the highest qualities, it would be almost impossible for a child to realize it: not having experienced the *absence* of something makes it difficult to recognize its *presence*. Whichever the case, looking for ideals is a high human privilege.

The fact that we look for ideal parents is not in any way to be interpreted as a criticism of our real parents. They did the best they could, having been brought up by their parents, under circumstances mostly unknown to us. Have we thought or tried to imagine how our parents were as newborn babies, as children, as adolescents? How *their* parents were acting and feeling? That time-space seems to us more distant than the moon—after all, we have seen the moon and we have seen *living* human beings walking on it. The records of our parents' infancy and childhood are scant in comparison, generally nonexistent. To criticize our parents, of whom we have such incomplete knowledge, such a one-sided view, would be unjust and unintelligent.

Laura Huxley
Between Heaven and Earth
Farrar, Straus & Giroux
1975   320 pp. $8.95

Am I Parent Material?

Here are some additional questions for you to consider before you deal with the important decision of whether to have a child. . . .

These questions are designed to raise ideas that you may not have thought about. There are no right answers and no grades—your answers are right for you and may help you decide whether you want to be a parent. Because we all change, your answers to some of these questions may change two, five, even ten years from now.

You *do* have a choice. Check out what you know and give it some thought. Then do what seems right for you.

Have my partner and I really talked about becoming parents?

1. Does my partner want to have a child? Have we talked about our reasons?

2. Could we give a child a good home? Is our relationship a happy and strong one?

3. Are we both ready to give our time and energy to raising a child?

4. Could we share our love with a child without jealousy?

5. What would happen if we separated after having a child, or if one of us should die?

6. Do my partner and I understand each other's feelings about religion, work, family, child raising, future goals? Do we feel pretty much the same way? Will children fit into these feelings, hopes and plans?

7. Suppose one of us wants a child and the other doesn't? Who decides?

Raising a child? What's there to know?

1. Do I like children? When I'm around children for a while, what do I think or feel about having one around all the time?

2. Do I enjoy teaching others?

3. Is it easy for me to tell other people what I want, or need, or what I expect of them?

4. Do I want to give a child the love s(he) needs? Is loving easy for me?

5. Am I patient enough to deal with the noise and the confusion and the twenty-four-hours-a-day responsibility? What kind of time and space do I need for myself?

6. What do I do when I get angry or upset? Would I take things out on my child if I lost my temper?

7. What does discipline mean to me? What does freedom, or setting limits, or giving space mean?

What is being too strict, or not strict enough? Would I want a perfect child?

8. How do I get along with my parents? What will I do to avoid the mistakes my parents made?

9. How would I take care of my child's health and safety? How do I take care of my own?

10. What if I have a child and find out I made a wrong decision?

(Prepared by Carole Goldman, Executive Director of the National Alliance for Optional Parenthood, 2010 Massachusetts Avenue N.W., Washington, D.C. 20036)

Costs of Children

Parents can raise loving and happy children with a variety of incomes. Money alone is not what is important in raising a child. A realistic assessment of your finances may be necessary, followed by a plan which is realistic.

We need to address the modeling parents do in the way they value and handle money. Personal awareness is important, as the way we consumers manage our dollars and communicate needs and priorities to each other may be mirrored by our children. Some of us operate as spendthrifts and others are overcautious; meanwhile, our children are taking it all in and reproducing our attitudes and behavior.

In this era of increasing inflation you should take a hard look at your financial situation, especially if you plan to stop working. Hospital births can cost anywhere from $750–$2,500 (depending on your area of the country and the type of services you opt for). Home births can range from moderate cost and up to $1,000.

Consider also that a baby may mean moving because of inadequate space or because your neighborhood isn't right for children. Calculate the mover's costs and the other costs of relocating.

Having the right insurance can help avoid financial problems. Tracy Hochner, in *Pregnancy and Childbirth*, recommends that it may be wise to take out a separate Comprehensive Major Medical Policy in advance of your pregnancy. Be sure that if you buy it through your employer and you stop working that you can convert to an individual policy and continue payments. Hochner warns: "Be sure that the policy covers all catastrophic health expenses: with a maximum of $20,000 or more. It should cover all complications of pregnancy, including the care of the unborn child and the newborn baby from birth. There should be no exclusion for laboratory fees, X-ray, anesthesiology, equipment, drugs, ambulance, or consultation fees."

Pregnancy and Childbirth: The Complete Guide for a New Life
Tracy Hochner
Avon
1979   689 pp. $6.95

This comprehensive book fills the need for a balanced presentation of all the aspects and options of pregnancy and birth. It is easy to read, medically accurate, and maintains a steadfast objectivity about the many volatile, controversial issues surrounding pregnancy and birth. Hochner provides the reader with down-to-earth questions and answers on such topics as: deciding to have a baby, financial considerations, prenatal testing, difficulties in conceiving, choosing a childbirth method, postnatal depression, sexuality, how to fix up your baby's room and choosing a pediatrician. She also includes a fetal development chart, vitamin chart, dangerous drug list, immunization calendar, listings of child health service regional offices, and much more.

First of all, let us consider what having a family actually costs you. The minimum amounts for essentials for a family continue to climb each year. Depending on where you live and how much you must manage on, the costs will vary widely.

You may begin by making a budget based on your income, expenses, additional costs of having a child, food, clothing, equipment, baby-sitters, toys.

Fill in Amounts for a Sample Budget

(Estimate your expenses)

Housing _____

Food _____

Clothing _____

Medical _____

Insurance _____

Transportation _____

Taxes _____

*Miscellaneous _____

Total _____

---

*Miscellaneous expenses might include: tuition for you and/or your children, union dues, laundry, vacation expenses, furniture payments, gifts, spending money for you and your mate, entertainment, babysitters, toys, etc.

Some of the Costs of Having a Baby

(During pregnancy)
Doctor office visits _____
Insurance _____
Maternity clothing _____
Midwife or hospital delivery _____
(After delivery)
Doctor office visits (mother and baby) _____
Baby clothing _____
Baby furniture _____
Total _____

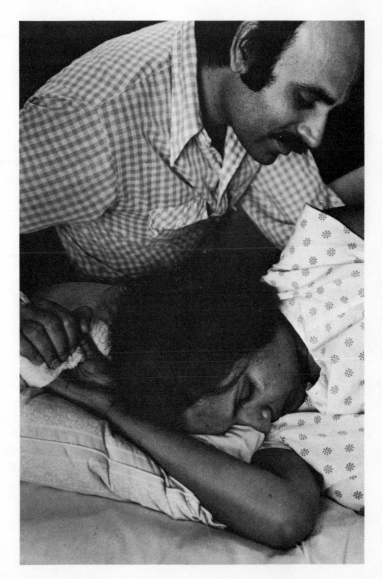

Begin to Explore and Discover Now, Before You Have a Child

Your Body

- dance
- yoga
- running
- tennis
- sports
- swimming

Your Mind

- reading
- talking and sharing with others
- pursuing educational goals
- career development

A Baby? Maybe
Elizabeth Whelan
Bobbs Merrill
1975   237 pp. $10.00

This book guides you in one of the most fateful decisions of your life. The author describes her own experience in deciding about parenting. Whelan spent a great deal of time interviewing couples who were both confirmed parents and nonparents. The book offers you an opportunity to examine your own parenthood puzzle.

If you're confused about the maybe of having a baby, be assured you're not alone. A lot of other people are confused with you. These days it's becoming more and more common to raise questions about this all-important issue. And some questions don't give rise to answers before they've given rise to more questions. Even if you're fairly sure you've made up your mind, you're likely to rehash why you decided one way or the other.

How to Bring Up a Child Without Spending a Fortune
Lee Edwards Benning
Doubleday (Dolphin)
1976   317 pp. $2.95

Ms. Benning has researched and produced guidelines on how to minimize the expenses involved in raising a child to the age of eighteen. With good humor, she presents commonsense advice on selecting clothing, food, furnishing the nursery, selecting a doctor, lessening the bills, toys, and schools.

SOME WAYS TO GET MORE THAN YOUR MONEY'S WORTH

1. *Start sewing. Make family clothing or draperies yourself. You can save from 35 percent to 50 percent of the cost of store-bought accessories.*

2. *Start a hand-me-down program with your friends and relatives. When kids outgrow their clothes, just start passing them around and ask that relatives and friends do the same. You can get some nice outfits this way.*

3. *Try good, old-fashioned do-it-yourself foods instead of pre-cooked or premixed.*

4. *Use a price gadget that determines cost per pound or unit when you food shop. It can tell you the best buys in a grocery store. It will help you compare prices and see whether you're getting cheated. You can find price comparers—simple or fancy—in your local department store.*

5. *Cut costs on recipes by using nonfat dry milk and water instead of milk, margarine instead of butter, skimping on the amount of ingredients when possible.*

Pregnancy

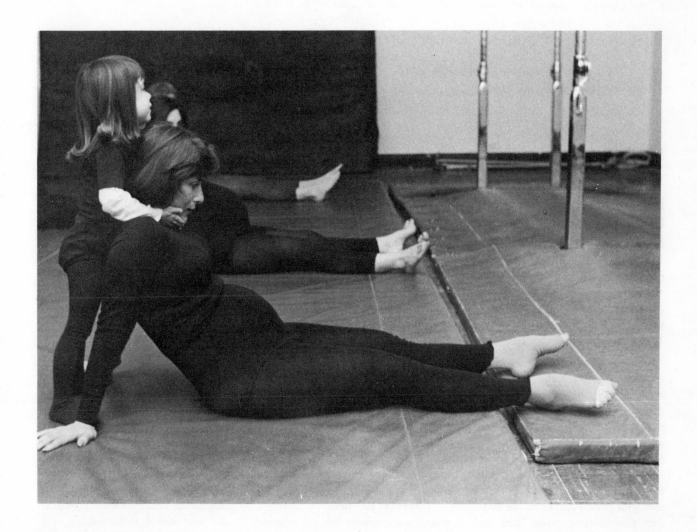

Discover Yourself

Many interests can be pursued as a parent and can provide for an enriching experience for you and your family. The point of self-exploration prior to parenthood is to give you an opportunity to get in touch with who you are as a person before you decide who you want to be as a parent.

Some Useful Resources in Self-Development

- est (Erhard Seminars Training)
- Actualizations
- yoga
- meditation
- contact your religious leader
- talk with a social worker
- enroll in courses in personal growth and development at a community college or community agency or organization
- see a psychologist or talk with friends, parents, teachers or your doctor.

To Experience Children, You May Want To Consider:

- volunteering to care for a friend's child
- joining Big Brothers or Big Sisters
- volunteering to assist with a scout troup or other organized group
- tutoring a child
- volunteering at a local childcare center or preschool

Books and Courses to Help You as an Individual

Est, 60 Hours That Transform Your Life
Adelaide Bry
Harper & Row
1976   96 pp. $1.95

Bry explains the specifics of est training—a method of introspection which teaches new approaches to living. Est participants, through the training, learn new ways to understand themselves and others.

Once we can detach ourselves from the belief that children must love and need parents all the time, and that parents must love and want the children always, once we accept that all feelings and experiences between parents and children are acceptable, then we can free ourselves and our children from guilt and dishonesty, and allow ourselves simply to be together. We can only love each other really when we can let each other be who we really are.

Your Erroneous Zones, Bold and Simple Techniques for Taking Charge of Your Unhealthy Behavior Patterns
Wayne Dyer
Funk and Wagnalls
1976   200 pp. $2.25

Dyer explores love: relationships, useless emotions, breaking barriers, changing the habit of procrastination, getting rid of anger and how to operate from "a clear place."

Dyer says "love" is only a word, and stresses the importance of allowing those you care for to be what they choose for themselves without any insistence that they satisfy you. By loving yourself, by feeling that you are important, worthy and beautiful, you won't need others to reinforce your value.

Actualizations: You Don't Have to Rehearse to Be Yourself
Stewart Emery
Doubleday (Dolphin)
1977   222 pp. $4.95

What I see many of us want from our children is for them not to be a problem. We call it being well-behaved. Well, for the most part, the way we see that children can cease being a problem is by being dead but still moving. When you stop to think about it, the adage that children should be seen and not heard is incredibly suppressive. We live in a society that is populated by adults who were told as children, "sit down and shut up," and "you should be ashamed of yourself"—"what's the matter with you anyway?"

CHILDREN AND PARENTS—WHAT THEY WANT MOST

Children want little more than to make a contribution to their parents' lives and will do literally anything to accomplish that. I remember vividly that in my own childhood I wanted to find out more than anything else how to do things in a way that would make my parents' lives incredibly wonderful. It was the context for everything I did, for a while.

I remember too that most, if not all the things I was told to do, seemed totally irrelevant to my purpose in life. What I wanted to do was not just find out about things, although that was useful. What I really wanted to learn about was how all the thousands and thousands of things I learned each day could help me to participate and contribute to life, which meant, of course, family life—my parents and me. If I could just arrange my experience in the right way, I could contribute, matter, make a difference in the lives of those I loved—my parents and my brothers and sister.

Of course, I also remember the frustration I experienced when most of the advice and counsel my parents gave me told me almost nothing about this vital concern. It seemed that most of the things they thought were important—staying out of the street, chewing my food, etc.—were irrelevant. Just not useful. Didn't they know what I was trying to figure out? Reluctantly, after many attempts to keep the hope alive, I concluded, almost in despair that they didn't know, that they had filled their lives with lots of rules about the right and wrong way to be, but apparently weren't working on what I was working on, which now years later, I would call contextualizing my experience of living.

If communication between us had been complete, which is what we both wanted, we might have found out then what we have since found out—that my parents were doing exactly what I was doing, attempting to contribute to me what they wanted most to contribute to me—the wisdom which would enable me to live a good life.

I have since "found out"—I would now say observed—that all parents and all children want precisely this— to contribute to the lives of those they love. Two things I know for sure are:

1. All I need do to have my child's fondest wish come true is acknowledge his or her intention for my life to be magnificent.

2. All my child needs to do to have his or her fondest wish come true is accept my intention for his or her life to be magnificent.

There is space for real satisfaction for parents and children who *know* each other so intimately.

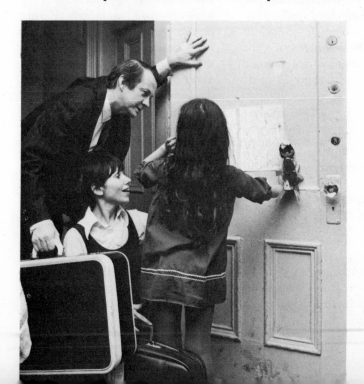

Werner Erhard
founder of est
Erhard Seminars Training

Sharing Roles
Working and Parenting

Ellen Peck, author of *The Baby Trap* (G. P. Putnam's Sons) and co-founder of the Consortium on Parenthood, offers some questions for a working woman who is considering having a baby. They are similar to those given in the last chapter under "Am I Parent Material?"

(1) Do I care about my job? (2) Do I care about maintaining or improving my present standard of affluence? (3) Do I have illusions about parenthood? (4) Do I have illusions about combining parenthood with my job? (5) Do I genuinely like and enjoy children of all ages? (6) Have I thought about the implications of parenthood deeply and carefully?

Can you continue working while you are pregnant? How does your employer provide for pregnancy and returning to work? Many women can juggle marriage, motherhood and a career, although it is often detrimental and exhausting. Being "Supermom" is not an easy task—child care is not readily available and is limited by inadequate numbers of licensed facilities. Finding a good baby-sitter is often difficult. (Child-care arrangements are discussed later in this sourcebook.) If you are able to have a full-time assistant at home, have a boss who is humane, a baby who is cooperative and a husband who is totally supportive, you have it made.

The Future of Marriage
Jesse Bernard
Bantam Books
1973   367 pp. $2.75

Bernard covers marriage today, past and future. The author feels that stereotyped thinking defines or limits the possibility of choices. The role of the housewife and mother, both in terms of self-perception and the perception of others, is one of the more important areas discussed.

Bernard explores the "should I have children" question, saying that:

Parents undoubtedly do love their children, but parenthood is not for everyone a fully rewarding experience. When, in addition, there is no special praise forthcoming for having children, there will be less socially induced sense of frustration for not having them. The wave of the future does not, however, seem to be childlessness, so much, of course, as just smaller families.

In an article entitled "Becoming a Mother, Should I" (*Working Woman*, July 1977), Amy Gross writes:

You have established yourself in a job that is meaty enough to engage you and you can rest at that plateau for the next few years, letting your career carry you along on its own energy. Some mothers do not want the responsibility of taking care of a child all day every day. They say, "I love Saturdays, having the whole day together, but by Sunday, I'm ready to go back to the office." This split between office and family, which has defined men's lives, is disturbing to some women.

Preparing for Parenthood
Lee Salk
Bantam Books
1975   211 pp. $1.95

Salk takes a firm stand on the position that parenthood means both motherhood and fatherhood —being a parent is not solely a female responsibility.

While bringing up children is an enormous task entailing a lot of hard work and much tedious activity, there are also tremendous pleasures involved. Males raising a child and influencing the kind of person he or she will be. . . .

With the confirmation of his wife's pregnancy, the father should begin participating actively in learning the same things that the mother learns about prenatal care and childrearing practices. . . . I have observed that fathers who are present when their children are born generally have a far greater sense of the importance of fatherhood than those who are excluded during the dramatic moment.

To date, little has been done to provide flexible working hours for parents of children under the ages of three; little effort has been made to accept family needs as being at least as important as the needs of industry or government; little effort has been made to provide the kind of parent education that is necessary to prepare people for the enormous responsibility of bringing another human being into this world. . . .

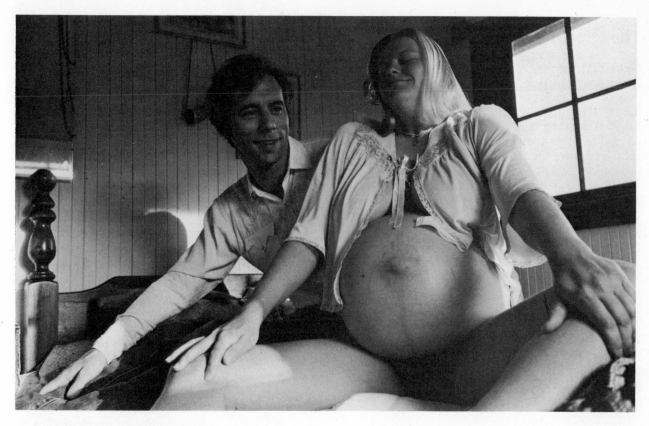

Rooming-in arrangements (for childbirth) also encourage the kind of early contact between a father and his family that serves to get fathers really involved in childrearing. The more contact the father has with his baby during the hospital stay, the easier it will be for the whole family when the new baby comes home. If, in the hospital, the father held his baby, burped his baby, and cared for him in other ways, the father's resulting sense of confidence will bring him increased joy in being a parent and his experience will lighten the load on his wife when she needs help later on. Many hospitals offer classes to mothers on bathing, feeding and dressing babies during their hospital stay. I think another set of these very same classes should be made available to fathers because I am convinced that it is far better for a hospital to teach these skills to fathers than to expect a new mother to teach the father after the baby gets home.

So, You're Going to Be a New Father
Administration for Children, Youth and Families
U.S. Government Printing Office
Publication No. (OCS) 73-28
1973   35 pp.   50¢

A simple, thorough discussion for expectant fathers of what to expect during pregnancy.

The mother needs to be protected against falls and similar injuries, but she does not need to be kept from normal activity, unless that includes sky diving or operating a jackhammer. . . .

Expectant Fathers
Sam Bittman and Sue Rosenberg Zalk
Hawthorn Books
1979   277 pp. $12.95

Child-rearing used to be a strictly female province, and the needs of the father who wanted to be an active participant in the pregnancy were ignored. This book explores the feelings, defenses and changes in the man involved in a pregnancy. Chapters deal with sex, jealousy, in-laws, fathers' rights, labor, home birth and more.

Parenting is not a solo routine unless necessity forces it to be. It can be a team effort, a partnership that requires discussion and even practice to smooth out patterns well in advance of the birth of the baby.

The Older Mother

New York gynecologists and obstetricians David James and Frederick Silverman estimate that 15 percent of their practice consists of women over forty having their first babies. "All our over-forties took pains to develop in their careers, then married and wanted to fulfill the motherhood role. And having a child revitalizes them—you don't feel that you're becoming menopausal," says James.

However, a woman of thirty-five has a one-in-200 chance of having a child born with Down's syndrome (mongolism). A woman of thirty-seven has a one-in-100 chance, a woman of forty one in 50, and a woman of forty-four one in 20.

Amniocentesis, a test that determines if the child will be born with any birth defects, is being used routinely on women over thirty-five. James says, "Today a woman over forty gets much more concerned prenatal care. She undergoes more frequent testing. Consequently, she has a very good chance of having a healthy child and ending up healthy as a mother."

The psychological prognosis is also good. Eleanor Rutstein, a New York clinical psychologist and an older mother herself, says, "An older mother may be more secure in mothering than a younger one. If she decides to have a child, it's because she wants it very much. It's often easier for older mothers to be more sensitive to the needs of a child. This sensitivity often comes with maturity and wisdom and an acceptance of who you are."

Up Against the Clock: Career Women Speak on the Choice to Have Children
Marilyn Fabe and Norma Wikler
Warner Books
1980   291 pp. $2.75

Nearly one million women now in their 30's are approaching their biological deadline for having children. Fabe and Wikler provide one forum on the pros and cons of having children for women over thirty. Interviews with ten women who have made their decisions examine combining children and careers, going it alone as a single mother, choosing to be childless, and making up your mind. Practical questions are explored: What about my biological clock? How will a child affect my relationship with my mate? Can I successfully raise a child and still move forward in my career? What are the costs of raising children? What is proper day care? What about adoption?

Difficult as the choice of motherhood may be, it should be confronted head-on. Clearly, it is better to reach an enlightened decision by grappling with the complex problems involved than to risk finding oneself childless by "default" or in a "panic pregnancy."

The Pregnancy After 30 Workbook
Gail Sforza Brewer
Rodale Press
1978   233 pp. $8.95

Brewer offers a comprehensive program for the mother-to-be over thirty. Contributions from a physiotherapist, psychiatrist, obstetrician, natural-childbirth instructor, nursing mother and psychologist map out a program which covers the "No-Risk" Pregnancy Diet, exercises, emotional aspects, risks and what to do about them, breast-feeding, cesareans and other topics pertinent to the mother over thirty.

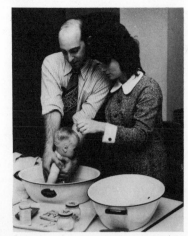

For example, the mother over thirty often has a well-established career and wants to keep it, and to her, nursing and full-time motherhood, even for a short time, may seem a great disadvantage. For those mothers who will nurse only with resentment, bottle-feeding offers a better solution.

I had to go back to work six weeks after my son was born. At first I came home at lunchtime to nurse him; later I found a babysitter near work and nursed him there. It worked out very well.

You Are Not Too Old to Have a Baby
Jane Price
Penguin Books
1977   147 pp. $2.95

Dispels many myths about late childbearing and presents an encouraging, yet honest discussion of the medical risks involved and the problems of the working mother.

CONSCIOUS CONCEPTION

When the decision to create a human life is taken, conscious conception is often experienced. As one woman expressed it, "You feel both the tranquil and dynamic waiting of the egg and the compelling race, the fundamental need of the sperm. You feel the sperm wiggling upstream, daring and overcoming all obstacles. It is very beautiful to feel the duality of egg and sperm, and the explosive 'becoming one'—like a burst of illuminated energy to match the most effulgent sunburst you have ever witnessed."

By consciously experiencing the moment of conception, women may bring about an evolutionary leap as momentous as the transformation which took place when we grew from four-legged to erect posture.

How do we know what tremendous enrichment a human being may derive from the attention and love bestowed upon him at the moment of conception?

Jean Houston
Listening to the Body
Delacorte
1978   249 pp. $4.95

Pregnancy and Mother Care

You should prepare early to get your body into the best possible condition prior to becoming pregnant. If you are overweight, it is important to discuss reducing with your doctor. Diet, rest and other personal habits are very important; exercise, refrain from smoking cigarettes, drinking alcohol, taking drugs, and the like. After all, the body, for the first nine months, is the home of the unborn child, and it is through the placenta that the child is nourished. It is essential, therefore, that the condition of the body be as well tuned as possible.

The combination of wanting a child and adequate preparation is the key to having normal, healthy babies.

During Pregnancy

- eat well
- get plenty of rest
- exercise
- do not take any drugs unless prescribed by doctor
- read
- talk to other mothers and fathers
- learn about the care of a baby
- spend time with a friend's or neighbor's baby as often as you can

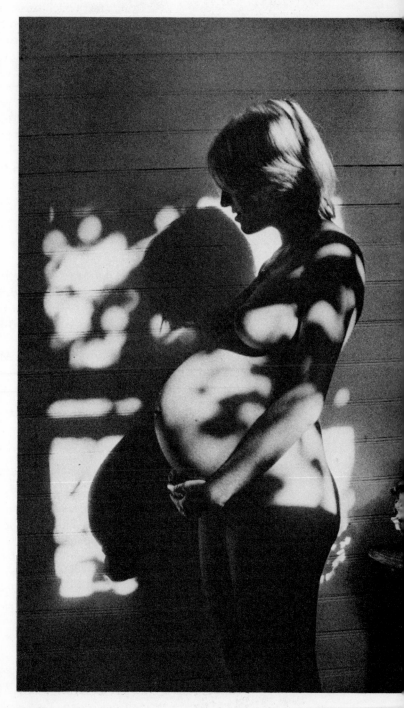

The Single Mother

A Guide to Pregnancy and Parenthood for Women on Their Own
Patricia Ashdown-Sharp
Vintage Books
1977   200 pp. $3.95

This comprehensive guide tells you how to make certain you are pregnant, arrange for birth, put a child up for adoption or in a foster home, find the financial and emotional assistance available to single mothers in your state, choose the best contraceptive for you and much more.

As with everything else, there is a system to pregnancy and parenthood outside marriage. With sufficient information, you can learn how to make that system work for you, or help change the system where you find it operating against you and others in a similar position.

Life Before Birth
Ashley Montagu
New American Library
1955   248 pp. $1.95

The author, a renowned anthropologist, says "life begins, not at birth, but at conception, and what happens in the interval between conception and birth is very much more important to our subsequent growth and development than we have, until recently, realized." He deals with such topics as nutrition, maternal age, drugs, disease, stress, radiation and X-rays.

A Child Is Born
Lennart Nilsson
Dell
1977   160 pp. $11.95

Expectant parents or wide-eyed students of the facts of life will love this colorful, easily read text which surveys the entire birth cycle of humans. Starting with the union of the two parent cells and progressing through fetal development, the author parallels the internal development with external events, such as prenatal care and how to prepare for the baby. The fetus is revealed in unique *in utero* photographs yielding vivid detail. The author says that "For the first time, people outside the research laboratories are able to share this knowledge."

A Motherhood Book: Adventures in Pregnancy, Birth, and Being a Mother
Joan Wiener and Joyce Glick
Macmillan
1974   126 pp. $1.95

This book is about motherhood as seen through the lives of two women and their experiences during and after pregnancy. The authors have included a guide to information on natural childbirth, breast-feeding, prenatal and postnatal care.

In the midwife/mother relationships I am familiar with, the emphasis is placed on cooperation, a joint effort of the midwife and the woman in labor. They are doing something together. Whereas in most deliveries by doctors, the relationship is authority/layman— the doctor is doing something to the mother, who, in a good many cases even today is still induced, anesthetized, barely functioning.

Joyce said if she had been aware of this factor before Danielle's birth, she would have sought an alternative. "If I'd have known my childbirth was only going to last a couple of hours, I probably would have forgotten the whole trip of rushing off to a hospital, having some uptight nurse sticking her fingers up me while I was having a contraction and just have laid back in my vegetable garden, Marc at my side, maybe a few close friends, sunshine, good vibes, and have had a much more 'natural' birth. But while I was pregnant, I was magnetized. I followed the crowd to a doctor I'd heard of who would deliver a baby without using drugs and this was the right way for me to have it done at the time. I hadn't heard of midwifery at the time or much about home delivery."

Pregnancy, Birth and You
Linda B. Jenkins
Published by Linda Jenkins
1978   110 pp. $3.95

An objective presentation of a wide variety of topics important to expectant couples: alternative birthing, traditional birth methods, fetal monitoring and often-ignored subjects such as sexual intimacy during pregnancy. Also included are a useful bibliography, diagrams, and summary charts of anesthesia, labor and delivery.

Touching is essential to life and living. While a delightful aid to relaxation, it can also be a source of sexual gratification. . . . How wasteful to lose the beautiful moments of pregnancy which may occur only once or twice during a lifetime. Use this time to the fullest to enjoy the growing child resulting from your intimacy.

Pregnancy, Birth and Family Planning
Alan F. Guttmacher
New American Library (Signet)
1973   407 pp. $2.50

A complete, direct volume, this paperback's coverage starts with the moment of conception and ends with the basics of newborn care.

A Season to Be Born
Suzanne Arms
Harper & Row
1973   112 pp. $4.50

This light, airy picture essay shares the feelings and a few woman-thoughts during pregnancy and the birth of Molly.

I wrote Mother all about my interest in Natural Childbirth. She thinks I'm crazy. "Any kind doctor," she says, "would want to put you out so you wouldn't suffer."

Feeling lumpy today. Lopsided. I always thought pregnant tummies were perfectly spherical. Well sometimes it's just not so.

It's a nice feeling knowing that this baby is one thing in my life that I can't force or organize or schedule. I just have to let it happen. The baby isn't going to be born till it's ready. I'd like my whole life to be like that.

See Appendix film resources for information on Suzanne Arms' film.

A Shared Journey—The Birth of a Child
Donni Betts
Celestial Arts
1977   74 pp. $3.95

This book addresses the great complexity of feelings which surround the birth of a child. With remarkable clarity and warmth, Donni Betts creates a portrait of her

pregnancy—"the emotional highs and lows, the seemingly inexplicable fears, and excited anticipation that envelop and sometimes overwhelm a woman expecting her first child."

That New Baby: An Open Family Book for Parents and Children Together
Sarah Bonnett Stein
Walker
1974   46 pp. $6.95

This book was developed in cooperation with the Center for Preventive Psychiatry; it is designed with texts and photographs for the adult and the child, all aimed at helping a child adjust to the addition of a new family member.

Sooner or later a child asks: "Who do you love the most?" It is honest to tell your child that is a question no mother, no father, can answer. Mommies and daddies don't love one child more than another. They love each the most in a different way. They notice what each child is like; they help him grow into the kind of person he is best at. And that is what they love.

David, We're Pregnant!
Lynn Johnson
Meadowbrook Press
1975   107 pp. $3.45

Lynn Johnson reveals a lighthearted view of pregnancy and birth in this cartoon collection. Every facet—from sex, morning sickness and postpartum soreness to settling in as a family—is covered.

Making Love During Pregnancy
Elisabeth Bing and Libby Coleman
Bantam Books
1977   165 pp. $5.95

Taken by trimester, sexual activity of expectant couples is revealed through brief personal accounts.

Every couple should discuss sexual activities during their pregnancy with their doctor; in fact, communicating during this period is of utmost importance.

Prenatal Care
U.S. Government Printing Office
1973   72 pp.   75¢

A pamphlet for pregnant women covering personal hygiene, health maintenance, physical symptoms, mood changes, complications, being in the hospital, giving birth and taking care of the newborn baby.

In The Beginning: Your Baby's Brain Before Birth
Mortimer G. Rosen and Lynn Rosen
New American Library (Plume)
1975   143 pp. $3.95

Chapters detailing the physiologic development of the brain, how the environment affects the fetus's brain, the effects of different delivery methods and the infant's life after birth make this book fascinating reading, providing

. . . information which will remove fears and ignorance, . . . information that will make the first nine months of life not only more knowledgeable, but also more enjoyable. And, it is our desire to interest patients and physicians in more study and concern with in utero growth and development of the brain prior to birth.

Chromosome 21 and its Association with Down's Syndrome
March of Dimes Birth Defects Foundation

This free pamphlet, which explains the relationship between cellular irregularities and Down's syndrome, a common birth defect, also illustrates the physical effects of this disease.

Your Baby's Sex: Now You Can Choose
David M. Rorvik and Landrum B. Shettles
Bantam Books
1971 114 pp. $1.95

This work is a comprehensive home guide to assist parents in choosing their children's sex prior to pregnancy.

A method of sex selection has been developed and is at our disposal. For the first time in all time, parents have the opportunity to make a scientific attempt with a justifiably high expectation of success. The procedures involved are safe and simple, and nothing about them is morally or ethically objectionable.

For Children

We're Going to Have a Baby
Doris Wild Helmering and John William Helmering
Abingdon
1978 130 pp. $6.95

A well-written, colorfully illustrated story for young children. "With the announcement of the coming of a new baby in the home, many children experience a myriad of feelings. This book is written to

let your child know that all feelings, both positive and negative, are okay."

My Childbirth Coloring Book
Laurence K. Scott and David Baze
Academy Press
1978 32 pp. $2.95

Happy, lively drawings for young children to color join a clear, natural-sounding narrative presenting the basic facts of life from a child's point of view. A short glossary explains unfamiliar words in simple language. For example:

ovum: a mature female cell capable of joining with a sperm to produce a baby; genitals: the parts of people's bodies that help create babies.

Making Babies
Sarah Bonnett Stein
Walker
1974 47 pp. $7.95

Making Babies is an educational book with a unique format. One narrative is aimed at helping the parents understand and deal with the perceptions a young child may have about reproduction; the second, in larger, child-sized print, explains the fundamentals of reproduction to young children. Stein assumes that the book's effectiveness is limited without the extra parental insight to anticipate certain questions and perplexities on the child's part. For example,

Each of these pictures shows dogs enjoying each other's company in one way or another. Talk to your child about each one. If you get to one that bothers you, try not to slur over it. If more formal words like "intercourse" feel awkward, you can use "make love" to mean the same thing.

For further information you can contact the following organizations (addresses are in Appendix A)

- American Association of Marriage and Family Counselors
- American Home Economics Association
- American National Red Cross
- Federation of Planned Parenthood of America, Inc.
- International Transactional Analysis Association
- Jewish Board of Family and Children's Services
- National Council on Family Relations
- National Forum of Catholic Parent Organizations
- Profession of Parenting Institute
- U.S. Department of Health and Human Services
- United Synagogue of America

These magazines carry relevant articles of interest to parents (See Appendix B)

- *Marriage and Family Living*
- *Parents' Magazine*
- *Redbook*
- *Working Mother*
- *Working Woman*
- *Young Children*
- *Young Mother*

Drugs, Diet, X-Rays and Illness

During the first trimester of pregnancy, the developing baby is most sensitive to drugs, X-rays, disease, lack of essential nutrients and medications. Drugs taken by a pregnant woman can cause abnormalities in the baby such as blindness, deafness, malformations and small size. Women who take Valium are four times more likely to have babies with cleft lips or cleft palates. Thalidomide was a drug which created malformations in babies. Babies can be born addicted to medication.

Spinal injections given to relieve a mother's pain or discomfort during labor pass through the placenta to the baby and may interfere with early bonding processes so necessary following the birth. A year after delivery, babies whose mothers received medication during labor showed poorer performance on standard tests than babies born from undrugged mothers.

The fetus depends on the mother for all vitamins, minerals and nutrients. Severe protein shortages in early pregnancies have caused fetal brain damage. The mother also confers on her baby immunity to a number of diseases. Antibodies are manufactured by her immune system and circulate in the baby's bloodstream as well.

During pregnancy, a woman undergoes many physical, emotional and metabolic changes, which influence her attitudes and feelings toward her pregnancy. These changes largely determine her experience. Good health and serenity are particularly vital during this time and bear a direct relationship to the new life developing within.

Be Good to Your Baby Before It Is Born
March of Dimes Birth Defects Foundation
1977   20 pp.   free

Keeping well during pregnancy, feeling good about yourself, exercise and care of the body, rest and sleep, bathing, care of teeth, smoking, alcohol, clothing and makeup, travel and weight gain are the concerns of this pamphlet, which suggests:

Get sufficient sleep during the night, have rest periods during the day. Be sure to lie down with your feet up as much as possible; wear a good brassiere with support that is not binding; wear comfortable clothing; exercise (do yoga and stretching exercises); take warm baths every day; take care of your teeth during early pregnancy; quit smoking long before you become pregnant as it is essential to your well-being and the well-being of your child; do not drink alcohol or coffee during the pregnancy, as it is damaging to your new child's health and well-being. This is a wonderful time to make comfortable clothing for yourself—your maternity clothes can be attractive; walking and swimming are particularly good exercises, as they help digestion and circulation; take trips as often as you wish; be careful about crossing your legs so that the circulation won't be cut off.

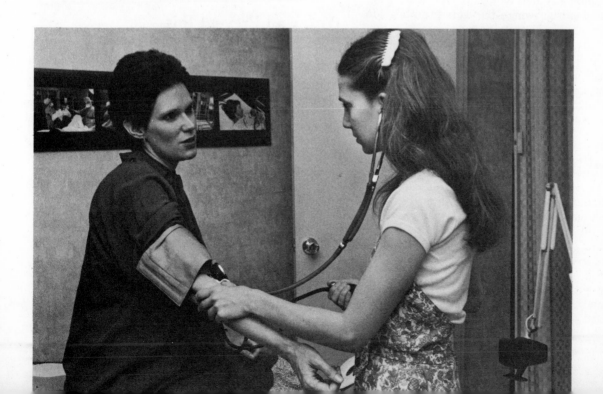

When You Drink, Your Unborn Baby Does, Too*

When you're pregnant your unborn baby receives nourishment from you. What you eat, he eats. What you drink, he drinks.

So if you have a drink—beer, wine, or hard liquor—your unborn baby has a drink too. And because he is so small, he is affected twice as fast as you are.

That's the immediate effect. But alcohol can also have serious long-lasting effects on an unborn baby.

How Alcohol Damages Unborn Babies

Scientists have found that many children born to women who drink excessively while pregnant have a pattern of physical and mental birth defects. They call the more severe problems the "fetal alcohol syndrome."

Growth deficiency is one of the most prominent symptoms. Affected babies are abnormally small at birth, especially in head size. Unlike many small newborns, these youngsters never catch up to normal growth.

Most affected youngsters have small brains and show degrees of mental deficiency. Many are jittery and poorly coordinated, and have short attention spans and behavioral problems. Evidence to date shows that their IQs do not improve with age.

Many Babies Are at Risk

Fetal alcohol syndrome is a very real problem in the United States today. It is estimated that there are more than one million alcoholic women of childbearing age. And the number is growing—particularly among adolescents.

Babies of teen-agers who drink heavily are in double jeopardy. They may be born too small or too soon because their mother's bodies are not mature enough to meet the demands of pregnancy. If they also are subjected to excessive alcohol from their mothers, they may suffer some symptoms of fetal alcohol syndrome.

We Need to Know More . . .

Scientists know that, as with other things pregnant women eat and drink, alcohol passes through the placenta, the organ which nourishes the unborn baby. The drink the baby gets is as strong as the one the mother takes.

It is believed that the alcohol adversely affects the baby's fast-growing tissues, either killing cells or slowing their growth. Because the brain develops throughout pregnancy, it stands to reason that it is the organ most affected by maternal drinking.

Is It Fair to Force Your Baby to Smoke Cigarettes?

Babies who are born undersized and underweight can be off to a bad start. A follow-up study of 17,000 British children who were born in the same week showed that newborns who were "small for date" had more educational and behavioral problems in later life compared with those of normal birth weight. At age seven, youngsters who were undersized infants had poorer social adjustments in the family and school.

Nevil Butler of the University of Bristol is now completing further followups on these 17,000 youngsters at age 11. According to Butler, one of the major factors influencing the size of the newborn was cigarette smoking by the pregnant woman. The crucial period in the pregnancy was the last five months. There was no difference in low-weight babies and stillbirths between women who did not smoke cigarettes and women who smoked for the first four months. However, if women continued smoking for the last five months, a significant difference occurred in the number of undersized infants as well as babies born dead.

Recent experiments with pregnant rats have also shown that fetuses removed from mother rats who were exposed to cigarette smoke were not only undersized but had smaller brains. Though the human brains were not measured in the Butler research, one of the characteristics of a "small for date" baby is a head circumference of below normal size. Another characteristic of small infants is a high rate of oxygen consumption for body weight.

You Can Prevent this Birth Defect

Fetal alcohol syndrome is a tragedy. An even worse tragedy is that it *doesn't have to happen!*

If you are a woman of childbearing age, *you can prevent* birth defects caused by excessive use of alcohol.

If you're pregnant, don't drink. If you drink heavily, don't become pregnant.

If you can't stop drinking on your own, seek help before you become pregnant.

---

* Reprinted with permission of March of Dimes Birth Defects Foundation.

A Nutritious Balanced Diet During Pregnancy

Every day of the week you and your baby must have:

- one quart of milk (any kind will do; whole milk, low-fat, skim, powdered skim, or buttermilk; whole milk is best)
- one (or two) eggs
- one or two servings of fish or seafood, liver, chicken, lean beef, lamb or pork, beans, any kind of cheese
- one or two good servings of fresh green leafy vegetables (the darker green the better)
- a generous portion (or two) of fresh citrus fruits and/or freshly opened can of tomato juice, lemon juice, lime juice, orange or grapefruit juice
- one pat of butter or margarine (more if you can stand the calories)
- other fruits and vegetables (approximately 6 helpings per day)
- after you are sure you are going to have all the above, enough whole-grain bread or toast (no preservatives; sweetener—honey) to produce energy for the day's work (and none extra to make you overweight)

Also include

- one serving of whole-grain cereal such as oatmeal or granola
- one yellow- or orange-colored fruit or vegetable five times a week
- liver once a week
- whole baked potato three times a week

These Drugs Could Harm Your Unborn Baby *Do Not Use**

alcohol
antacids
aspirin
cigarettes
coffee
hormones
iodides
laxatives
medicated salves
nose drops
ointments

*Unless prescribed by your doctor.

Minestrone (8 servings)*

Minestrone can be an exceptionally pretty soup if you use a variety of vegetables. Start with the basic soup and vary by using any number of fresh, frozen, or canned vegetables. Add them so they will be just done at serving time. Chopped greens and sliced zucchini are especially attractive tasty additions. Be sure you add them only a few minutes before the soup is done in order to preserve the flavors, color, consistency, and nutrients.

2 cups dry beans
2 quarts water or stock
1 pinch rosemary
1 minced clove of garlic
salt, pepper
meat scraps or pieces of Italian sausage (optional)
½ cup grated cheese
1 tablespoon olive oil
1 cup high protein macaroni
vegetables as desired.

Soak beans 12 hours. Put to boil in the water or stock for 2 hours. Add rosemary, garlic, salt and pepper, meat scraps, cheese, and olive oil. Start adding vegetables and macaroni according to cooking time needed. It is desirable to add at least 1 chopped tomato for color and flavor. Serve with grated cheese.

Creative Tossed Salad (any number)*

Tossed salad is my favorite contribution to any meal. I never make it exactly the same because I have no set recipe. It is invariably a success whether I concoct the dressing right on the salad or whether I make it separately (for a picnic or potluck supper) and add it. With the addition of cheese, meat, hard cooked eggs, etc., it makes a filling luncheon main dish. Use any of the following ingredients in any combination (you should have some type of green as a base). You can use up leftovers in an attractive, tasty and nutritious way.

lettuce	chopped cooked meat
endive or escarole	shredded chicken
Chinese cabbage	cubed Cheddar cheese
carrots	well-drained cottage cheese
onions	marinated artichokes
parsley	chunks of tuna
cauliflower	sardines
fresh mushrooms	green or red sweet peppers
cooked green beans	zucchini
tomatoes	spinach

* Recipes from *Nourishing Your Unborn Child: Nutrition and Natural Foods in Pregnancy* Phyllis Williams, 1974. Nash Publishers, $7.95

Athletics During Pregnancy

Common sense is your best guide when pursuing athletics during pregnancy. The first three months are the riskiest for your health and that of the fetus, so you should be careful of heavy exercise: skiing, horseback riding, fencing and similar activities. Walking and swimming (be careful on the steps) are two favorite activities of pregnant women.

Research has shown that women in good physical condition have faster and easier deliveries, gain only twenty-five to thirty pounds, experience few lower back pains and have very fast recoveries. Aside from these obvious physical benefits, exercise also aids our spirits, helping us combat depression and fatigue.

In addition, you should wear elastic stockings whenever possible and lie with your feet up when you are resting. If you notice spotting or are having pains, contact your doctor immediately.

Various basic exercises to strengthen, make delivery easier and avoid chronic postnatal problems are included in this section and are found in several recommended books. Walk as much as possible and be sure also to get plenty of rest with your feet up.

For more information, *Ms.* magazine has a good article on athletics during pregnancy in its July 1978 issue.

Prenatal Exercises*

1. TAILOR SIT (whenever possible)
    This is best described as sitting "Indian style." Do this whenever possible (sit at the coffee table for dinner, etc.). This is a comfortable position for labor and it will also help to stretch the muscles of your inner thighs so that you will be able to get your legs wide apart for the birth of your baby. This will also help to throw your heavy uterus forward and out instead of allowing it to press heavily on your other pelvic organs.

2. SQUATTING (at least 15 per day)
    Place your legs wide apart, feet pointing straight ahead. Bend at the waist, swing your bottom under and down to the floor with your body between your legs and your knees by your armpits. To rise, raise your bottom first while you are still bent at the waist, straighten up. When lifting heavy objects, rise up straight and let your leg muscles do the lifting instead of your back. This is the position that you will assume for birth (except, of course, you won't be standing). If you stretch your muscles slowly now, you won't be sore after your baby is born. Remember, you must get your legs wide apart to allow the baby to pass easily—the wider you can get them, the easier your birth will be.

3. PELVIC ROCKING (40 mid-morning, 40 mid-afternoon, 80 just before bed)
    Get on hands and knees. Place hands directly under shoulders and knees directly under hips. Rock your pelvis, SLOWLY. To do this, point your tailbone toward the ceiling. Next, slowly tuck your tailbone under (think of a dog tucking his tail). While you are rocking your pelvis, your upper back should stay relatively straight—only your waist and lower back should move. This exercise is designed to lift your uterus out of the pelvic cavity and throw it forward, where it belongs.

4. REST AND SLEEP POSITION (whenever lying down)
    This is the same as the side relaxation position which is described below. Avoid lying on your back. It will allow your heavy uterus to press on the veins and arteries which supply the placenta and hinder the circulation to it and baby. Use this position whenever you rest or sleep. You will find that it is extremely comfortable, especially as your uterus gets bigger.

5. LEG SEPARATIONS (10 separations per day)
    Lie on your back, but propped up at a 45° angle. Bend your knees comfortably and put feet flat on the floor. Have coach apply MODERATE pressure to the outsides of your knees. Separate them as far toward the floor as possible. Remove pressure and bring them back together. This will help to strengthen the muscle which opens your legs.

6. KEGEL (250 per day only 20–25 at a time to be effective)
    These are also called vaginal contractions. The kegel muscle is a hammock-like structure slung between your pubic bone in the front and your coccyx, or tailbone, in the back. (Its real name is therefore, the pubococcygeal muscle.) There are three openings in the muscle: one for the urethra, one for the vagina, and one for the rectum. The best way to find this muscle at first is to try to stop the flow when you are urinating. (Don't be alarmed if you can't do it at first—most of us have never exercised it because we are unaware of its importance. Control will come with practice.) Once you have identified the muscle, you will be able to contract and release it at any time. Do this exercise whenever you think of it.

---

*from Lisa Frank, childbirth educator.

7. SIDE RELAXATION

Lie on your side. Place one pillow under your head. Your bottom arm should be behind you, your top arm in front. Both legs should be slightly flexed. Place a second pillow under your top knee for support. Your tummy should be resting on the bed. Learn to like this position. It is one of the best for labor and is the most relaxing. It allows every part of your body to be properly supported without pressure points to disturb your comfort. Remember, good relaxation is 75% of the key to an easier labor.

8. ROLF LIFT

Lie on your back on the floor with your legs extended. Use your lower abdominal muscles to slowly draw up your legs until your knees are comfortably flexed and your feet are flat on the floor. Feet and knees should be slightly separated. Rock your pelvis so that the small of your back presses into the floor. Hold the pelvic rock position and lift your bottom and lower back off the floor until you are supported by your shoulders and feet. VERY SLOWLY lower your back onto the floor again, one vertebra at a time. Un-rock your pelvis. Rock and lift again for a total of five times. Let your lower abdominal muscles extend your legs again. This will help to strengthen your abdominal muscles to support your uterus which we are throwing forward with the pelvic rocking. It will also strengthen your back muscles and help to prevent the swayback and backache of late pregnancy.

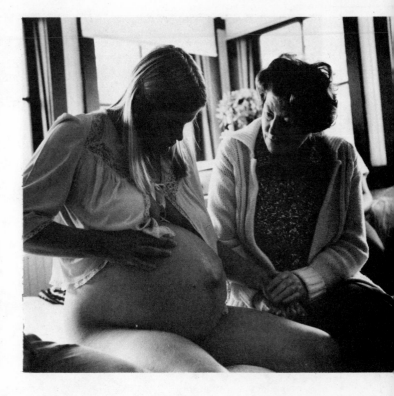

Optional Exercises for Comfort

1. LACTATION EXERCISE (for heartburn)

Tailor sit on the floor, arms and hands at your side, back straight. Take a deep breath as you slowly bring your arms up, cross them over your chest, and lower them, still extended, outward and back so that your arms are out to the side, hands touching the floor at a line about even with your hips but extended away from them. Inhale again as you swing your still extended arms toward the back as though you were going to touch your thumbs together. Swing them from the side to the back three times as you inhale the one time. Exhale again as you return your arms comfortably to your sides. Repeat this as many times as you wish. It may not eliminate your heartburn altogether but it will help.

2. BENT LEG ELEVATION (for swelling or tired achy legs)

Lie on your back in front of a couch, chair or bed. Your bottom should be about 12 inches from it. Rest your legs on the chair for as long as you like. A good rule of thumb is about 5 minutes for each hour you've been on your feet. Be sure to pelvic rock when you finish, to increase circulation again.

3. FOOT CIRCLES (for swollen ankles)

Get in the same position as for LEG SEPARATIONS. Place the calf of one leg on the opposite knee about at the midpoint of your lower leg. Point your toes and circle. Go around 8 times. Change legs. Be sure that as you point your toes in the different directions, you always make your circles toward the inside to avoid cramps in the calves.

REMEMBER: Simply KNOWING these exercises will not help to make your birth easier—you must DO them regularly.

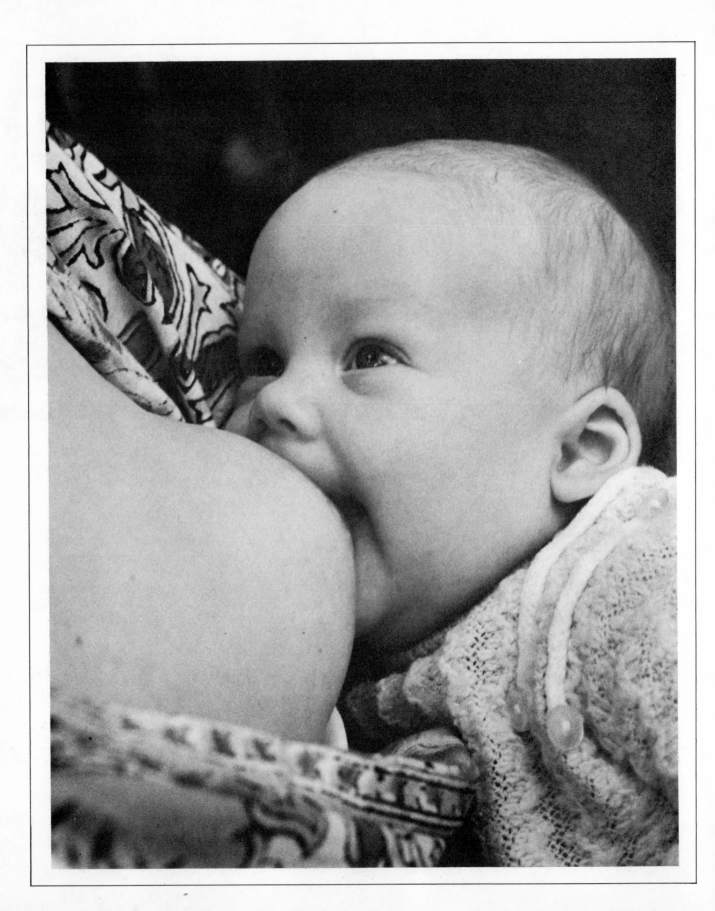

Birth

THE RELATIONSHIP BETWEEN MOTHER AND CHILD

During the three trimesters of pregnancy, the mother has a vital physical relationship with her unborn child. This physical relationship fosters an increasing psychological and emotional relationship between mother and infant. As the infant is born and the umbilical cord cut, the physical relationship then shifts to a psycho-emotional relationship, which is as necessary to the infant's future survival as the previous physical one.

The first three months of the newborn's life we are calling the Fourth Trimester to indicate the importance of this period for the mother to have a strong and healthy relationship with her infant. Just as the unborn child depends on the mother's health for survival during pregnancy, the newborn depends upon the special bond of "maternal attachment" (i.e., the mother's ability and desire to identify her child as her own and desirable) during the first three months of life to provide his physical, social and psycho-emotional needs. This lays the groundwork for an ongoing relationship that will continue to meet the infant's needs as it grows and develops.

The development of maternal attachment early is equally important for the mother. Her needs in relation to her baby include identification of the newborn as her own, her being pleased with the infant's appearance and behavior, feeling pleasure at caring for the child and feeling confident in her ability to be a mother.

The shift from physical to psycho-emotional dependence occurs at birth, and it is during this time and in the first few days of "getting acquainted" after birth that the crucial quality of maternal attachment is formed. The process is usually natural and progresses in an orderly manner with the mother first wanting to see her child, to touch it, to hold it close to her body and then to care for it. Disrupting this process (e.g., due to the birth of a premature infant or a sick infant that must be placed immediately in an intensive care nursery, birth of a deformed baby, a difficult delivery, a mother's postpartum illness, etc.) can alter the natural progression of attachment of mother to infant. An alteration in this process can result in a mother feeling less confident in her care of her infant, in a mother developing angry or rejecting feelings toward her infant or in the mother developing feelings of detachment ("He doesn't seem to be my baby").

In all the concern for assuring a mother's physical health during the three trimesters of pregnancy, it must not be overlooked that the essential work of pregnancy is not complete; the "Fourth Trimester" should be remembered as a time for establishing perhaps the whole character of the mother-child relationship. Mothers need to see their infants at birth, to touch them, to hold them. Separation of newborns from their mothers immediately at birth or for long periods of time, oversedation of mothers during delivery and lack of opportunity for mothers to care for their babies during the early postpartum period should be discouraged if not eliminated whenever possible.

Lois Chandler
Nurse, Parent, Educator

Having Your Baby— Choosing a Method

Having a baby is one of the most exciting and fulfilling moments of your life. Of course, having a baby is just the first step in becoming a parent. The preparations for birth are very important for you and the baby, your husband and the rest of the family. Together, you have an opportunity to prepare for and to plan the kind of birth you most want to have—whether at home or in the hospital, with a doctor or midwife or both assisting you, and with your husband, family, or friends present. Of course, sudden emergencies do come up, and your plans may change. But initially, it is good to have a plan that is going to be the most satisfying to you.

Many hospitals today have birth center clinics, which offer an opportunity for the family to be together, with the birth taking place under soft lights in a calm and quiet atmosphere. Whether you decide on a specific birth process or not, you will want to prepare yourself as much as possible and to have a guide with you; the guide could be your husband, midwife and/ or a doctor. We have included suggestions on how young children can share in the birth experience and even some exercises for the father and mother to enjoy together.

It is advisable to visit the hospital, talk with your doctor about her methods and approach, find out if she is willing to work with a midwife, ascertain whether the midwife can be present during the entire delivery, find out the preferences of your mate as to the kind of experience he would prefer and ready yourself by learning all you can about childbirth.

Giving birth can take anywhere from four to twelve hours or longer. It is important that you are relaxed and comfortable and as informed as possible about what is going on. After all, you are simply the vehicle for the baby's birth; the baby will let you know when it's ready to arrive. You need to assist the baby by staying as calm as possible, creating an atmosphere in which you feel comfortable and having the love and support you need around you. You can make the whole experience an exciting and enjoyable one.

One of the most satisfactory ways to prepare is to read as much as possible about childbirth—look at the alternatives that are currently available and decide which process suits your own style. You will find numerous books to assist you in learning about birth; and you can also study and take classes.

Perhaps the most important question to ask yourself is: "What is the best possible environment my child can be born into?" You should strive for a situation in which your family can be with you, since it is the supportive connection in this early period that is so important.

THE VALUE OF HOME BIRTH

The pregnant woman in America today actually knows little more about her coming birth than the child in the street. She can probably recount many stories about other people's births, including at least one chilling tale of a friend who supposedly "wouldn't be alive today" if it had not been for a quick-thinking obstetrician who intervened to save the day. But information about what really goes on inside the hospital stops at the front door. . . . Childbirth is one of the most profound, personal experiences a woman can have. Yet our present system of uninformed care does not allow her the freedom to choose her own way of birth and reclaim the experience as her own. . . .

By making home birth seem totally unreasonable, physicians are robbing American women of a vital choice in the function of their own bodies.

Doctors fail to point out that there are many arguments against routine hospitalization for birth. Besides the threat of damage to mother and infant, hospital birth causes strain in the average family's budget, enforces rigid separation of family members and of mother and child after birth, and results in long isolation of mother and infant from siblings, all of which place unusual strain upon the healthy family unit. Since birth is a time of emotional crisis and change, hospital-created strain upon an already strained family can be enough to weaken even the strongest ties.

But the greatest problem in the controversy over home versus hospital birth is that these arguments tend to polarize groups into factions of absolute belief in one place or the other. Midwives continue to stress that neither can be made so safe as to guarantee that every mother and every child will survive the process. Just as no device or medical interference has yet been created to insure total safety in any process of life, so does birth always entail a small degree of risk.

Home birth is thus a natural choice, not for all couples but for many couples, and today doctors either deal honestly with this fact or avoid the issue entirely and forget they are in a service profession. Home birth is a safe choice for healthy women who consciously prepare for birth, who receive careful prenatal care and screening, and who call in a skilled attendant to assist them. The only reasonable argument left today that can be stated against home birth is that it is too simple and inexpensive a solution for such a complex society as ours. And perhaps that is the real reason why home birth is no longer a choice in America.

Since it has been proven time and time again that over 90% of all births are completely normal and require no medical attention beyond the first prenatal examinations, and since statistics of home births in other countries compare favorably to hospital statistics in the United States, there is no reason for the medical community or governmental agencies to fight the emergence of practicing midwives today. Their continuation to do so can only be attributed to feelings of personal and professional threat from women—and some men—whose intention is only to assist nature, not to practice medicine.

That a profession which considers itself so advanced, because of the very medical technology and procedures that are ruining the birth process for thousands of women across the nation, should so callously dispense with the very birth attendants who can reclaim the process for women and make it safer as well, is no less than a shameful indictment of the medical fraternity in the United States today.

Suzanne Arms
Immaculate Deception
Bantam Books
1977 398 pp. $2.95

GRANDMA COMES OF AGE

What does the well-groomed grandma wear to attend the birth of her second grandchild on a commune in California? I asked myself in my air-conditioned upper eastside New York apartment. In fact, what prompted me to accept the invitation to be present at a home birth, when the only births I have ever attended were those of my own two daughters at Doctors Hospital, the obstetrician's answer to the Plaza Hotel?

. . . . . Two years ago I had managed to avoid confronting the realities of a home delivery. (The only home delivery I had dealt with successfully was the Sunday edition of the *New York Times!*) Thus, Jeremy, Nancy's firstborn, had come into the world unaided by an M.D. and unabetted by me.

. . . . . It's 2:30 and David can see the black-haired head emerging from Nancy's birth canal. He refers to the baby as "she." He surely knows it will be a girl. He embraces Nancy, massages her back and generally conducts himself in such as way as to raise a question as to who is having the baby. It's obvious. *They* are having the baby. The same way it was conceived it will be birthed; together and with love. How does he know just what to do? I always thought that poppas waited outside to be told of the birth of their offspring. Birth was a matter for *women*. Oh, everything is cascading down. All the myths and beliefs.

Cynthia Lewin
Author, Grandmother

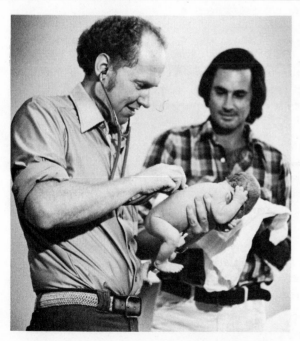

ON THE THRESHOLD

We must behave with the most enormous respect toward this instant of birth, this fragile moment.

The baby is between two worlds. On a threshold. Hesitating.

Do not hurry. Do not press. Allow this child to enter.

What an extraordinary thing: this little creature, no longer a fetus, not yet a newborn baby.

This little creature is no longer inside his mother, yet she's still breathing for them both.

An elusive, ephemeral moment.

Leave this child. Alone.

Because this child is free—and frightened.

Don't intrude: stay back. Let time pass.

Grant this moment its slowness, and its gravity.

Frederick Leboyer
Birth Without Violence
Alfred A. Knopf
1975 115 pp. $8.95

THE PREGNANT PATIENT'S BILL OF RIGHTS*

American parents are becoming increasingly aware that well-intentioned health professionals do not always have scientific data to support common American obstetrical practices and that many of these practices are carried out primarily because they are part of medical and hospital tradition. In the last forty years many artificial practices have been introduced which have changed childbirth from a physiological event to a very complicated medical procedure in which all kinds of drugs are used and procedures carried out, sometimes unnecessarily, and many of them potentially damaging for the baby and even for the mother. A growing body of research makes it alarmingly clear that every aspect of traditional American hospital care during labor and delivery must now be questioned as to its possible effect on the future well-being of both the obstetric patient and her unborn child.

One in every 35 children born in the United States today will eventually be diagnosed as retarded; in 75% of these cases there is no familial or genetic predisposing factor. One in every 10 to 17 children has been found to have some form of brain dysfunction or learning disability requiring special treatment. Such statistics are not confined to the lower socioeconomic group but cut across all segments of American society.

New concerns are being raised by childbearing women because no one knows what degree of oxygen depletion, head compression, or traction by forceps the unborn or newborn infant can tolerate before that child sustains permanent brain damage or dysfunction. The recent findings regarding the cancer-related drug diethylstilbestrol have alerted the public to the fact that neither the approval of a drug by the U.S. Food and Drug Administration nor the fact that a drug is prescribed by a physician serves as a guarantee that a drug or medication is safe for the mother or her unborn child. In fact, the American Academy of Pediatrics' Committee on Drugs has recently stated that there is no drug, whether prescription or over-the-counter remedy, which has been proven safe for the unborn child.

The Pregnant Patient has the right to participate in decisions involving her well-being and that of her unborn child, unless there is a clearcut medical emergency that prevents her participation. In addition to the rights set forth in the American Hospital Association's "Patient's Bill of Rights" (which has also been adopted by the New York City Department of Health) the Pregnant Patient, because she represents TWO patients rather than one, should be recognized as having the additional rights listed below.

1. *The Pregnant Patient has the right*, prior to the administration of any drug or procedure, to be informed by the health professional caring for her of any potential direct or indirect effects, risks or hazards to herself or to her unborn or newborn infant which may result from the use of a drug or procedure prescribed for or administered to her during pregnancy, labor, birth or lactation.

2. *The Pregnant Patient has the right*, prior to the proposed therapy, to be informed, not only of the benefits, risks and hazards of the proposed therapy but also of known alternative therapy, such as available childbirth education classes which could help to prepare the Pregnant Patient physically and mentally to cope with the discomfort or stress of pregnancy and the experience of childbirth, thereby reducing or eliminating her need for drugs and obstetric intervention. She should be offered such information early in her pregnancy in order that she may make a reasoned decision.

3. *The Pregnant Patient has the right*, prior to the administration of any drug, to be informed by the health professional who is prescribing or administering the drug to her that any drug which she receives during pregnancy, labor and birth, no matter how or when the drug is taken or administered, may adversely affect her unborn baby, directly or indirectly, and that there is no drug or chemical which has been proven safe for the unborn child.

4. *The Pregnant Patient has the right* if Cesarean section is anticipated, to be informed prior to the administration of any drug, and preferably prior to her hospitalization, that minimizing her and, in turn, her baby's intake of nonessential pre-operative medicine will benefit her baby.

5. *The Pregnant Patient has the right*, prior to the administration of a drug or procedure, to be informed of the areas of uncertainty if there is NO properly controlled follow-up research which has established the safety of the drug or procedure with regard to its direct and/or indirect effects on the physiological, mental and neurological development of the child exposed, via the mother, to the drug or procedure during pregnancy, labor, birth or lactation (this would apply to virtually all drugs and the vast majority of obstetric procedures).

6. *The Pregnant Patient has the right*, prior to the administration of any drug, to be informed of the brand name and generic name of the drug in order that she may advise the health professional of any past adverse reaction to the drug.

7. *The Pregnant Patient has the right* to determine for herself, without pressure from her attendant, whether she will accept the risks inherent in the proposed therapy or refuse a drug or procedure.

8. *The Pregnant Patient has the right* to know the name and qualifications of the individual administering a medication or procedure to her during labor or birth.

9. *The Pregnant Patient has the right* to be informed, prior to the administration of any procedure, whether that procedure is being administered to her for her or her baby's benefit (medically indicated) or as an elective procedure (for convenience, teaching purposes or research).

10. *The Pregnant Patient has the right* to be accompanied during the stress of labor and birth by someone she cares for, and to whom she looks for emotional comfort and encouragement.

11. *The Pregnant Patient has the right* after appropriate medical consultation to choose a position for labor and for birth which is least stressful to her baby and to herself.

12. *The Obstetric Patient has the right* to have her baby cared for at her bedside if her baby is normal, and to feed her baby according to her baby's needs rather than according to hospital regimen.

13. *The Obstetric Patient has the right* to be informed in writing of the name of the person who actually delivered her baby and the professional qualifications of that person. This information should also be on the birth certificate.

14. *The Obstetric Patient has the right* to be informed if there is any known or indicated aspect of her or her baby's care or condition which may cause her or her baby later difficulty or problems.

15. *The Obstetric Patient* has the right to have her and her baby's hospital medical records complete, accurate and legible and to have their records, including Nurses' Notes, retained by the hospital until the child reaches at least the age of majority, or, alternatively, to have the records offered to her before they are destroyed.

16. *The Obstetric Patient*, both during and after her hospital stay, has the right to have access to her complete hospital medical records, including Nurses' Notes, and to receive a copy upon payment of a reasonable fee and without incurring the expense of retaining an attorney.

It is the obstetric patient and her baby, not the health professional, who must sustain any trauma or injury resulting from the use of a drug or obstetric procedure. The observation of the rights listed above will not only permit the obstetric patient to participate in the decisions involving her and her baby's health care, but will help to protect the health professional and the hospital against litigation arising from resentment or misunderstanding on the part of the mother.

* Endorsed by the International Childbirth Education Association. Bulk orders: $.03 each plus $.40 postage and handling. For a complimentary copy send a stamped, self-addressed envelope to the Committee on Patients' Rights, Box 1900, New York, New York 10001.

THE ENVIRONMENT OF BIRTH

Childbirth must be practiced as an art, assisted by science; for the creation of a new human being is a conception of the heart and spirit as well as the body. It is an extra-ordinary state of consciousness, for everyone involved.

Our customs and our attitudes about childbearing reflect the way we feel about ourselves, our society and our world view and most important, affect the new baby coming to life. Life in the womb and the passage through the birth canal into autonomous life is the primal patterning experience affecting the child's behavior for many years thereafter, perhaps all of its days. Recently, we have been discovering through research in altered states of consciousness, the infinite amount of complex memories that we record, store and act out of that shape our lives. Some of those memories, as incredible as it may seem, are of conception, womb life and birth.

The childbearing year is also a crucial transitional period in the lives of the parents. Everything is changing for them: their self-image, their relationship with each other, the whole structure and focus of their lives. It is a crucial "rite of passage" for all involved. Most crucial for the baby but also for the parents who create the environment for these captive 9 months.

We are challenged to create a total environment for the pregnant year, a harmonious setting in which all the complex psychological, social and transpersonal dynamics as well as the physiological ones can be supported and facilitated. We need to design places in which the parents can be enfolded as they, too, are unfolding during the prenatal period, places where groups of pregnant parents can share the anxieties and joy of this time and ready themselves for the future parenting responsibilities. We need to design places in which we can celebrate *all* the aspects of this rite of passage.

Leni Schwartz
Environmental Psychologist

COUPLES' CHECKLIST

Hospital or Home Birth—should be done well before your due date:

Go to hospital and fill out all necessary pre-admittance forms, even if you are planning to have your baby at home. Take all necessary insurance forms in order to know what further financial arrangements must be made.

Choose your pediatrician and be sure he goes along with your plans to breastfeed. A doctor not in favor of breastfeeding will only make an unpleasant doctor-patient relationship.

Check out camera and make sure you have plenty of film and flashcubes.

If you are going to the hospital, be sure to have your suitcase packed well in advance of your due date. The last thing you want to be doing in labor is packing your bags!

Home Birth Only

plastic sheet
extra blankets and sheets
lots of grocery bags around the room
minimum of 20 Chux pads
beach chair

6–8 pillows
mirror
three bowls
wash rags
ice chips
frozen orange-juice bars
birthday cake and candles
champagne to celebrate
ear syringe
orance juice (preferably fresh squeezed)

Things to have for hospital or home birth:

Mom's	Baby's	Dad's
nightgowns	T-shirt	full gas tank
bathrobe	disposable	camera, film,
slippers	diapers	flashes
nursing bra	safety pins	watch
nursing pads	puddle pads	list of phone
warm socks	receiving	numbers
hair ribbon	blankets	
sanitary belt	going home	
chapstick or lip	outfit (if	
gloss	desired)	

Lisa Frank
Childbirth Educator

EMERGENCY BIRTH— (JUST IN CASE!)

When discussing emergency birth, we are assuming that it is just that—an *emergency!* The father, or other untrained person, should never attempt to deliver the baby without proper medical supervision. The process of childbirth, while a perfectly natural phenomenon, is surrounded by *potential* dangers. With proper medical supervision, these possible complications can easily be detected and treated; but without proper medical supervision, these complications can go undetected and place the mother and/or baby in serious danger.

Unattended births are risky, but occasionally the situation arises where a medical attendant is not available and the baby decides to make his appearance anyway. In our populated area, these occasions are rare indeed but they may occur—such as when the couple is on the way to the hospital, snowed in in the mountains, or on a boat in the middle of the ocean. Since the last two circumstances mentioned will be exceptionally rare, we will consider the first circumstance (the couple is on their way to the hospital and the baby won't wait).

If the father, or other untrained person, is forced to deliver the baby, use the following procedure:

1. *Stop the car!*—If the mother experiences the burning, stretching sensation of crowning, and you are not fairly close to the hospital, it is a safe assumption that you probably won't make it before the birth. (If you are close, and can probably make it, continue to the hospital and pull into the emergency entrance. Honk your horn and the emergency room staff will come to you.)

   It is important that you stop the car! Don't attempt a one-handed delivery at 90 miles per hour. Your wife needs your assistance. Be sure to pull the car completely out of the flow of traffic.

2. *Make her comfortable!*—This may be difficult in some cars; however, if you have a back seat, put her there. In either case, have her turn sideways on the seat and lean against the side of the car. (This way the baby will emerge over the seat— remember it's slippery—and not over a drop to the floor.) Be sure to get her slacks and/or panties completely off. You need room to maneuver and she needs to be able to get her legs wide apart to facilitate the birth and help to prevent tearing.

3. *Have her BLOW throughout the entire birth!*— This will help to prevent tearing of the perineum and/or vaginal tissues during the birth. The force of the contraction alone is adequate to push the baby out. The additional force of the mother's pushing may cause a tear because the birth will be fast and uncontrolled. A slow, controlled birth is best.

4. *Let the baby's head deliver slowly and by itself!* —Do not try to pull on the head or twist or turn it. After the baby's head delivers, there will usually (but not always) be a wait and the body will deliver with the next contraction. While you are waiting, be sure to keep the baby's face out of the amniotic fluid that will be puddled by the mother's hips. The best way to accomplish this is to have the mother keep her pelvis tilted *up*.

5. *If the shoulders do not deliver within the next two or three contractions, check for the cord around the neck!*—Although the doctor does this routinely, it is best that the untrained attendant not do it unless necessary because the attendant does not have sterile gloves and the chance for infection is increased. To check for the cord around the neck, gently insert *one* finger beside the neck and feel for the cord. If it is there, you may try to pull it *gently* (*not* with force) over the head. If it won't pull over the head, try to slip it over the shoulder and it will slip down as the body is born. If the cord is not around the neck and the shoulders still will not come (after 2 or 3 contractions), the mother may give a *gentle* push to help deliver them.

6. *Once the top shoulder slides under the pubic bone, the rest of the body follows very quickly!* —Remember that the baby will be very slippery from the amniotic fluid and the vernix (outer coating). Be sure to hold it securely! *Support the baby's head only, and hold onto the body.*

7. *Keep the baby WARM!*—Babies lose body temperature very easily and this could lead to respiratory problems, so be sure to keep him warm once he is born. Wrap him in anything handy that is relatively clean—a receiving blanket, your shirt, anything.

8. *Hold the baby head-down, and lower than the placenta until the cord stops pulsing!*—There is extra baby-blood in the placenta which the baby needs. As long as the blood flow is open (the cord is pulsing) this extra blood will drain by gravity flow to the baby. You can tell if the cord is pulsing by observing it (immediately after the birth it is firm and bluish-white colored; as the pulsing stops, it becomes limp and paler-white) and by feeling it with your fingers.

9. *Put the baby to breast!*—After the cord stops pulsing, if it is long enough, put the baby to breast and have the mother nurse him. This will cause the uterus to contract and the placenta to separate and to deliver. If the cord is not long enough to put the baby to breast, place the baby on the mother's abdomen, have her caress the baby with one hand and hand express the colostrum with the other. Be sure the baby is kept WARM!

10. *If the baby is having difficulty breathing*—By holding the baby head-down following the birth, the mucus and fluid should have easily drained from his lungs and throat. However, there may be more mucus in his mouth. If this is the case, use *one* finger to *sweep* the mouth. Start at the side, in one cheek, and sweep in a circular motion to the back of the throat, and on to the other cheek on the other side, and then forward and out. Do not stick your finger down his throat, this could only drive the mucus deeper. If the baby still is not breathing, begin Mouth-to-Mouth Resuscitation. (Remember to cover the baby's mouth *and* nose completely and breathe very *gently*—just the puff of air that you can hold in your cheeks—at the rate of about 20–30 breaths per minute.)

11. *Deliver the placenta!*—Do *not* pull on the cord! The placenta will separate and deliver spontaneously, within 5–10 minutes, if the mother is nursing or hand-stimulating the nipples because of the oxytocin being released into her blood stream. After the placenta separates, there will be a flow of blood from the vagina, and the cord will visibly push forward. After this happens, watch for the placenta to "crown" at the outlet of the birth canal. When you can see the placenta, you can gently pull on the cord to deliver it. If there is resistance to your pull, *stop* and wait a minute or so, and then try again. You could also have the mother give a gentle push to expel the placenta.

12. *Wrap the baby and the placenta together!*—Do not attempt to cut the cord—it isn't necessary. Place the placenta next to the baby and wrap them together to keep the baby warm. Continue nursing the baby to keep the uterus firmly contracted and prevent hemorrhage!

13. *Continue to the hospital!*—Don't make the mistake of thinking that just because the baby has been born you don't need a doctor!! It is important that you continue on to the hospital! The doctor will want to check your wife for possible tearing, stitches, and retained placenta. He will want to cut the cord and examine the baby. Just pull up to the emergency entrance and honk the horn—the emergency room staff will come to get both mother and baby. Depending on your individual preference, and your doctor's recommendation, you may choose to go home immediately, stay for a brief period of observation, or stay for a day or so.

Remember, babies that are coming are seldom a problem; it is babies that won't come that cause problems. If you do find yourself in the situation of having to deliver your own baby, don't panic. A clear head is the most important thing for the attendant. Babies come! And, if they don't, you have time to get to the hospital!

If you forget everything else—remember these two Cardinal Principles and it will be unlikely that you will ever get into any trouble:

1. *Do as little as possible; and when in doubt, do nothing!!* It is far better to do nothing than to do something and do it wrong! Just be there to supervise and catch the baby. Then keep it *warm* and keep the uterus *contracted* (by nursing or hand-stimulation of the nipple). Then go to the hospital.

2. *Don't touch the perineum!!* Your hands are not sterile and, at the time of childbirth, the mother is very open to infection—either through a tear or at the placental site. A germ that is introduced at the outlet of the birth canal can quickly make its way up the birth canal, through the cervix and into the uterus.

If you find yourself delivering your baby—

1. Relax,
2. Keep your head,
3. Do what you can to help,
4. Continue to the hospital,
5. Congratulate yourself on a job well done, and
6. *Enjoy* one of life's most precious experiences.

Lisa Frank,
Childbirth Educator

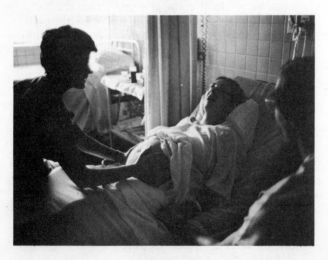

Labor

When the fetus has completed approximately 280 days (40 weeks) in the uterus, the birth process begins.

The first stage of labor may last from two to sixteen hours or more; the uterus contracts at regular intervals; the cervix slowly dilates to allow the baby to pass into the birth canal. Uterine contractions are faint, and gradually increase.

The second stage. The baby passes headfirst down the vagina; lasts a few minutes. For the first baby this stage generally lasts an hour; but the time varies greatly.

The expulsive stage of labor involves bearing down during contractions. General anesthesia may interfere; father's presence may help mother relax during contractions and enables parents to be involved as a couple.

The third stage. The placenta is expelled. Lasts a few minutes. Drugs may be given to the mother to relieve pain; these drugs may pass through the placenta to the baby and interfere in the first few days by causing a drugged condition.

Birth Without Violence
Frederick Leboyer
Alfred A. Knopf
1975   115 pp. $8.95

Sensitively spelling out how an infant must perceive birth, Dr. Leboyer details his technique based on patience, gentle handling, serenity and warm, tactile sensations for the newborn. His poetic style and nontechnical manner appeal to our own senses in a way that really registers. His viewpoint is a must for expectant parents about to make the first decisions affecting the well-being of their child.

A word about the hands holding the child: It is through our hands that we speak to the child, that we communicate. Touching is the primary language. The child knows if the hands are loving, or if they are careless or worse if they are rejecting. . .

Childbirth At Home
Marion Sousa
Bantam Books
1976   211 pp. $1.95

Well researched from the fields of biology, sociology and anthropology, this absorbing discussion of childbirth at home concludes that "our national custom of confining normal births to the hospital is definitely unhealthy and possibly dangerous." Principal reasons given for the dangers are increased exposure to infection at a time when the mother's body is very vulnerable and various questionable procedures taken to hasten birth in a busy hospital.

Childbirth Without Fear
Grantly Dick-Read
Harper & Row
1979   402 pp. $2.95

Approaching childbirth as a positive experience free from suffering, Dr. Dick-Read shows how careful prenatal observation and instruction can prevent most of the fears and dangers of childbirth. He was responsible for introducing the idea of natural childbirth in the 1940's in Great Britain. Well-illustrated chapters discuss such things as prenatal health, education, physical fitness, breathing and care of the newborn.

When the prepared woman who has just experienced natural childbirth is asked: "What is the most difficult part you experienced?" she doesn't mention the actual birth! She invariably replies,

"The most difficult time came just before I was taken into the birth room," usually adding something like, "That back pain was really getting to me, but not the birth. The birth was exciting and I wouldn't have missed it for anything!"

Having A Cesarean Baby
Richard Hausknecht and Joan Rattner Heilman
E. P. Dutton
1978   201 pp. $4.95

This book details the entire cesarean birth experience—from pregnancy until well after the mother and baby are safely home. It tells how a cesarean birth can be as gratifying and emotionally fulfilling as any other and provides vital information about the reasons for having a cesarean, anesthesia, delivery, risks of a cesarean birth, choosing a doctor and hospital and more.

Though one out of every six infants in the United States is born by cesarean section today, cesarean birth is not only "different" and, to some people, "unnatural," but also involves physical discomfort and a recovery period that does not accompany vaginal birth.

The Home Birth Book
Charlotte and Fred Ward
Doubleday (Dolphin)
1977   149 pp. $5.95

This anthology of essays includes various first-person accounts of home birth, as well as contributions from experts. Ashley Montagu discusses how hospitals tend to "dehumanize the mother-child relationship—the very relationship out of which all humanity grows," concluding that certainly babies should be born at home, "for that is where they belong."

Labor and Delivery: An Observer's Diary (What You Should Know About Today's Childbirth)
Constance A. Bean
Doubleday
1977   203 pp. $7.95

From the introduction by Gerald Cohen:

For the first time, to my knowledge, here is a compilation of many labor and delivery room experiences handled beautifully, sensitively and artistically by a dedicated woman whose love for her fellow human beings and interest in the subject are quite evident. The dramatic events involved in the labor and delivery of many lives are accurately depicted.

Methods of Childbirth
Constance A. Bean
Doubleday (Dolphin)
1974   194 pp. $2.50

Bean discusses natural childbirth vs. childbirth under anesthesia and covers topics from pain and how to control it to postnatal care.

The most difficult part of labor comes near the end of the first stage as the cervix dilates the last three centimeters out of the ten

centimeters of total dilation. It is called transition. Transition does not last longer than an hour and there is a space of time between contractions. It feels different from the preceding part of the labor. The contractions are about to change into the bearing-down kind of contractions of the second stage. They are frequent and intense. Although transition can be welcomed because birth is near, childbirth classes always give special attention to practical help in promoting comfort for transition. Occasionally a woman reports that she was not aware of transition and never used her transition techniques, but this experience is not common.

Psychology of Childbirth
Aidan MacFarland
Harvard University Press
1977   140 pp. $2.95

MacFarland writes that:

birth is of course only one part of a continually unfolding relationship from conception onward, first between the baby and the mother, the father, and the environment in general.

Especially interesting is the discussion of the psychological variables in the first encounter between the newborn and its parents, and the lasting effects that this encounter may have on the family relationship.

Six Practical Lessons For An Easier Childbirth
Elisabeth Bing
Bantam Books
1967   128 pp. $1.25

Helpful, informative book on the Lamaze method of psychoprophylactic childbirth, complete with photographs and drawings which illustrate the method (including

the muscular-control program) in detail.

We are often asked to give statistics about our method. Many physicians want to know whether birth injuries, prematurity, hemorrhaging, etc. can be reduced by using this method. Studies made in France and many other countries show that the psychoprophylactic method does reduce these complications. But there is one important factor that cannot be measured statistically. That is: How does a rewarding experience in childbirth enhance a young couple's relationship with each other? How does the feeling of achievement, of having collaborated in the performance of a difficult job, such as giving birth, affect the husband and wife who have worked hard together toward this goal?

Spiritual Midwifery
Ina May Gaskin
The Farm
1978   475 pp. $8.50

This fine book gives numerous personal accounts of "birthing," plus technical information on midwifery skills. Gaskin lives on The Farm in Tennessee and embraces both Eastern and Western philosophies.

It was my first baby, after several years of trying to get pregnant. We had finally gotten unattached to having our own genetic kid, and applied to adopt an orphan. I conceived within the next seven to ten days.

I flashed on all the mothers around the world who must be having babies at the same time, and felt telepathic with them. Then I felt it all go back in time to include all mothers. It just felt like giving birth is such a pure, eternal thing always happening somewhere, always Holy.

Baby

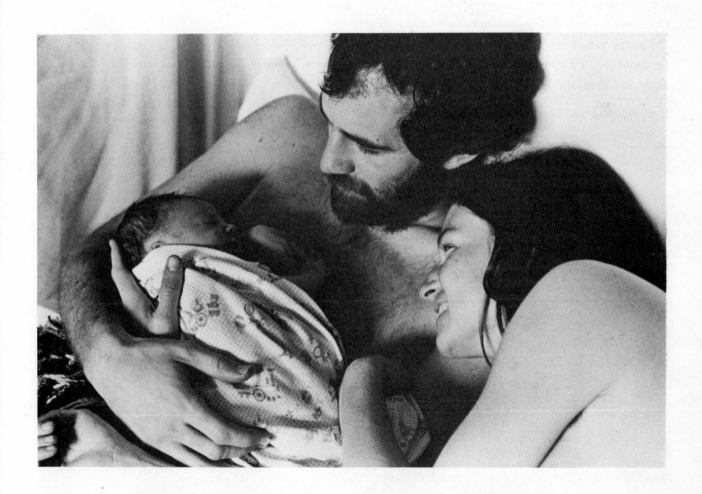

INFANT CARE

Welcoming the new baby (or babies) is a most exciting event. From the moment of birth and throughout the first days and weeks, how the baby is treated is critical to its growth and development. Nurturing of the infant when touching, feeding, playing, washing, diapering and so on conveys the joy of its arrival felt by both parents.

For multiple births (twins, triplets or more) the new challenges are compounded, but manageable with cooperation and assistance from your spouse and others in the family.

TEN PRINCIPLES FOR RELATING TO INFANTS

Do involve the baby in things that concern him. Don't work around him or distract him to get the job done faster.

Do invest in quality time when you are totally available to the infant. Don't settle for constant time together when you are only "half there."

Do learn the baby's system of communication and teach him yours. Don't underestimate his ability to communicate.

Do invest in time and energy to build a total person. Don't strive just to "make the baby smart."

Do respect the baby as an individual. Don't treat him as a cute, empty-headed doll to be manipulated.

Do be honest about your feelings. Don't pretend to feel something that you don't.

Do model the behavior you want to teach. Don't preach.

Do let the baby learn to solve his own problems. Don't take away valuable learning opportunities from him.

Do build security by teaching trust. Don't teach distrust by being undependable.

Do worry about the quality of development in each stage. Don't rush the baby to reach developmental milestones.

Janet Gonzalez-Mena
Director
Neighborhood Child Care Program

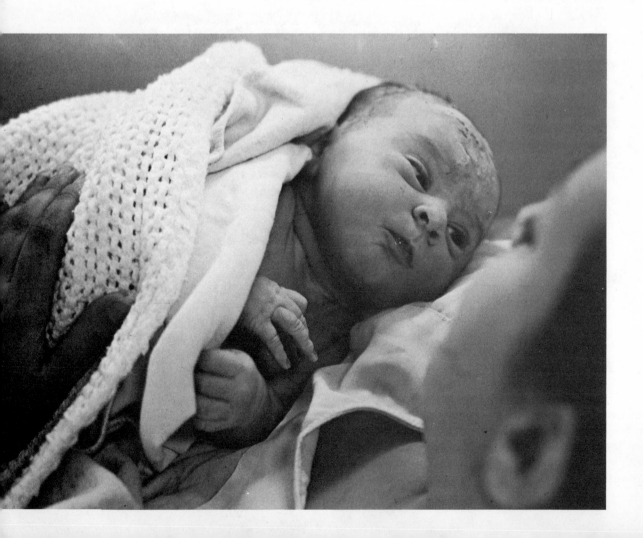

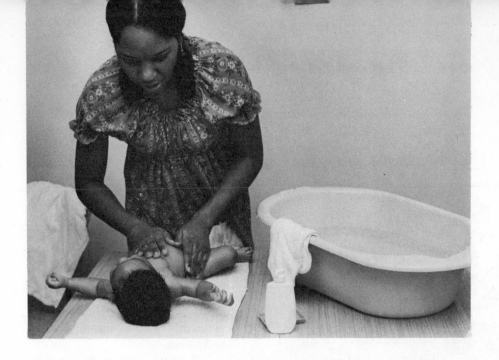

Sample Baby Announcement

IT'S A _____:

OUR BABY'S NAME: _____

TIME BORN: _____ WEIGHT: _____ LENGTH: _____

COLOR OF HAIR: _____ COLOR OF EYES: _____

OUR COMMENTS: _____

A List of Persons You Want to Write or Call
After the Birth

Name	Address	Phone No.
_____	_____	_____
_____	_____	_____
_____	_____	_____
_____	_____	_____
_____	_____	_____
_____	_____	_____
_____	_____	_____
_____	_____	_____
_____	_____	_____

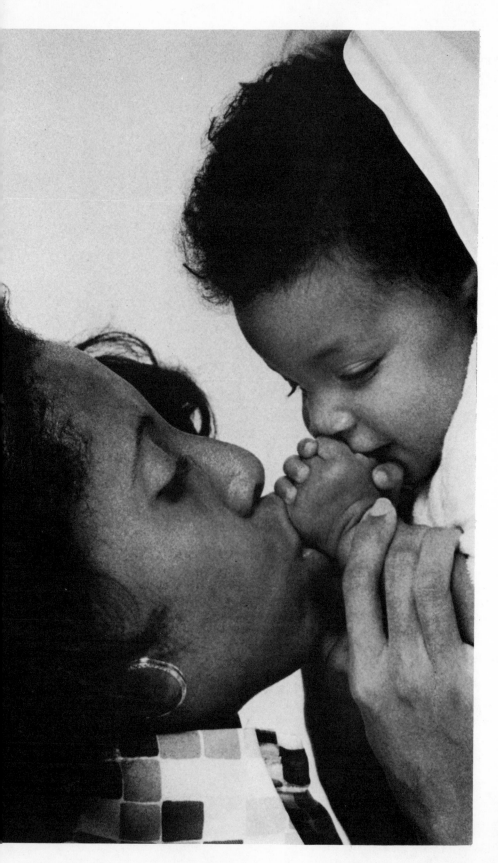

Baby Names

Name Your Baby
Lareina Rule
Bantam Books
1980   224 pp. $1.95

This paperback lists over 6,500 names for children along with the origins, meanings and nicknames.

A short given name coupled with a short surname often sounds harsh or insignificant. A short name is more euphonious and harmonious with a two- or three-syllable family name. If you like a longer, two- or three-syllable first name, such as Bradley or Meredith, it will sound better with a short, one-syllable last name, for example Bradley Jones or Meredith Brown.

New Age Baby Name Book
Sue Browder
Workman Publishing
1978   270 pp. $3.95

An interesting book with a wide variety of names to choose from.

Americans are constantly creating new names which reflect changing cultural consciousness, and these, too, have been collected from recent newspaper birth columns. You may want to use the names exactly as they are listed, or you may decide to use them as a base for creating a totally personalized name, in which case How to Create a Name and parts of Choosing an Ethnic Name will give you pointers on making up a name on your own.

Breast-Feeding

Breast-feeding has become popular with many new mothers as an improved way to feed, and be close to, the infant. The reasons for this, and the cautions are described here, and more on the subject is found in the later section called "Feeding and Nutrition of the Young Baby."

BENEFITS OF BREAST-FEEDING

The rest of the family, too, must be considered in the breast-feeding decision. Do they suffer? No! Fathers derive great satisfaction from seeing their wives "give" with such obvious joy to their precious newborn. Brothers and sisters benefit too. The hormones secreted during lactation make a woman more "motherly" and this carries over to the other children as well as the baby. Nursing provides the ideal time for reading to the toddler, for long, quiet talks, for snuggling with mommy, too, and feeling her love. The other children are not left out—there is more time to spend with them. And, sitting quietly with mommy and the new baby provides the opportunity for older children to get to know the baby, to touch and stroke him, to develop love for this newcomer.

Breast-feeding is truly a family experience. But, it doesn't tie the family down. It makes the family far more mobile. It's so easy to travel with a nursing baby—you just pick up a diaper and go. There are no cumbersome bottles or warmers to be concerned about. The baby's food is ever-present, handy, just the right temperature. And with the aid of a poncho or a well-placed blanket, baby can nurse happily anywhere.

Women who have bottle-fed and then breast-fed are unanimous in saying that breast-feeding is happier, easier, more relaxed. But breast-feeding is not merely a woman's physiological function. It is an emotional experience which reaches to the depths of her being, comfort, pleasure, joy, peace, love and a sense of oneness with this precious new part of her life.

The nursing mother is fulfilled biologically and emotionally. This is the total woman; truly liberated. She is free—from formula making, bottle sterilizing and warming, schedules, baby's food allergies and digestive upsets. And yet, she is bound too; bound in love to this tiny person, this gift from God, who will reap the benefits of her love for the rest of his life.

Lisa Frank
Childbirth Educator

BASIC INFORMATION
(from La Leche League's *Nipple Care* brochure)

Concepts

- Mothering through breastfeeding is the most natural and effective way of understanding and satisfying the needs of the baby.
- Mother and baby need to be together early and often to establish a satisfying relationship and an adequate milk supply.
- The baby has a basic need for his mother's presence which is as intense as his need for food. This need remains even though his mother may be absent for a period of time for needs or reasons of her own.
- For the healthy, full-term baby breast milk is the only food necessary until baby shows signs of needing solids, about the middle of the first year after birth.
- Breast milk is the superior infant food.
- Ideally the breastfeeding relationship will continue until the baby outgrows the need.
- Alert and active participation by the mother in childbirth is a help in getting breastfeeding off to a good start.
- The father's role in the breastfeeding relationship is one of provider, protector, helpmate, and companion to the mother; by thus supporting her he enables her to mother the baby more completely.
- Good nutrition means eating a well-balanced and varied diet of foods in as close to their natural state as possible.
- Ideally, discipline is based on loving guidance.

Advice

- Be together early and often.
- Nurse as soon after delivery as possible.
- Learn to nurse from different positions.
- Offer both breasts at each feeding.
- Feed baby as often as demanded. The more your baby wants, the greater supply of milk available.
- Be sure to drink a lot of liquids.
- If soreness occurs feed the baby as frequently as possible from the nipple that is not sore.
- Heal sore nipple by exposure to air, sun, hydrous lanolin, ice if needed before nursing to reduce soreness.
- Fatigue and tension work against adequate supply of milk.

From La Leche League's Statement of Policy:

We believe that breastfeeding is best for baby. We believe also that it is the ideal way to initiate good parent-child relationships and to strengthen the family and hence the whole fabric of our society. The many other advantages of breastfeeding, both physical and psychological, are in a sense fringe benefits. . . .

We hope to foster a deeper understanding and acceptance of the mother's special vocation in life—its sacrifices as well as its rewards. But we do not attempt to define the perfect mother, rather keeping the focus on good MOTHERING—the understanding and satisfying of the needs of the baby and the growing child with the loving help and support of the husband and father. . . .

As we grow in the understanding that to be a mother is to be the person who is most concerned with understanding and satisfying the needs of the child, we appreciate the value of helping each other to see the kind of needs our children have, and how best to help toward fulfilling them. We believe that mothering through breastfeeding is the most natural and effective way for a mother to fulfill the infant's needs.

Nicotine in Breast Milk

University of California researchers have noted that nicotine collects in the breast fluids of women smokers, whether or not they are nursing.

Dr. Nicholas Petrakis, a cancer epidemiologist at the UC Medical School in San Francisco, said studies have shown that nursing mothers' milk can contain over a hundred substances from outside the body, such as aspirin, antibiotics, pesticides and nicotine. They pass out of the mothers' bodies and into the babies during breast-feeding.

Breast Milk and DDT

Although most medical studies have shown that the breast-fed baby is more resistant to disease, the discovery of contamination of breast milk with dangerous chemicals such as DDT has raised questions about the wisdom of breast-feeding.

"I don't think I'd tell nursing mothers to make any changes in their breast-feeding now," said Dr. David Rahl, director of the National Institute of Environmental Health Sciences.

La Leche also noted that the U.S. Food and Drug Administration tests have found contaminants, including lead, in formula.

NEW MOTHERHOOD

Today's isolated nuclear family can be a difficult setting for parenting. It affords little of the support systems that traditional extended families have provided: role modeling, shared experience, and in general, a haven from the physical and emotional stresses of parenting. My personal experience with new motherhood reflects these issues.

My daughter Alison was born in Los Angeles on September 21, 1974. After years of medical school, a residency in adult and child psychiatry, and the initiation of a private practice all had gone smoothly in my life. I expected no less of motherhood. I had attended a Lamaze course, had read some books on infant care, and had taken great care in selecting a pediatrician. I worked until my due date, and planned on resuming work part-time soon after childbirth.

The stress of a complicated labor and delivery, delay in rooming-in, and an uncomfortable two-day hospital stay were outweighed by my joy at being the mother of this beautiful little girl. I could not wait to take her home and begin caring for her. When I arrived home from the hospital, a housekeeper whom I had hired cancelled at the last minute, my husband went back to work, and I was home alone with Alison. I changed her, washed her, held her, nursed her on demand, and slept with her at my side. I was filled with wonder at this magnificent, perfect little creature. I assured my mother in Toronto who wanted to fly out to Los Angeles to help me, that I could do it myself. After 10 days of increasing exhaustion, I realized I couldn't. I called my mother who came out and took over.

What I had not realized was that my new role had no built-in support. For the first time in my life I had difficulty coping. Mothering was a totally new experience for me. My former life structure was suddenly replaced by a new rhythm over which I had little control. I had to let go of all my patterns, and allow myself to be governed by Alison and her needs. My mother helped me bridge the gap. She nurtured me both by taking care of practical needs such as food shopping and cooking, and by sharing with me the care of Alison. She also taught me, both explicitly and by example, many things about baby care. My mother and I developed a new connection. By the time she left two weeks later, I was able to assume the mothering role with renewed energy and pleasure. I then resumed my psychiatric practice on a limited basis of 4 to 8 hours a week, with my primary focus still being on Alison.

Now I began to look to other women for understanding, companionship and shared experience. My daughter and motherhood became a connection for me to other women and to my own identity as a woman and total person. I discovered my inner rhythms as I tuned in to Alison. Our relationship began to have a sharing and flow.

As Alison grew older, I discovered the interdependent need for and community of parents, teachers, and other child care givers.

My experience has shown me that parenting takes place best in a supportive community. This can take the form of extended family, friends, or organized groups such as play groups, day care centers, or nursery schools. The natural life cycle transition from child to parent does not occur naturally in our present culture. Our high schools and colleges prepare us for professions or careers, not for parenting. Fortunately, a new consciousness is evolving, one that is reflected in this *Whole Child Sourcebook.* An emphasis on human values, on the importance of individual growth and development, on higher consciousness, and the discovery and nurturing of our inner child have all contributed to an openness, individually and collectively, and to a recognition that we are all part of a community of humankind. We grow together.

Hyla Cass
Psychiatrist

Postpartum Depression

"Nearly every woman has problems during the first few months of being a mother," said Gideon G. Panter, assistant clinical professor of obstetrics and gynecology at the New York Hospital–Cornell Medical Center.

"No matter how mature the father is, he too will likely become depressed," said Panter. "Expectant fathers begin to face the blues a couple of months before the baby is born. The expectant mother gets most of the attention. Men need to keep constructive during this period. A new activity, hobby, sport can fill that attention gap."

Panter continued, "Suddenly, when the baby arrives, both parents are neglected. This is the time when parents should receive gifts, not the baby."

One good way to avoid or reduce postpartum depression and to return to prepregnancy figure is to exercise. Walk every day and follow the suggested exercises.

Remember to watch your diet as your successful breast-feeding depends on your own good health and well-being.

Getting Back Into Shape

Some physicians suggest that you start exercises to strengthen your muscles within a few days after you have had your baby. This is on an individual basis and depends upon your condition and how your doctor feels about exercises. Getting up out of bed and moving around is almost always all right and helps strengthen your muscles. Nothing strenuous should be done until after the red bleeding has stopped.

Lying on your abdomen may help your uterus return to normal position. The exercises shown are commonly done but check with your doctor to see if they are all right for you to do.

Standing

Try to stand with your lower back flat. When you work standing up, use a footrest to raise your legs alternately to help relieve swayback. Never lean forward without bending your knees. Ladies take note: shoes with moderate heels strain the back less than those with high spike heels.

Lifting

Make sure you lift properly. Bend your knees and use your leg muscles to lift. Keep a wide base of support. Hold objects close to body as you stand. Keep back flat.

Exercise 1

Begin on 1st day or as instructed. Take in and expel 5 breaths, breathing deeply as though from abdomen.

Exercise 2

1st day, or as instructed. From position shown in Exercise 1, move arms out from the sides, with elbows stiff. Raise over head, bringing hands together. Return arms to the sides. Pause. Repeat 5 times.

Exercise 3

3rd day, or as instructed. While lying flat on back, head unsupported by pillows, raise head to touch chin to chest. Don't move any other part of body. Repeat 10 times.

Exercise 4

5th day or as instructed. Raise leg as high as possible, with toes pointed in line with leg, and knee unbent. Lower leg slowly, making use of abdominal muscles. Do not use hands. Alternate with right and left leg, exercising each 5 times. Later on, raise both legs at once, gradually increasing the height.

These and other helpful exercises can be found in *Essential Exercises for the Childbearing Years*, Elizabeth Noble, Houghton Mifflin, 1976, 180 pp., $4.95.

Baby's Development

Babies differ enormously in temperament and prevailing mood. Each has her own way. One baby will be placid and easygoing and sleep through practically anything. Another baby will be sensitive to the slightest noise or change around her, waking up startled as you tiptoe out of the room. She may even be hard to hold because she wiggles and squirms so much. She may resent being held at all, while the placid baby relaxes comfortably in your arms and takes everything in stride. Then there are babies who seem to need a lot of attention and are most happy when being held and fussed over. Enjoy your baby for what she is and don't feel she should be like another baby.

Each baby follows her very own timetable. Variations in development are natural, so she may develop more slowly than other babies in certain areas. Even though things are going well, we suggest that you check with your doctor. There are many factors that influence a baby's personal and social development. Whenever you are worried about the way your child behaves—about what she will or will not do—it is important to obtain professional advice. Your doctor and pediatric nurse are best qualified to determine if your baby's physical and mental growth are proceeding well.

If there are any special problems, such as difficulties with vision, hearing, coordination or feet, early treatment can make the problem much less serious and may even correct it entirely.

How to Keep Your Child Fit from Birth to Six
Bonnie Prudden
Harper & Row
1964   242 pp. $13.95

A manual showing how to exercise the new baby and prepare him to move well and grow healthily. The author describes how to teach infants to swim; exercises for five- and six-year-olds; and how to organize a physical-fitness program that can be continued throughout life.

I believe now that once a child learns to use his body correctly (and that's what basic exercises teach) he continues in daily action of any kind to use it correctly.

How Babies Talk
Peggy Daly Pizzo
Day Care Council
1974   85 pp. $4.95

Pizzo explains in simple language and drawings the process of learning communication skills. An appendix includes research notes and a bibliography of books by experts on child development.

While she has been learning to talk, the baby has also been learning to understand what her family means when they talk to her! Many times a day, from the time when she was just a few weeks old, her parents have talked to her and named things for her.

TECHNIQUES FOR INFANT MASSAGE

We take for granted the sensation of our own bodies sliding into the sheets when we go to bed at night, but consider the experience of the newly born baby for whom every sensation, every movement is a new experience. He needs the stimuli—coming as he has from the weightless environment of the womb—with which to experience his own body. Providing your baby with gentle massage is an awakening for him of his kinesthetic sense.

Of course babies organize their sensory input on their own. It all works; there is nothing to worry about. However if parents are willing to do massage with their baby, they will learn more about him and will provide a framework of sensory integration in which normal development can occur.

There is an actual sharing of energy, an energy connection between you and your baby. It includes the sense of pressure, of heat and a joining of energy fields between two bodies. Relish what you do with your baby, knowing that through your knowledgeable touching, you are providing him with an organizing principle that will allow him to come more fully into his own potential, his own faculty. You are also assisting him in being able to release whatever excess energy there is in the baby's structure. Part of an infant's frustration in life is that he has minimal movement available to him—he doesn't have a lot of ways to express his energy.

The way this massage is done is by following the pattern of the body's own development. This pattern begins with the head and moves toward the feet; and from the back, at the spine, around to the front of the trunk. Using your fingertips in a slow stroking motion, apply gentle pressure, always moving the tissues in the direction of the body's own developmental pattern—head to toe, back to front. Work along the spine, lengthening it from the head down. You can think of babies as being somewhat unfinished when they arrive in the world. Their development begins in the womb and continues long after birth, with some areas being more developed than others. An example of a relatively undeveloped area is the hips and legs. The legs flop over to the sides in the beginning, but long before they are ready to walk, you may bring the legs around to the front so that they are lying straight. Align them and gently bend them toward the chest, working them up and down in imitation of a walking pattern. Alternate with one leg, then the other, then both together. This begins to organize the whole pattern of the leg. The same thing can be done with the arms.

It is interesting to note that babies can develop tension very early in their necks and shoulders from the effort of holding up their heads. The effect may be a very short neck, or the neck disappearing as the shoulders are pulled up in the baby's effort to master this movement. So don't forget to massage this area each time you work with your baby.

When he is a little older, you will want to assist the baby in his experience of balance in a field of gravity. Ultimately that's what he needs to do in order to move. Provide him with gadgets to pull up on and to stand upright. Balance the baby on his feet, holding him at the armpits and giving him the experience of vertical alignment by bringing his weight down onto his feet. This gives the baby the biofeedback he needs in order to let him know where he's going.

The body is an instrument needing to be practiced. Your massage is an education in the use of energy, of how to go with gravity rather than against it, of how to balance your baby's body with ease. Your touch and massage will provide him with a sense of security about being in the world so that it becomes a supportive place in which to grow—that it is, after all, okay to be here.

Joseph Heller
Trainer, Heller Method

Infant massage is an art. Like any art we first build our foundation by learning techniques. Once the techniques become mastered they can be forgotten, then the massage will flow from your hands gracefully, effortlessly and effectively.

The child is to be completely naked, so provide a warm, safe place. If outdoors be sure to shade your baby's head. Choose a time when you can be relaxed and totally uninterrupted with the child for 10–20 minutes. Always massage when s/he has an empty stomach. Dr. Leboyer recommends that the morning bath be given after the massage; others prefer to give it just before nap or bedtime. It is important to sit on the floor with the spine erect and wise to pad your lap with a thick towel. You should use oil—apricot (odorless), castor (amazing healing properties), coconut, olive, almond, etc.; to prevent rancidity keep refrigerated when not using. In winter you may want to heat the oil in a small metal container; always be sure to warm the oil in your hands before applying it to the baby's skin.

Now you are ready to begin the massage. As the giver of this beneficial art you will need to be extremely sensitive to this new being's responses. Often the infants will cry a little in the beginning, this may merely be their way of speaking with you and they should soon quiet down and enjoy it.

With warm oil begin with the baby's chest. Move slowly and evenly up towards the shoulders, as if you are spreading the pages of an open book. Come back to the middle and repeat this move several times. Now your hands will work one after the other. Your right hand starts from your baby's flank, and moves across the chest towards the opposite shoulder. The moment this right hand reaches the shoulder, your left begins its motion, from the opposite side of your baby's abdomen, moving across the chest until it reaches its opposite shoulder. Then the right hand, starting again . . . and on, and on, like waves . . . never accelerate the movement, keep it slow, regular and consistent . . . the pressure of your hands will instinctively become stronger.

Now turn your baby on one side and begin to massage the arm. Supposing you start with the baby's left arm; your left hand holding the wrist, extend the arm. Your right hand grasps the shoulder and slowly moves up the arm with a "milking" motion. The moment your right hand reaches the wrist, your left hand, which has been holding it, is free and grasps the shoulder; repeat this several times. Your hands have been working one after the other, now they will work together. They both grasp the shoulder with a twisting and squeezing motion; moving circularly and in opposite directions, move towards the hand. Repeat this several times, ending each arm by working the wrist and hand, both of which are very important and take a little longer. Both of your hands hold the baby's wrist, your thumbs (one working after the other) massage the palm, working towards the fingers. Once this is completed, massage the fingers, unfolding them again and again. Now turn the baby to its opposite side and repeat all of this with the other arm.

Return the baby to his/her back. Both of your hands will move in an alternating rhythm, massaging the belly. Starting from the base of the chest, move downwards towards yourself, as if to empty the stomach. To fully relax the abdomen, grasp the feet and stretch the legs upward, thus deepening your massage.

For the legs, use the same techniques you did with the arms, although s/he may remain on her/his back. Ankles are as important as the wrists, so give them some special attention. Finish with the feet, using your thumbs first, then your palm.

Now you are going to massage your baby's back, which is perhaps the most important of all. Place the baby across your lap with its head to your left. First massage across the back with your hands rhythmically synchronized, although moving in opposite directions. Start near the head and work down the back, ending over the buttocks. Now your right hand holds the baby's buttocks firmly while your left hand moves alone, down along the spine. The more slowly you move, the stronger the sensations; move with continuity and full concentration. Then with your right hand grasp the baby's feet, so your left hand goes right on down to the extended heels in one sweeping motion.

The back massage is complete. It was the most important part of all, as the tensions are easily released at this young and tender age. As time goes by the release becomes more and more difficult, often "turning the proudest of living creatures into inner cripples."

Turn your baby onto its back and, using the tips of your fingers, move sideways along the eyebrows. Then, with your thumbs working together, gently move up the sides of the nose and over the eyelids. Now move down and slightly sideways, sliding along the nose and out towards the corners of the mouth, gently stretching the mouth outwards. Many babies find this intrusive at first, but if done so they can develop a tolerance for the sensation, they will soon give in to this delightful new experience.

The massage is concluded with three stretching exercises or asanas. To begin with, grasp your baby's hands or fingers with yours, fold both arms over and onto the chest, release, then unfold them, stretching them out, like unfolding bird wings. In the same way, grasp one foot and the opposite hand; make them cross each other. The baby will be able to touch foot to shoulder, hand to buttocks. Last, but not least, the padmasana, or lotus position. Grasping both feet, bring both legs up and cross them over the abdomen, giving them a good stretch, then back to where you started, stretching the legs out in this direction. Repeat this gentle folding and unfolding several times.

Claudia Lyman
Infant Massage Instructor

Loving Hands: The Traditional Indian Art of Baby Massage
Frederick Leboyer
Alfred A. Knopf
1976   139 pp. $8.95

In his previous work, *Birth Without Violence*, Dr. Leboyer decried women's lack of spontaneity and knowledge of how to touch their infants. Now he provides the necessary instructions through clear black-and-white photos and simple explanations of exactly how to touch baby by massage. The technique described is traditionally East Indian, with a sari-clad woman demonstrating on her baby. Even the technique is described in Leboyer's poetic style, helping keep in view the esthetic purpose of the massage, which is

Feeding the baby with touches, giving food to their skins and their backs, . . . just as important as filling their stomachs.

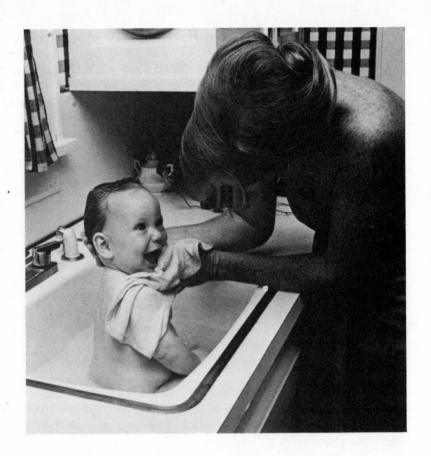

Bathing Your Baby*

Sponge baths are recommended until the umbilical cord has dropped off and the site has healed.

For baby's tub bath, assemble items needed within easy reach.

- Linens:
    Soft washcloth
    Small soft towel for drying
    Large soft baby towel (for baby to lie on)
- Tray items:
    Cake of mild soap
    Baby powder (or cornstarch)
    Baby lotion
    Cotton balls
- Clothing:
    Diapers, pins, shirt, nightgown
    Allow an extra diaper in setting out baby's needs at bath time.

---
*from *Infant Care*, Children's Bureau Publications, U.S. Department of Health and Human Services, U.S. Government Printing Office

- Equipment:
    Tub containing three inches of comfortably warm water (test with your elbow)

Using comfortably warm water, bathe your baby before a feeding in a room that is warm and free from drafts. Lower the baby to a sitting position in the water, supporting the head and back with your hand and arm.

The corners of the eyes may be cleansed with a soft cotton ball and cool water. The area around the mouth can be cleansed with a soft, damp tissue or cloth. Clean the external parts of the nose and ears with a moist cotton ball. Do not attempt to clean inside the nose or ears.

Wash baby's hair and body gently with a mild soap and washcloth. Be sure to wash the areas between folds of skin. Thoroughly rinse off all the soap, and lift baby from the bath. With a soft towel, dry the hair and skin.

Some babies quickly learn to enjoy their baths and it becomes a daily pleasure.

Layette and Nursery Needs

- diapers   3–4 dozen (1 dozen if you use diaper service)
- disposable diapers   1–2 boxes
- diaper pins
- waterproof pants   2
- shirts   4–6
- sleepers/gowns   4–6
- sweaters/sacques   2
- booties/socks   2 pair
- receiving blankets   4–6
- stretch suits   4
- coat and hat
- bibs   6
- carriage blanket
- stroller or carriage
- portable seat
- sling carrier or baby backpack
- bottles (4 oz. and 8 oz.) and nipples
- bottle brush
- measuring cup
- feeding spoons
- thermal bag
- mild soap
- baby shampoo
- baby lotion or oil
- baby powder
- cotton balls
- crib or bassinette
- waterproof mattress
- waterproof pads   4–6
- crib sheets   3–4
- crib blankets   2

Suggested Sleep and Bedding Choices

- bassinette   A bassinette or portable bassinette is good for a new baby. They are movable, portable and cozy for a new infant. Can be moved into parents' room if needed. Several sizes available.
- bassinette liner
- bassinette mattress
- bassinette sheets

or

- portable crib   Portable cribs are often used in lieu of bassinettes as they last longer.
- portable crib mattress
- portable crib bumper guard
- portable crib sheets

or

- six-year crib   Many parents use six-year crib from the start. If properly equipped with bumper guard, there is no reason why this is not feasible. Buy top-quality mattress only. This is one item where saving does not pay.
- six-year mattress
- six-year bumper guard
- six-year sheets   Fitted sheets are easier to manage.
- receiving blankets   Available in flannel, knit or thermal.
- lap pads   Use between baby and sheet. Place in diaper area.
- waterproof flannel sheeting   Size depends on size of bed. You can buy it by the yard.
- crib blankets   Size 40 × 60 is best. Thermal blankets are safest.

Extras

- Zip-A-Quilt   Bag converts to crib quilt. Often a gift item.
- shawl   Typical gift.
- crib quilts   Typical gift.

Equipment

- infant seat type carrier   Very practical. Must be adjustable.
- car seat   Essential for baby's safety in auto. Reclining models available. Must meet government standards for child safety.
- portable bassinette   Buy early if you plan to use it instead of bassinette. Bassinette sheets fit pad.
- carriage   Many carriages now lift out and make portable beds, and some convert to strollers. Carriages are still the best protection for tiny baby.
- carriage mattress
- carriage sheet
- carriage net

or

- reclining stroller   Many parents buy strollers right away, skipping carriages altogether.
and
- stroller napper pad
- cloth carrier   For carrying infant. Keeps baby snug and comfortable.

Suggested

- chest or dresser-chest
- playpen   Buy early, get more use.
- high chair   Some convert to youth chair.

or

- feeding table   Gives baby more space.

Extras

- walker
- jumper seat
- swing   Doorway type or on stand.
- nursery lamp   Typical gift.
- diaper stacker   Convenient, also typical gift.
- insulated diaper bag   A must! A typical gift.

For help in assembling a layette and buying clothing, toys, furniture and other items, call The Children's Design Center (within the U.S. (800) 833-4655, in New York State (800) 342-4774). This mail-order house carries a wide range of baby needs and will assemble, wrap and ship a ready-made baby shower. One of the greatest boons of this toll-free service is the complete consumer information and safety updates that are an integral part of the philosophy of The Children's Design Center. For catalogue ordering information see the Toys Section.

See also Appendix D—Clothing and Equipment Suppliers.

Safety Equipment—Basic

- night light   Good to have right away for your own protection and easier night feeding.
- electric plug-ups   Vital when baby starts crawling around the house.
- electric safety plates
- door locks   For doors you don't want baby to be able to open.
- safety doorknobs   For doors you don't want baby to be able to open.
- gates   Measure your doors first. Some gates are stationary, others movable.
- cabinet locks   To keep baby out of kitchen and bathroom cabinets.
- drawer stops   Prevents accidental opening of drawers.
- crib bumpers   To prevent head injuries.
- zippered harness   Secure baby in stroller or high chair. Keep a rein on toddler.

Toilet Training—Basic

- toilet seat adapter   If you can start your child on top of toilet.
- urine deflector   For boys.

or

- pottie chair and pot   For those who prefer to be closer to the ground.

or

- combination toilet seat and chair   Combines the two.
- step stool   Enables child to reach sink.

FIRST TWELVE MONTHS

Birth to 1 Month

Head sags forward when he is propped up. When lifted, head falls backward loosely. An object put in the hand will drop out. Stares indefinitely into space. Responds to loud noises and remains quiet when a bell is rung. Makes a humming noise when content. Stares at mother's face when nursing. Can lift head off bed and turn it from side to side. Body temperature regulator becomes steady.

2 Months

Coos and smiles. More responsive to adults. More alert facial expressions. Follows movements of people. Likes red and orange. Holds head up briefly when in prone position. Awake longer and may have eliminated 2 A.M. feeding. Notices light and associates sound with meaning (i.e., footsteps mean help).

3 Months

Rears head when prone. Sustains weight on forearms. Friendly but aware of strangers. Looks at hands. Smiles frequently and gurgles.

4 Months

Turns head to voice. Likes to hold head upright. Likes propped sitting position for no more than ten minutes. Smiles at sight of faces; very vocal. Laughs and looks at objects. Anticipates routine. Fingers are more nimble and busy. Plays with hands on chest, puts fingers and objects into mouth. May wake later in the morning and fuss in the late afternoon for attention, handling and change of position.

5 Months

Seeks the source of sounds. Will grasp objects. Suspicious of others. Pulls forward trying to sit up. Birth weight is usually doubled.

6 Months

Can roll to side. Grasps an object on sight. May begin creeping now through fifteen months. Puts things into mouth. May sit alone. Moves usually by wriggling and worming. Tries to pick up small objects.

7 Months

Grasps toes, rolls to prone position, gains sitting position with slight help. This process usually begins between now and nine months. Content to be alone long periods. First tooth usually appears now. Eager to use hands, banging objects and trying out senses in new ways. Sleep periods: two to three hours in the morning; one hour in the afternoon; twelve hours at night. Likes outdoor naps. Usually can wait half an hour or more for morning feeding. Pulls off booties and socks with joy. Beginning to be shy with strangers.

8 Months

Easily excited. Close interplay of laughing and crying. May say dada, mama, or similar syllables between now and ten months. Gets around easily creeping, crawling and wriggling.

9 Months

Soft spot on front of head begins to close and will usually be closed by eighteen months. Stands with help of crib or other handy object. Reaches, tastes, touches everything.

10–11 Months

Coughs to get attention. Probes with index finger to learn depth. Learns pat-a-cake and motion for bye-bye. Beginning to show temper in new ways. May cry during the night without waking or needing attention. Usually prefers to sleep indoors with shades drawn. Shows no food preferences. Afraid of strange voices. Uses various syllables such as ga-ga. He may have a verbal language all his own.

12 Months

Birth weight has tripled; about nine-inches gained in height. Sits well, stands while holding on, walks with help. May use occasional words and understands a great deal. Diet may be almost to the level of the common family diet with the exception of rich, heavy, spicy or fried foods. If family does not indulge in these foods, either, baby will join in family meals sooner. Appetite is moderate but interest in exploring the feel of food has emerged. Enjoys finger foods and participating in his own feeding. May have about six teeth now. Likes an audience and has a fine sense of humor. Imitates others and responds to rhythm. May begin to drop and throw, although parents should be prepared for mostly drop for a while! Between now and fifteen months, learns to feed self and walk with confidence.

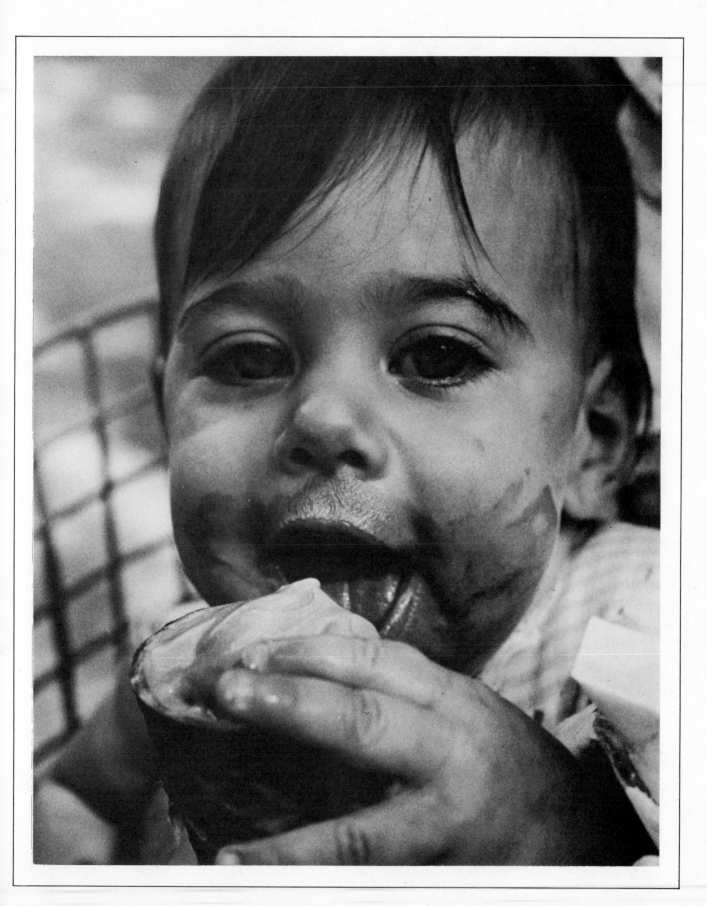

Tips on Baby Development/Care

6 Weeks

By this time your baby is becoming a social person who will respond to you by cooing and gurgling. This often starts so suddenly that you might miss it. By now he has usually been put on cereal. Start with rice cereal, as this is the easiest to digest. Mix 1 to 2 tablespoons of cereal with formula to the consistency of thin mashed potatoes twice a day.

2½ Months

Now he begins to develop rapidly. He is smiling and has well-developed head control. He can follow objects with his eyes from one side to the other. He can push with his feet if held erect. He should begin to sleep through the night.

You need not boil his water anymore. You can put him on all baby cereals and start fruit if you haven't already done so.

He will receive his first DPT (diptheria, pertussis and tetanus) and oral polio immunization at this office visit. You can help prevent or reduce reaction and fever by giving your baby half of a baby aspirin or Tylenol drops as directed by your physician. If he develops a fever or if he seems to be having much pain, apply a cool washcloth to the site of injection. Fever and pain should subside within twenty-four hours; if not, call your doctor. Comfort him as best you can during this period. Holding, rocking and the reassuring voice of mother can do wonders for pain, physical or emotional.

3½ Months

Your baby should be able to get by on three solid-food feedings per day, with an extra bottle of formula at bedtime. If not, don't panic. Your child may have unique needs which you need to listen for.

Until now, solid food has not been necessary. A whole new world will open up to you and your child in food variety. Go slowly with new foods. Introduce them and if rejected, don't force. This pace will give you a chance to see if your child has an allergic reaction to the food and will give your child a chance to adjust to new foods slowly.

He will receive his second DPT injection. Watch for fever or irritability and follow suggestions mentioned at his first injection at 2½ months.

It is important for you and your baby that he be sleeping through the night by now. Sometimes an evening bath helps prepare him for sleep as well as quiet music. If you choose this time for active play with him, he may not be able to settle down for sleep easily.

When he wakes up in the morning, don't hurry in to pick him up. Give him an opportunity to be alone for a while. This will pay off some Sunday morning when you would like a few minutes of extra sleep.

4½ Months

Your baby is becoming more independent and self-sufficient. She is able to hold her own bottle, which may be plastic if there is a chance of breaking and which is easier to hold. One of the reasons we began by being breast-fed as a species is so that mother would hold her baby for periods of time throughout the day, communicating her love and protection to the baby. Don't just hand your baby the bottle because she knows how to hold it and walk away. It is a trap many of us fall into easily, especially when we are tired, overworked or appear to have other priorities at the moment. When making your decision whether to hold the baby or hand her the bottle, listen to your needs and hers and make what seems to be a reasonable decision, noting how often you make the same decision and why. It gets you in touch with your parenting style and unmet needs, yours and hers.

At this age, your baby can vocalize pleasure and displeasure in new ways. You can give her a rattle as a toy. She will begin to respond to strangers. Now she will remember her doctor as the person who gave her that third DPT injection. This time she will also receive her second oral polio, which was skipped the month before.

She can start meat if she hasn't done so already. You may be interested in making your own baby foods. It can be fun, easy and very nutritious for your baby. There are two books which I recommend you read: *Feed Me! I'm Yours* and *Instant Baby Food* both described in the section, "Making Your Own Baby Food."

You can add fruit or vegetables to help flavor cereal and meat, which usually have a flat taste, especially the store-bought kind. How much she takes of each food is not important. Some days she will take more and some days less. Just offer food to her until she rejects it. Never force.

6 Months

Your baby is beginning to sit now and may be starting to creep. He bangs and shakes a rattle and transfers a toy from one hand to another. His language consists mainly of vowel sounds (e.g., "ah," eh"). He takes his feet to his mouth, and he reaches and pats his image in the mirror. His weight should be slightly more than double his birth weight.

Now is a good time to begin putting medicines and household items out of baby's reach if you haven't already done so. Keep your purse away from him, since it is likely to contain all sorts of unsafe "goodies."

You can augment his diet from strained baby foods to "junior" foods or make your own. This early nutritional pattern will have an impact upon his health later in life as well as now. If you make your own food or use table food as a base, beware of two ingredients to use sparingly: salt and sugar.

Your baby will receive his third oral polio immunization and won't receive any more immunizations until he is over a year of age.

7½ Months

Your baby probably has cut his first tooth by now or, if not, he will shortly. This may alter his sleeping pattern temporarily. He may become cranky and not feed as successfully as he has been. You may begin to offer him finger foods now. Sometimes the pressure of Zwieback toast or other food on the gums eases the pain. Drugstores offer remedies also for teething that you may wish to explore as a last resort. Please remember that this is a natural process for your child. Comfort him as best you can.

Diaper rashes and diarrhea are quite common at this time. For the diaper rash, I suggest trying to leave the diaper off as much as possible to allow for air circulation. Use Vaseline, Desitin or other ointments when you put the diaper back on. For diarrhea, limit fruit and just let the bowels rest. It is important not to leave him in diapers soiled by diarrhea, as it may create a burning sensation to the baby. Limit the feedings, including liquids as much as possible. Clear liquids like slightly sweetened herb tea, Jell-O water (one package of Jell-O to one quart of water) or flat 7-Up are helpful. If tolerated, you may add rice cereal and bananas, a good binder. If this method doesn't help, call your doctor.

9 Months

Your baby will probably be able to pull to a standing position by now. She says "ma-ma" and "da-da" and responds to her name or nickname. She also responds to social play such as "pat-a-cake" or "peek-a-boo."

She can definitely begin to learn what is and is not acceptable. If she is reaching for objects she shouldn't touch, it is a good idea to show her what she *can* do rather than just show her what she *can't* do. Try not to laugh at her when you correct her, as this is a double message. She will be confused as to whether you really mean it or not.

At this age, you will notice that she will begin to imitate. This is an important period of development. Your child will look to older siblings, often imitating their behavior. Be aware that the older child has emotional needs. The more mobile the baby, the more the sibling will feel impingement upon his territory. This includes attention from parents and others, as well as loss of position as the cute baby of the family.

Many table foods can now be added to the diet. The best ones to start with are hamburger, potato and scrambled eggs. Encourage her to feed herself. Be prepared for a messy operation. It takes time to learn, and we all have our own pace. Don't push the baby to be proficient faster than she is ready, able and willing. If you do push, you may promote a feeling of failure, and she may not try new experiences as readily.

12 Months

Now he may be walking. Don't hurry this process, because it necessitates much personal discipline and control. If he is preferring to walk rather than crawl, then I would buy some "first walker" shoes. They will protect his feet and facilitate his walking. Some of the best companies for shoes are Stride-Rite, Buster Brown, Edwards and Jumping Jacks. They all have a reputation for taking their time while fitting your child. These shoes also give good ankle support and have stiff but flexible soles.

He may be able to say a few words by one year of age. You can encourage him, adding to his vocabulary by having him repeat words after you in the form of a game. He may enjoy it. Do this especially if he is asking for something by pointing to it with his finger. He will delight in imitating the sounds. If he reproduces the sound incorrectly, don't say no and correctly pronounce it. *No* is often associated with failure. Just repeat the sound again and be patient. Imagine yourself learning a new language, trying to make the sounds correctly. This is a good time to get out the tape recorder and camera, recording for posterity!

His style of play has diversified. He will take great joy in playing with your Tupperware in the bathtub, your pots and pans in the kitchen and your magazines in the living room. Now grandparents can bring him all sorts of toys.

In order that your child have safe toys that last, you can develop a toy list for grandparents and others who gift-give at holiday time and on birthdays. They will be grateful for the information.

Toys should be selected for the appropriate age of the child, safety, use and, of course, price. Plan your toy list carefully. You will save money over a period of time and your child will feel more successful playing with toys that do not consistently break. Refer to Appendix E for information and recommendations.

The doctor will give him a tuberculosis test, which he will get periodically. On his next visit, at fifteen months, he will be immunized against measles, mumps and German measles (Rubella) with one injection. If your baby has no serious problems, your doctor will probably see him two to three times during the second year of development. Be sure to share any problems you are having in managing your baby's health needs, so that the physician can work with you in meeting health-care needs. Having a tuned-in physician can also do wonders for your mental health.

Adapted from
new-parent guide created by
Ron Goldman
Pediatrician

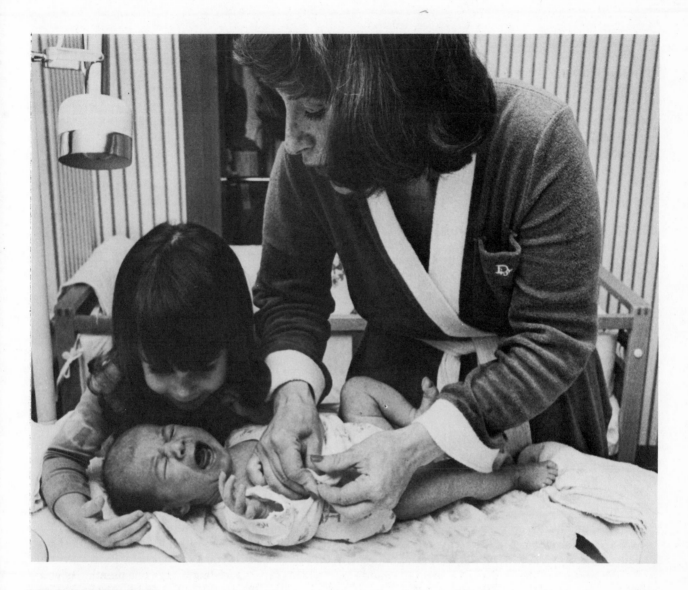

ON DIAPERING

Let us consider the process of diapering. While being diapered, the baby is close to the carer, sees her (or his) face, feels her touch, hears her voice, and learns to anticipate and know her. If the carer perceives diapering as a chore, she will try to do it fast and efficiently, putting an object into the baby's hand to distract him or her from the activity. There is little eye contact or communication as the carer concentrates on the lower half of the body. If the infant cries or objects, the carer hurries faster telling the baby, "We will be through with this in no time, and then we can play together."

Yet, what opportunities were lost! These caring times could be prime quality times for both participants.

Magda Gerber
Resources for Infant Educators

FEEDING AND NUTRITION FOR THE YOUNG BABY

The development of good mental and physical health is related to the ways mothers and fathers provide their newborn infant with nurturance. Nurturance includes meeting the infant's needs for love and for nutritious foods.

The feeding patterns of early infancy are tailored to fit the infant's hunger and sleep patterns. The baby learns to trust the special adults in his/her family to meet his/her general needs based on the way the baby receives nurturance. During the first month of life the baby's source of nutrition is milk, either breast milk or formula. Feedings should be pleasant times for the baby and the parents.

Tips about Infant Feeding

- Your baby knows how much milk his/her body needs and can handle at a feeding. Newborns tend to cry when they are hungry and will usually go back to sleep when their needs for milk and sucking are satisfied.
- Sucking is an important newborn instinct. The strength of the suck varies in each baby. Full-term babies have a stronger suck than premature babies.
- All newborns lose weight in the first few days. Most babies who get an adequate amount of milk will regain this weight in a few days. It takes two or three days longer for the breast-fed baby to regain weight. This is because the mother's breast milk supply isn't well established until the baby is four to six days old.
- Each baby gains weight at his/her own pace. During the first three months, babies tend to gain two pounds per month.
- Milk, either breast or formula, provides all the nutrients the baby needs during the first two to four months of life. When the mother's diet contains adequate nutritious foods, including vitamins and minerals, breast milk supplies all the nutrients and calories a baby needs.
- The feeding schedule and the amount of milk needed by your baby depend on the baby's size, the strength of the suck, quality of appetite, sleep-awake patterns, and the baby's need for calories to supply energy for growth and development. Some parents prefer to feed the baby every 3–4 hours; others prefer to feed the baby on demand. Flexibility in schedules is most important in the early weeks as you and your baby form a sense of fit and satisfaction. Many babies give up the middle of the night (2 A.M.) feeding by age one month. As your baby settles into a routine, the length of hours between feedings tends to stretch out to about four hour intervals during the day and evening.
- Typical feeding schedules for the first few months are:

1 week–1 month	4–5 ounces	in 6–8 feedings/24 hours
1 month–3 months	5–6 ounces	in 5–6 feedings/24 hours
3 months–7 months	6–8 ounces	in 4–5 feedings/24 hours

- Water (plain, no sugar added) should be offered to the baby between feedings in small amounts, about 2–3 ounces.
- Babies do not need solid foods before age three months. The baby's doctor or pediatric nurse practitioner will help you to decide when and how to add solids to the baby's diet.

Where to Go for More Information

The following companies put out brief pamphlets which are available FREE through doctors' offices, public health nurses and pediatric or well baby clinics:

- Ross Laboratories: "Breast Feeding Baby," "How to Fix Your Baby's Formula," "Como Preparar la Fórmula de su Bebé," "Your Milk Sensitive Infant," "Acerca de su Bebé, que no Tolera la Leche"
- Mead-Johnson Labs: "Breast Feeding your Baby"
- Roerig (C. Pfizer): "Handbook of Infant Formulas"
- Beech-Nut Baby Foods: "Happy Mealtimes for Your Baby," "Horas de Comida Felices Para Su Bebé"
- Johnson & Johnson: "Baby's Eating and Sleeping Habits"

New mothers usually have many questions about feeding their babies. In most hospitals, the nurses who take care of you and your baby can be very helpful in showing you and talking about techniques of nursing or bottle feeding and burping your baby. Other mothers are also good sources of information about feeding techniques. When a mother is in a comfortable position herself and holding her baby comfortably, feedings tend to be relaxed, pleasant and satisfying for the mother and the baby.

Georgia Millor
Nursing Instructor

VITAMINS AND FLUORIDE

If your baby is on Enfamil or any other commercial formula there is no need for him to take vitamins, since these formulas are fortified with the necessary amount of vitamins already.

If you are breast feeding or if you are using evaporated milk not vitamin fortified, then your baby should be on Tri-Vi-Flor drops daily. Also, if you switch your baby to whole milk before 6 to 8 months, you should begin vitamins then and continue until he reaches that age (6 to 8 months).

The use of fluoride has been shown conclusively to help prevent tooth decay. If your area does not have fluoridated water, it is a good idea to take vitamins with fluoride. After your baby stops his vitamins . . . give him fluoride . . . until he is 8 to 10 years old.

Ron Goldman
Pediatrician

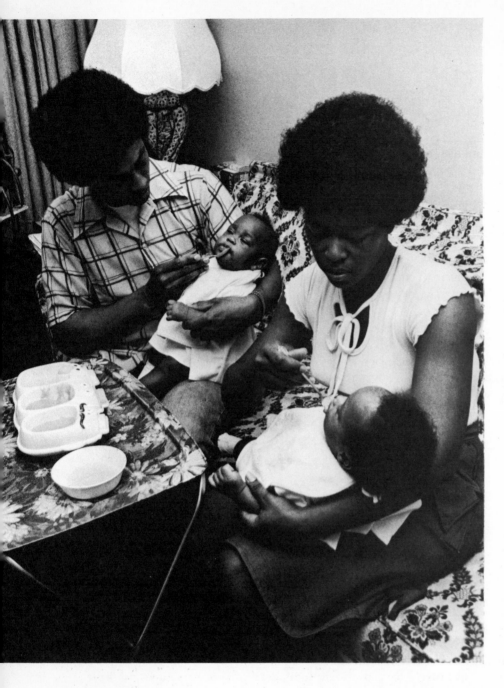

Making Your Own Baby Food

Instant Baby Food
Linda McDonald
Oaklawn Press
1976   112 pp. $3.95

Many parents like to make their own baby food and do so with a good food blender or a table-model food grinder. Food can be ground immediately after cooking, then served. Babies like stewed fruit, cooked vegetables, tender potatoes and boiled rice. Whole-grain nut cereals and yogurt and fruit are also recommended. Buy supplies in large quantities, thus saving money. Buy food without sugar and avoid commercially prepared foods that have cream or carbohydrates in them. Buy plain meat. Baby food is convenient and easy to prepare, and making your own makes a lot of sense, both in terms of cost and nutrition.

Feed Me, I'm Yours
Vicki Lansky
Bantam Books
1981   153 pp. $2.95

This book of recipes for your child's meals from infancy on was written by six mothers, all members of the Childbirth Education Association of Minneapolis–St. Paul, a nonprofit organization that prepares couples for a rewarding childbirth experience. Even to the adult reader, some of the recipes are mouth-watering and appealing. They are wholesome, nutritious and made with natural ingredients. Processed baby foods are wonderful for traveling, but *Feed Me, I'm Yours* offers

an alternative that is not as time-consuming and difficult as you might think . . .

Babies are particularly susceptible to digestive upsets, so it is important to remember that when you make your own baby's food, proper handling is necessary.

Stomach, Intestinal, Urinary and Genital Disorders

So many different things are quickly reflected in the digestive system, bowels or urine. A mild cold may depress the appetite, cause diarrhea or more frequent urination. A more serious illness can do the same. Check with the doctor when anything unusual appears. Treatment will vary with the cause, not the symptoms.

Diarrhea in a small child is of great concern, because it can so quickly lead to loss of water and imbalance of salts in the body. Diarrhea may be a symptom of dysentery caused by specific organisms, which are usually spread by careless handling of the baby's milk. However, diarrhea is more often the result of irritation from food, allergy or other illness. Do not give the baby with diarrhea too much fluid. Care for diarrhea lasting more than 24 hours should be supervised by a doctor.

Constipation is seldom serious. Parents mean different things by the word *constipation.* Some mean that the baby does not have a daily bowel movement. This is normal for some babies. Some mean that the baby strains at producing a stool. All babies strain during the first two or three months of life as they gradually stretch the anal opening. They look uncomfortable, but they are all right. They do not need a laxative. Some seem to like the parent to hold a hand under their feet so they can flex their knees and shove their feet against the hand.

Some parents use the word to describe hard, dry stools. Usually this type of constipation can be controlled by increasing fluids or making other minor changes in the baby's diet. If the baby is on formula, it may help to change to dark corn syrup or brown sugar in making it. See that he gets foods which aid in keeping the bowels soft, such as fruits and vegetables. Prunes and prune juice are good unless they happen to give the baby cramps.

The doctor can prescribe a safe regime for stubborn cases of constipation. While you wish to avoid subjecting a baby to painful bowel movements, the routine use of laxatives or enemas is never wise unless specially prescribed by a physician.

Foamy, frothy, foul-smelling bowel movements usually result from an inability to digest and absorb food properly. For malabsorptive disease, often called celiac disease, you'll need the doctor's help in planning a diet.

Occasionally there will be an obstruction somewhere in the baby's digestive tract. One type is called pyloric stenosis, which is characterized by frequent vomiting so forceful that the regurgitated milk lands some distance from the baby's body. Vomiting results because the opening leading from the stomach to the intestine is narrowed unnaturally by a thick, tight wall, which fails to permit the food to pass through. Almost every baby will, on some occasion, lose a whole feeding. But forceful vomiting, increasing in frequency, should be investigated. If the baby's vomit contains green bile, another type of obstruction may be involved. Get immediate medical help.

Once in a while, in a baby from three to six months of age or older, a segment of the bowel will fold in on itself, cutting off the passageway. The baby will scream in pain and pull up his legs. When the pain goes away, though, he seems well or possibly pale or listless. Pain may return, next time with vomiting. The bowel movement, when it occurs, may be dark with blood. This condition, known as intussusception, requires immediate medical attention.

Any unusual appearance of the baby's urine should be investigated. A kidney infection, called pyelitis, may cause the baby to have fever and appear quite sick. He's cross as can be and is quite miserable. There may or may not be vomiting. Loss of appetite is characteristic. The doctor will make the diagnosis from examination of the child's urine. Pyelitis is more common in girls than boys, perhaps because the urethral tract of girls is shorter and infection can reach the kidney more easily.

A discharge from the vagina of a little girl is normal in the first few weeks of life, but anytime thereafter, a discharge of any kind may indicate a mild or serious infection. Consult your doctor.

Learning, Play and First Toys

Play is a very important way your baby learns about himself or herself and the world. Through play, your baby will learn to use his body and his mind.

Your baby learns step by step. She learns to hold her head up before she learns to roll over. She learns to roll over before she can sit. She learns to sit before she can stand and stand before she can walk. Your baby learns to listen to your voice before she can talk.

By learning to do small things first, your baby is getting ready to do and learn bigger things later.

Your baby's growth and learning is like building a tower of blocks. Each little block is one step your baby has learned. Each block helps build the next block. All the blocks together can be a healthy child ready for successful learning in school.

Be sure that your youngster is ready for a particular toy. Avoid toys that are too complicated for him to use unassisted. Also avoid toys that are too big. An over-sized teddy bear or other stuffed toy may prove frightening to a small child. Toys that are too little are not wise choices either. Toys that have lasting value over the many stages of interest and development are the best purchases. Brief descriptions of some of the more popular toys for babies have been given here. You will find shopping for baby much easier if you familiarize yourself with what is available.

Good toys that will entertain and stay useful during your child's changing interests—things that will aid in his development—are worth buying. One well-constructed toy that will satisfy a need is far more meaningful than a lot of cute little toys that come apart when they're supposed to stay together.

Music box animals, made of soft fuzzy material, molded vinyl teething toys that are easy to grasp and mouth, fingered teething balls that have lots of little fingers protruding from the surface for baby to chew on, and wooden rattles with rounded edges that are sturdy and completely safe are all good.

Toys for First Year

Toys to bite, shake, hold, drop, look at or listen to. Washable, large enough so that they can't be swallowed; painted with nonpoisonous paint. Oilcloth or soft animals; colored wood or plastic beads; rattles; transparent, rubber, or sponge balls; teething rings, hanging objects to look at, clothespins, spools on string, blocks, cup and spoon, pie pan, box with cover.

See also the Toys section in Part II and Appendix E—Toys and Toy Manufacturers and Suppliers.

Teaching an Infant to Swim
Virginia Hunt Newman
Harcourt Brace Jovanovich
1977   116 pp. $2.45

"According to the National Safety Council, more two-year-old children drown than any other age up to five!" Safety is the primary consideration in teaching a child to swim, which could begin at age four months or simply whenever the child is ready. Health, fun and "a strong body, coordination, and a good appetite" are other benefits praised by the author. Special problems, particular swim techniques, safety rules and games are also discussed.

How to Play With Your Baby
Athina Aston
Fountain Publishing Co.
1976   119 pp. $5.95

An interesting guidebook for parents endeavoring to enter the child's world of sensory exploration. The formative years from birth to twenty-four months are explored through the various stages of development. Preverbal communication and a playful, productive atmosphere are stressed as essential to a child's growth and to a parent's increased understanding of it.

Watching your baby will be one of your greatest joys. Knowing something about the sequence of his development will help you to meet his needs. Each stage of development follows a progressive pattern that has never varied since prehistoric time. When your baby jumps at a sudden sound or shakes a rattle, he is doing what babies have done throughout history.

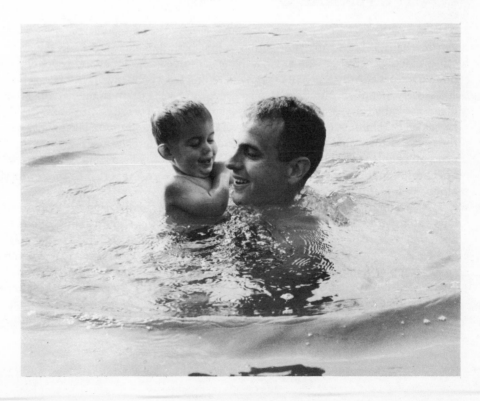

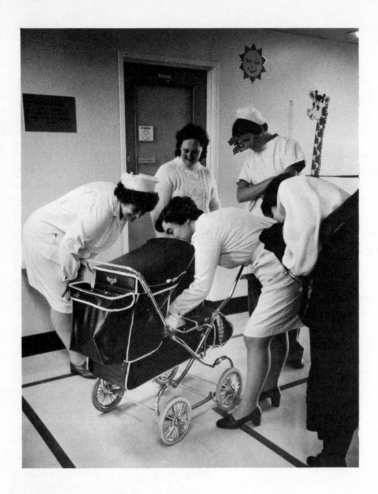

LOVE POTENTIAL OF THE BABY

When a baby is born parents are often in that period of their life when the greatest involvement is with career, self-discovery, necessity of making a living, unsolved emotional and psychological problems, etc.; and they are often overloaded with work, worries, and failing self-confidence. The child is invariably the victim, because he is still closely identified with the parents. The lack of self-esteem in the parents often imprints, directs and ruins the life of the baby for years, sometimes for all of his life. Generally, the parent does not realize the imprinting power he has on the child: our purpose is to make the parent or parenting person aware of his own needs, of the needs of the baby, of their differences, of the impact that the difference in size has on the baby (how would we like to depend on people some 15 feet tall?). Too often we are mindless giants, unaware of the baby's defenselessness and openness to motion, sound, touch, food, attitudes, words, mood. The sum of these is to a child what ground and air are to a plant.

A vast amount of love potential in people past the childbearing age lies unused. Often these people have been hurt and frustrated. Suspicion and fear keep the well of love tightly shut. Babies have the instantaneous power to open that well, to elicit that love which longs to express itself. Taking a baby to any public place, such as a market or a park, will make this evident: people with stern faces, self-absorbed and downhearted, light up at the sight of a child, dropping fears and defenses. This love potential should be channeled to the benefit of all: to the person who might not have a suitable channel, to the parents, who are often overworked, emotionally and physically undernourished and needing rest and direction; above all it would be to the advantage of the child who, having come into a welcoming and sane world would make it a better place, now and tomorrow.

Virginia Satir
Author, Counselor

Peoplemaking
Virginia Satir
Science and Behavior Publications
1975   305 pp. $5.95

Satir deals with every aspect of communication within a family —parent-to-parent and parent-to-child. Both the positive and negative aspects of nurturing the family are explored. Satir emphasizes fostering feelings of self-worth.

The Birth Order Factor
Lucille Forer and Henry Still
Pocket Books
1977   298 pp. $2.25

Drawing on case histories, Forer discusses the effects of birth order —and interplay with brothers and sisters—upon personality development and behavior.

. . . each role imposes specific challenges, offers specific opportunities, and fosters special skills and attitudes.

Good Things for Babies
Sandy Jones
Houghton Mifflin
1980   115 pp. $6.95

This consumer sourcebook of well-designed, safe products for babies gives instructions on how to shop and what to look for in such items as backpacks, shoes, playpens, toys, nursery decorations, and so on.

A thoughtful Grandma will buy baby everyday clothes that are comfortable and easily laundered rather than ornate laces and dresses, which often have scratchy, uncomfortable seams. Dresses are particularly unsuitable for the baby who is trying to crawl. Then too, a dress may be worn only once or

twice before it's outgrown or out of season, whereas the same money might be more wisely invested in blankets, shirts, and everyday things that will remain useful longer. Most of the ornate sweaters, hats and booties that are given as shower gifts are poor choices for tiny babies.

Everything You Need To Know About Babies
Linda McDonald
Oaklawn Press
1978   187 pp. $5.95

This guide to physical care of infants, from dental and foot-care information to clothing and baby products also lists services and organizations related to baby care as well as helpful publications.

For foot problems there is a better, fairly sturdy sneaker that is constructed with more rubber and with a stiffer canvas than the conventional sneaker. Some sneakers are so well made that they support the foot almost as well as an oxford. There is even a brand of sneaker made entirely out of leather. Children with weak feet should wear the better brands. If a child wears sneakers, he should change them regularly. Let him have as many as three pairs and give each pair a day or two rest between wearings.

Dr. Miriam Stoppard's Book of Baby Care
Miriam Stoppard
Atheneum
1977   192 pp. $10.95

As a doctor and the mother of four children, Miriam Stoppard draws on a wealth of medical knowledge and firsthand experi-

ence to provide a candid, practical, informal guide to having and caring for a baby from conception to three years of age.

Expertise is about textbook babies, parenthood is about your baby. So let me tell you what this book is not. It is not a book of rules, and still less is it the baby equivalent of a service manual. It is not a set of solutions to a set of problems, nor it is a set of instructions. It is, however, an attempt to guide you in making your rules.

Teach Your Child to Talk
David R. Pushaw
Dantree Press
1977   248 pp. $5.95

Pushaw stresses language as the basis of human thought and the importance of parents' role in communication development. This book includes activities to help reading, to assist motor coordination and to develop a healthy self-image and positive family relationship.

Around your baby's sixth month or a little earlier, you will hear him repeating syllables. He will make a sound consisting of a consonant followed by a vowel and repeat it over and over. It may sound like "ba ba, ba, ba" or "me, me, me." This is called babbling. Babies seem to enjoy both feeling and listening to what happens when they say these sounds over and over. This is useful. They need to associate the sound they make with the good feeling that goes with it. This helps them remember how to make it again. Babbling gives them this practice.

PART II

Raising Your Child

Abortion   After-School Activities   Away From Home
Abuse of Children   Alternative Schools
Adoption   Art

ABORTION. SEE BIRTH CONTROL.

ABUSE OF CHILDREN

See also Communication; Discipline; Rights of Children.

As frustration builds in parents they often direct verbal or physical anger at their children. To rid yourself of this anger, you must get to the source of it. Anger may come from many sources. For example, insufficient love and affection from your own parents can cause resentment which you may inadvertently direct at your children. Beware of taking your anger out on your children.

Children need you to understand that they are sometimes cranky, irritable, demanding and uncooperative. It is imperative that when the children express anger or displeasure, you do not respond in the same way. Go into another room and take a few minutes off to calm down. If you feel angry to the point that you feel you will hurt your child, pick up the phone and ask the operator for the local counseling service that you know can respond to your needs—or your child's pediatrician or a friend who will understand. Ideally every parent should have someone to call when he or she is angry or upset.

Many communities have set up "warm-lines," for just that pur-pose, with a number you can call at any time to obtain helpful counsel from an understanding, trained person.

Unfortunately, sometimes the people we need to talk with are not immediately available. In the meantime, close your eyes and relax, and think about something that you and your child enjoy doing together. Remember—frustration is normal. You are not wrong for feeling anger. Rather we can hit a pillow to vent our upset or cry, and not react to our child directly.

We must also look at the diets of our children, the amount of noise and upset they are exposed to and the state of our own lives before we blame our children for their emotions. Before responding in a negative way, attempt to find support within yourself or from people you can turn to.

No Language But a Cry
Richard D'Ambrosio
Doubleday
1970   252 pp. $8.95

This is a factual account of twelve-year-old Laura, who withdrew from the world after being physically deformed, brutally abused and nearly burned alive by her parents, and who, through psychoanalysis, coupled with patience, tenderness and imagination, learned to use language skills and become a functioning human being.

It is an unnerving experience to find oneself face to face with another human being who is alive, but not really living, who can feel but is not really feeling, who can think but is not really thinking. In those first moments between us the silence was deafening. It seemed something tangible, embracing the room, flowing out into the hallway and swelling through the entire institution—something I had to conquer. And in that spirit I reasoned that, if Laura couldn't talk to me, I would at least talk to her.

Web of Violence
Jean Renvoize
Routledge and Kegan Paul
1978   236 pp. $11.50

Who are the people who hurt each other? The author presents a vivid account of the feelings and problems of battering parents; of people who "rough up and assault." The author deals with child abuse, violent husbands and wives and incest, and looks into the psychological roots of people who react violently.

It doesn't much matter whom we consider the victim to be—the offender has in his or her time been victim too. Battered baby grown up to be battering father or mother, battered wife relating again and again to the wrong man, maladjusted adult sexually assaulting a loved child: all are victims and all sooner or later will be offenders, even if their offense is one of omission rather than commission. Inadequate, immature, insecure people can cause as much emotional damage to those they live with and give birth to as any aggressive, overbearing bully.

A

Organizations (See Appendix A)

Local:

California Children's Lobby

Parent Preschool Resource Center of the National Capitol Region

San Francisco Child Abuse Council

National:

Administration for Children, Youth and Families

American Association of Marriage and Family Counselors

Children's Defense Fund

Coalition for Children and Youth

Education Development Center

National Child Labor Committee

National Committee for Prevention of Child Abuse

See Appendix C for Films and Audio-Visual Aids

ADOPTION AND FOSTER PARENTING

See also Stepparenting.

IF YOU ARE THINKING ABOUT ADOPTION . . . THERE ARE CERTAIN THINGS YOU SHOULD KNOW

1. There are not as many babies available for adoption as there are families who want to adopt them. More unmarried women who used to place their babies for adoption are now deciding to keep them. If you wish to adopt a baby, you should begin the process now; waits of two to four years for a healthy infant are not unusual.

2. Consider adopting an older child or one with a handicap. There are over 100,000 older and handicapped children waiting for parents at the same time prospective adoptive families wait for babies. The children are as deserving, lovable and rewarding as a baby. Forty-seven states offer some financial help with medical and other adoption-related expenses. If you would like to know more about these children, please write to:

   ARENA's WAITING CHILDREN
   67 Irving Place
   New York, N.Y. 10003

3. Be careful about *how* you adopt. It is preferable to use an agency licensed in your state. Contact your division of social services for an up-to-date list of those approved organizations in your area. If you are considering adopting a child without an agency's help, you should see your lawyer about your state's requirements. Adoption is a legal as well as a social process; the rights of all parties must be safeguarded. Adoptive parent organizations can help answer your questions and provide support before and after adoption. For the name of one nearest you, please contact:

   NORTH AMERICAN COUNCIL ON ADOPTABLE CHILDREN
   1346 Connecticut Avenue, N.W.
   Washington, D.C. 20013

If You Have Already Adopted

Parenting a child through adoption is as rich and rewarding an experience as parenting a child you have borne. But it is different. Not recognizing this difference can lead to problems. Overemphasizing the difference has its own set of problems.

A

It is not helpful to deny the fact that the child was adopted. You cannot keep this secret successfully. When your son or daughter learns the truth, he or she may infer that there is something so bad about adoption, it cannot be discussed. Worse, concealment tells the child you cannot be trusted to tell the truth about important matters.

Sometimes parents are so zealous about disclosure, however, that they highlight the fact of adoption at every turn. Many stress the fact that their adopted child was "chosen." Overemphasizing the specialness of adoption may lead your child and others to wonder if you're really trying to convince yourself. Nor, in many cases, is it true that parents *are* able to choose one child in particular, although it has sometimes been possible to state a preference for the sex of a child to be adopted. Where a family is formed by having children biologically *and* by adoption, stressing the "chosenness" of the adopted youngster can make the children who were born to you feel inferior.

Adoption should be treated as a natural process. It is helpful to explain it to your child as you explain how babies are born and families are formed. If you are comfortable in explaining sex and reproduction, you will not have trouble explaining how your child grew inside another mother's body. It may be advisable for you to consult your local adoption or family-service agency for assistance if you find these issues difficult to discuss. You may also find the following books helpful:

- Berman, Claire. *We Take This Child: A Candid Look at Modern Adoption.* Doubleday, 1974. Interviews and case histories are used in a general review of the adoption scene today.

- Jewett, Claudia L. *Adopting the Older Child.* Harvard Common Press, 1978. Excellent reading for anyone considering the adoption of an older child.

- McNamara, Joan. *The Adoption Advisor.* Hawthorn, 1975. An overview of the adoption process, with helpful information for parents.

- For children: Livingston, Carole. *Why Was I Adopted?* Lyle Stuart, 1978. This book, for children 6–10, provides an excellent opportunity for parents and children to discuss adoption together.

Elizabeth Cole
Director, North American Center on Adoption

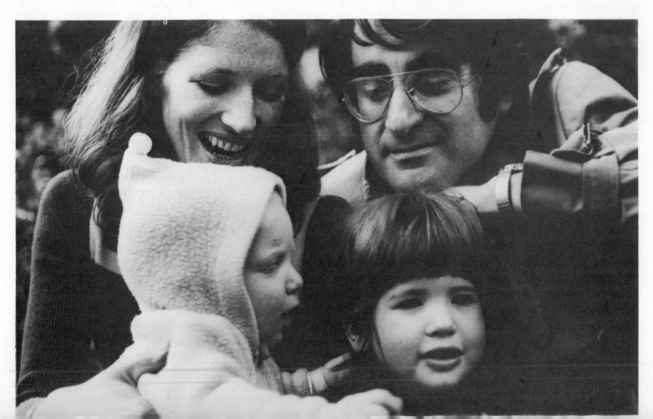

A

Foster Parenting

For a variety of reasons, a child sometimes needs a foster family. Foster-child care is an important responsibility that should be taken on with a great deal of consideration. Children need particularly loving support at a time when they or their biological parents are in the midst of a crisis. Every social service and health department offers a foster-care program; if you are interested in becoming a foster parent, contact these offices. The Education Development Center discussed in Appendix A can give you information as well.

Adoption—Is it for You?
Colette Taube Dywasuk
Harper & Row
1973   158 pp. $6.95

Adoption yesterday and today are discussed, and the author gives suggestions to help the reader decide whether or not he or she should consider adopting a child. Dywasuk explains how to weigh risks, evaluate consequences and adjust when the adopted child grows up. Names and addresses of adoptive-parents' organizations are included.

Your child's attitude toward the facts of adoption will be conditioned by you. If you feel you are his parents, you'll be able to discuss his adoption without anxiety, embarrassment, defensiveness, or apology.

Yours By Choice
Jane Rowe
Routledge and Kegan Paul
1971   148 pp. $4.50

A guide for those considering adoption, this book answers questions of heredity, illegitimacy and infertility and presents ways to help parents answer adopted children's questions regarding their origins.

What kind of children do you enjoy most and what is it about the others that you find trying? Do you like most of the children you meet, not only your relatives but the noisy little boys next door or the school children you see on the bus every morning? Or do you find yourselves criticizing the way these youngsters behave and feeling that if you were bringing them up they would behave better? It's as well to face realities here. Although it is certainly true that some parents do not handle their children as well as they might and that therefore these youngsters are more troublesome than they need to be, nevertheless the children you see around are almost certainly behaving much as the average child does all over the world. It isn't really too likely that the child you bring up will be any different, and when you get down to it, why should you want him to be?

Brothers Are All The Same
Mary Milgram
E. P. Dutton
1978   28 pp. $6.95

This book for very young children deals with two sisters who must contend with a neighbor, Rodney, who refuses to consider their adopted brother "real." Rodney is wrong about other things as well—he thinks there is only one

way to make a paper airplane. Eventually he comes to realize that there are many ways to make an airplane—and more than one way to get a brother or sister.

This is Joshie. He's my little brother and he's adopted. He's funny. He's a pest. And sometimes he's really dumb.

Is That Your Sister?
Catherine and Sherry Bunin
Pantheon Books
1976   35 pp. $4.95

This true story about interracial adoption by six-year-old Catherine and her mother is told in Catherine's own words. The book is filled with photographs of the entire Bunin family.

Sometimes when they see my mother, the kids ask, "Is that your mother?" I know why they ask me the questions, because my sister and my mother and I don't look anything alike. We don't have the same kind of skin or face or hair. I tell the kids that my sister and I are adopted. Then they ask, "What's adopted?"

Organizations (See Appendix A)

Child Welfare League of America
Education Development Center
North American Center on Adoption
U.S. Department of Health and Human Services

AFTER-SCHOOL ACTIVITIES

See also Creativity; Games and Activities; Playgrounds; Sports.

When the school day is over, children want to know that someone is there for them to share the day's lessons and adventures. They want to know that they can still check in with a responsible adult from time to time whether they are doing their homework, watching TV or playing with friends. Some parents are able to be at home when their children come home from school, and they can take the child to different activities—dancing lessons, nature studies, music lessons or trips to the dentist or doctor. Working parents who are not able to be home should make arrangements for after-school activities for their children. This may be an after-school program connected with a public school, a family day-care home nearby or a baby-sitter who lives near the school or home.

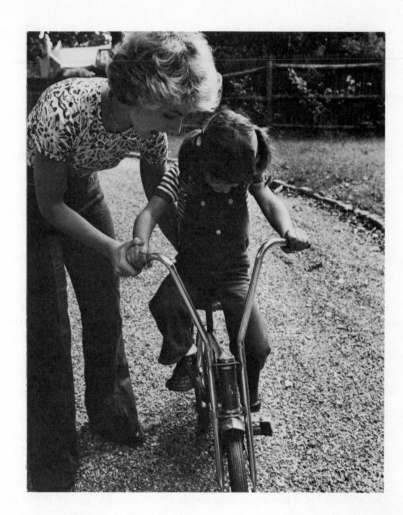

A

WHAT SCHOOL AGE CHILDREN ARE LIKE

School age children are far harder to handle than those of preschool age. These older children do not stay behind fences, they rebel against adult direction, and take delight in being rude and crude. On the other hand, they are exciting, venturesome, loving, creative, expansive, friendly, and pliable. . . . To develop in a healthy style and to be comfortable with the world take some sustained, invincible constancy in his life in the form of an adult or adults who provide the home base from which he ventures forth and to which he returns.

As the school age child progresses in the development of his physical, emotional, intellectual, and social self, the intervals between his need to touch a home base will be greater, but, until he is full grown, will not disappear entirely.

Preteens are "emancipated." At least they think so. And in many ways they are. But the sense of loneliness they feel when on their own is, perhaps, more devastating than the younger child's.

Preadolescence is the last stage of childhood, and its importance for the future of the child is immense. A good child care program will afford the maximum opportunity for meeting the preadolescent's normal growth needs. At this period in his life, neglect and loneliness will take their toll sooner or later, perhaps in mental illness, or in crime and delinquency, or in inadequate parenthood. . . .

Essentially, then, what every child needs is a spot in the world where he is welcomed every day by a familiar grownup—one who is glad to see him and who offers him the opportunity to be himself, to be protected when necessary against the hazards of living, to help him recoup the losses of the day and regain the sense of his own worth. This grownup may be a relative, neighbor, or friend who is in the child's own home or one who is outside of his home. But the child does not want to be engulfed by adults who commandeer him and make all his decisions. . . .

Successful Growing Requires a Balanced Routine

The years from 6 to about 10 are full of a growing feeling of importance. The child with good experiences senses his capacity to do things well. He starts to work hard at becoming good at something. School is one of the important doorways to helping him feel successful. However, the many hours and days outside of school also provide part of the foundation for the "grownup" feeling of importance and for belonging to the wider world. The struggle to achieve at this age prepares the child for the work world of the adult and for the capacity to cope with both progress and disappointment—the realities of life.

The key to successful growing through this age span is the balance between guidance and direction and expanding opportunities for independent thought and action. Each child will grow at a different pace. Some will learn more quickly than others, some will be more independent than others, some will master physical skills earlier than intellectual skills. Some will master nothing well if stable, understanding, supportive adults to emulate are missing or are in short supply. Much of a child's sense of importance, of feeling he has the ability to succeed, and of knowledge that he can learn comes from his playing with others his age in the street, on the playground, or in his own home with friends of his own choosing. . . .

The school age child has many needs which can and are met by a wide variety of community activities—through plans for the individual child, such as music or dance lessons, and through participation in agency or organizational programs such as the YWCA and YMCA, Boys' Clubs, Store Front Clubs, etc. But none of these can take the place of an adult who is responsible for a child before and after school, who talks with him when he is troubled by his friends or in trouble with his teacher, who helps him select the club or "Y" or swimming group or any of the other special things he likes to do on any given day, or sees to it that he has time to do nothing if he wishes. He is given freedom to play with another kid on the block, or to be a part of the neighborhood gang shooting marbles in the street; he does not have to go to a different club, group, or activity each day in order to find shelter and guidance.

From "School Age Child Care"
Gertrude Hoffman, U.S. Dept.
HEW, 1972 23 pp. 65¢

Organizations (See Appendix A)

American Alliance for Health, Physical Education and Recreation

American Red Cross

Boys' Clubs of America

Boy Scouts of America

Camp Fire Girls

Girls' Clubs of America

Girl Scouts of the United States of America

National Commission on Resources for Youth

local YMCA

local YWCA

ALTERNATIVE SCHOOLS

See also Education.

Over the years, public schools have received a great deal of criticism. Perhaps some of it is unfair, as any system is only as good as the people it serves and responds to.

If public or private school is not working for you or your child, an additional form of education is available: alternative schools. For the most part, these are developed and run by parents who group together much as a cooperative, and then hire a teacher or teach the children themselves. Often the school will run successfully and become a private school. But the philosophy may be more informal than the public-school program and allow more flexibility. Alternative schools will need the same kinds of materials that are used in public schools, but they might have additional kinds of activities not often found in the public schools.

Certainly the most important aspect of children's education is being with people who care about, love and respect them.

GROWING WITHOUT SCHOOLING*

Our newsletter is about ways in which people, young or old, can learn and do things, acquire skills, and find interesting and useful work, without having to go through the process of schooling. In part, it is about people who, during some of their own growing up, did not go to school, what they did instead and how they made a place for themselves in the world. Mostly, it is about people who want to take or keep their children out of school, and about what they might do instead, what problems come up, and how they cope with these. We hope, also, that children who are, right now, growing without schooling will let us know how they feel about this.

Growing Without Schooling, or *GWS* as we will call it from now on, will be in part an exchange. Much of what is in it, we hope, will come from its readers. In its pages people can talk about certain common ideas, needs, concerns, plans, and experiences. In time it may lead to many informal and personal networks of mutual help and support.

GWS comes out whenever we have enough material to make an interesting issue. This may at first be only three or four times a year. Later, as more people read it and send in material, it may come out as often as six times a year.

GWS will not be much concerned with schools, even alternative or free schools, except as they may enable people to keep their children out of school by (1) Calling their own home a school, or (2) enrolling their children, as some have already, in schools near or far which then approve a home study program. We will, however, be looking for ways in which people who want or need them can get school tickets—credits, certificates, degrees, diplomas, etc.—without having to spend time in school. And we will be very interested, as the schools and schools of education do not seem to be, in the act and art of teaching, that is, all the ways in which people, of all ages, in or out of school, can more effectively share information, ideas, and skills.

Subscriptions

GWS will be supported entirely by subscriptions, not by advertising, foundations, universities, or government grants, all of which are unreliable. We will do our best to print as much useful material as possible at the lowest possible cost. But we think it best that those who use a service should pay the cost of it. We also want those who work on *GWS* to be paid a decent wage, if only for the sake of staying power. People who work for nothing or for token wages soon grow tired of this and quit. We want this newsletter to come out as long as people feel a need for it. This can only happen if those who put it out do not have to do so at great personal sacrifice.

* Subscription $10.00 for six issues from Holt Associates (see Organizations)

On Social Change

A We are putting into practice a nickel and dime theory about social change, which is, that important and lasting social change always comes slowly, and only when people change their lives, not just their political beliefs or parties. It is a process, that takes place over a period of time. At one moment in history, with respect to a certain matter, 99% of a society think and act one way; 1% think and act very differently. Some time later, that 1% minority becomes 2%, then 5%, then 10, 20, 30, until someday it becomes the dominant majority, and the social change has taken place. Some may ask, "When did this social change take place?" There is no answer to these questions, except perhaps to say that any given social change begins the first time one person thinks of it.

I have come to understand, finally, and even to accept, that in almost everything I believe and care about I am a member of a minority in my own country, in most cases a very small minority. This is certainly true of all my ideas about children and education. We who do not believe in compulsory schooling, who believe that children want to learn about the world, are good at it, and can be trusted to do it, without much adult coercion or interference, are surely not more than 1% of the population and perhaps much less than that. And we are not likely to become the effective majority for many years, probably not in my lifetime, perhaps not in the lifetime of any readers of *GWS*.

John Holt
Educator, Author

Books

Private Independent Schools
Bunting and Lyon
Blue Book Publishers
1980   861 pp. $35.00

Lives of Children: The Story of the First Street School
George Dennison
Random House
1969   397 pp. $6.95

Instead of Education,
John Holt
E. P. Dutton
1976   250 pp. $8.95

Summerhill: A Radical Approach to Child Rearing
A. S. Neill
Pocket Books
1977   392 pp. $4.95

On Learning Social Change: Transcending the Totalitarian Classroom
Michael Rossman
Vintage Books
1972   384 pp. $2.45

Organizations (See Appendix A)

National Alternative Schools Program

For more information contact:

Holt Associates, 308 Boylston St., Boston, Mass. 02116

National Association for The Legal Support of Alternative Schools, Box 2823, Santa Fe, New Mexico 87501

National School Alternatives, 1289 Jewett St., Ann Arbor, Mich. 48104

Directories

New School Exchange, Pettigrew, Arkansas 72752

Department of Education, University of Massachusetts, Amherst, Mass. 01802

The Guide to Summer Camps, Summer Schools, Porter Sargent Publishers, 11 Beacon St., Boston, Mass. 02108

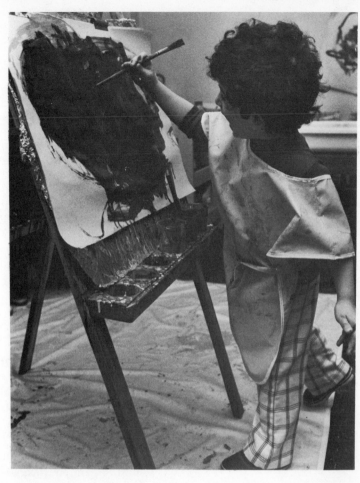

ART. SEE CREATIVE EXPRESSION.

AWAY FROM HOME—SCHOOL, CAMP AND OUTINGS

See also Camps.

You can prepare your child for her first solo experience away from home by creating opportunities to be without mother or father and with friends, relatives and schoolmates. You want to know that your child can function well in a new environment, so be sure she knows how to use the bathroom, how to wash her hands and has the basic skills of putting on shoes and rubbers, buttoning coats, zipping jackets and tying shoelaces. Make sure she has

clothing that is easy to get in and out of. When your child is comfortable, you make it easier for her to be away from home.

Children should carry identification with name, address and telephone number and be able to recognize their name on labels.

Before starting school or camp, your child needs a recent physical examination, a measles vaccination and vision and hearing tests. Be sure she has had a recent visit to the dentist.

Schoolchildren should know how to take turns, play fairly, to cooperate and still be able to stand up for their rights. Safety rules should be stressed, like looking both ways before crossing the street. Prepare your child for unfamiliar or unexpected situations: what to do when she misses the

school bus or what to do when she comes across a large, frightening dog.

How children feel when they are among others is important, but self-esteem is more important. To assist your child in her thinking and developing self-confidence, ask her how she would react to different problems and discuss them. Another good idea is to accompany your child to school or camp so that she feels comfortable during the trip and doesn't feel that you are abandoning her. Staying overnight with friends and grandparents is good preparation for being away from home.

BABY-SITTERS

See also Child Care; Nursery and Preschool Care.

Choosing a Baby-Sitter— An Important Task

One of the most important jobs a person can have is being responsible for someone else's child, yet parents too frequently hire a baby sitter at the last minute and know very little about her/him and fail to give her/him the proper instructions.

- It is important to choose a sitter wisely, whether it be aunt, grandfather, older sister, brother, neighbor, etc.

- If possible, pick the sitter from a family with whom you are acquainted.

- Know that he/she is reliable. Leave your child with a sitter who is feeling well and healthy.

- It is important that your sitter enjoy keeping children, for she/he is apt to be more attentive and cooperative with your instructions.

- Whether teenager or grandmother, the sitter you want should be capable of using good judgment—for example, never admitting a stranger to the house, never permitting dangerous play, never leaving a child alone even for a minute.

- Every sitter should be able to administer first aid for minor cuts and bruises.

- Ask the sitter to come at least 15 minutes ahead of time; this will give her/him time to read and hear your instructions and to get acquainted with your children.

Sitting Safely

If you have younger brothers and sisters at home, you probably feel confident and experienced. On the other hand, be frank about your qualifications. For instance, you won't want to accept a job caring for a young baby if you know nothing at all about infant care. It's best to gain your experience under a parent's supervision before taking full charge alone.

Safety Reminders for Different Ages

A good sitter watches both the child *and* the surroundings. Although no two children are exactly alike, there is a predictable pattern of development which can help to guide your care.

Babies up to 6 Months

A newborn needs close attention and protection. Make sure that the baby's face is free of covers, clothing or anything that might interfere with breathing. Take a look from time to time to make sure that the baby is resting comfortably, and also to see if more or fewer covers are needed. Even when adequately dressed and covered, a baby's hands usually stay cool. A better way to find out if the baby is warm enough is to feel arms, legs or neck.

Babies should never be left on anything from which they might fall. Make it a habit to keep the sides of the crib up when not tending the baby. A brand-new baby can move considerably by kicking and wriggling. Even an infant who appears to be unable to move much may surprise you—the moment your back is turned—by tumbling off a bed, sofa or table. So, never leave a baby unguarded even to get a fresh diaper or to answer the phone or doorbell.

From 6 to 12 Months

Between 6 and 12 months, babies can roll over, push backwards and forwards. They learn to sit, creep, crawl, and then pull up to standing. A crawling baby likes to get out of the playpen part of the time. It's the start of that "into everything" stage. When you let the baby out of the playpen, crib or highchair, be alert to all possible danger in the way—breakable bric-a-brac, matches and lighters on low tables and shelves, lamps and cords, electrical outlets, household cleansers and medicines. If a baby grabs a forbidden object, take it away matter-of-factly, and then divert attention to something else that's safe to have.

Ask Parents . . .

B

When you baby-sit, take along a small paper pad or notebook and write down pertinent information from parents. Here are the kinds of things you will want to know.

Where can I reach you? _____
(phone)

_____
(address)

What time will you be home? _____

Any special instructions? _____

_____

_____

_____

Necessary phone numbers?

Local emergency number _____

Doctor _____
(name)   (phone)

Neighbor _____
(name)   (phone)

Relative _____
(name)   (phone)

Police Department _____

Poison Control Center _____

Other _____

Remember not to tie up the phone with long conversations.

B

From 12 to 15 Months

At this age, a child's curiosity seems boundless. Babies need to roam and explore, but they also need limits. You have to keep an eye on them practically all the time. Be sure that safety gates at top and bottom of stairways are latched. Without these, you may have to bar the stair with a heavy chair, or what-have-you, to prevent climbing and falling.

A baby of this age usually likes to play with simple toys that can be taken apart and put together again. With several blocks, the baby can put one on top of the other and knock them down. You might build a block tower so that the baby can have fun toppling it over.

Around 2 Years

Two-year-olds are adventurous and independent. They know how to do many things and seldom sit still for a moment unless tired and sleepy. Turning a doorknob is a new skill which may mean trouble if, say, a cellar door is left unlocked. Or, in the blink of an eye, a child can be out the door and down the street! It happens all the time. So, besides being on the watch, make sure that doors leading to danger are locked or latched.

Suggestions for the Baby-Sitter*

- Be sure the parents give you full instructions. Follow the instructions carefully.

*Reprinted with permission of the American Academy of Pediatrics.

- **In case of illness or accident:** Call the parents. If they are unavailable, call their physician. If he is unavailable, call your physician.
- **In case of fire or smoke:** Get the children out of the house immediately, without stopping to dress them or to make a phone call.

  Take the children to the nearest neighbor, then call the fire department first, the parents second.
- Do not open the door to strangers. If you cannot identify a sound, call the police, then the parents.
- Never leave the children in the house alone, even for a minute.
- If a child awakens crying but does not feel feverish, tender loving care will usually quiet him. If all fails, call the parents.
- Remember that your primary job is to care for the children.

"Sitting Safely; for Baby Sitters" Metropolitan Life Insurance Co. 1978 15 pp. free

Here is an array of tips for baby-sitters that emphasizes safety and applies to charges of every age.

Besides alerting sitters to potential household dangers room-by-room, this covers every aspect of baby-sitting, from fee, hours, transportation to and from job, to where to find clothing and food for baby.

On-the-job performance caution:

- *Keep all doors locked and do not open unless parents tell you that a friend or relative is coming at a specific time.*

- *Never leave the children alone in the house.*
- *Stay awake, studying, reading or watching TV.*
- *Don't have friends in unless the child's parents agree to this.*
- *If you use the phone, make your conversations brief.*
- *Resist refrigerator raids. Parents usually tell you what's for you.*
- *If the baby can't sleep, just be calm and cheerful, letting him or her relax.*
- *Leave the house just as orderly as you found it. This means tidying up after yourself, and helping the child to put away toys.*
- *When you have to break a baby-sitting appointment, try to let the parents know well in advance.*

For Children

My Friend The Babysitter Jane Werner Watson, Robert E. Switser, J. Cotter Herschberg Western Publishing 1971 30 pp. $2.95

This book helps parents prepare young children for accepting temporary separation and having positive experiences with babysitters.

My friend the babysitter comes to stay when my mother goes away for a little while. I show my babysitter my books and my special toys. Sometimes I play with her. If I play by myself, I know she's there. If I go off by myself, I can come back and find her. That's nice to know. I have so much to do, and so many places to go!

BIRTH CONTROL

Several methods of birth control are available, and it is important to select the one that works best for you and your mate. Spacing children more than a year or two apart gives you a chance to heal and gives you and your baby time to get used to each other, and birth control can prevent unwanted pregnancies during these periods.

Abortion

The question of whether to terminate an embryo before or after three months of age is a controversial issue, both from a religious and an ethical point of view. Though opposition to abortion is great, from a practical, economic, social and psychological perspective, abortion is sometimes imperative. Responsibility for one's body and for the outcome of one's actions is essential. It is important to separate sex and procreation, recreation and responsibility. Teenagers, in particular, who become pregnant before they can be responsible for a young infant, are often endangering the life of that child.

These problems are not easily solved, but they should be respected and given consideration. Each individual must do what is in her heart, what is best for her situation, without judging or being judged by others.

Birth Control Book
Howard I. Shapiro
St. Martin's Press
1973 318 pp. $10

Shapiro's book is a guide to almost every type of pregnancy prevention, from diaphragm to vasectomy. There are suggestions on how to choose and use an IUD, how to apply recent advances in rhythm method and how the effects of a vasectomy can be reversed. Useful graphs, charts, illustrations, photographs and local organizations are included.

The diaphragm is an ideal contraceptive for women for whom accidental pregnancy would not be a physically, emotionally, or religiously devastating experience.

Women in their late forties, approaching the menopause, are well advised to use the diaphragm, since the chances of conception are lower at that age, while the dangers and side effects of the Pill and IUD are greater. The diaphragm is also an ideal contraceptive for a woman having infrequent intercourse. Taking birth control pills every day in anticipation of only an occasional sexual encounter appears to impose too high a risk on a woman. If you abstain from intercourse during the menstrual period because it is too messy, inserting the diaphragm over the cervix at that time solves the problem. Since the risk of pregnancy is minimal during the menstrual period, the diaphragm may be removed at your leisure over the next few hours following coitus.

Organizations (See Appendix A)

Planned Parenthood Federation of America

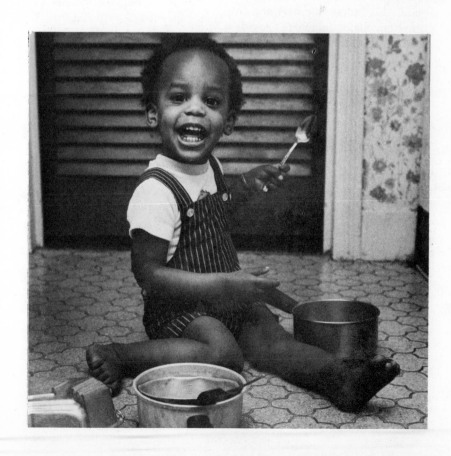

BIRTHDAYS AND PARTIES

B

Whether you have your child's birthday celebration at the beach, the circus, or in your own backyard, birthday parties can be fun, but they are trying for everyone. Advance planning can eliminate some of the potential problems.

Let your child help you. Kids can make up the guest list, design invitations, choose the food (ice cream, cake, icing!) and favors, plan the games and help decorate. Offer your suggestions if necessary. Keep your group small, and try to have a teenager or someone else assist you. If possible, have the party outdoors.

The party will be even more fun if you can make party hats and baskets and other decorations beforehand. Plan games. Children also like to sing and do rhythms together, to imitate animals and to draw and paint together. Provide each child with a small favor to take home; balloons or little toys are excellent. The day of the birthday party, plan a simple meal for the whole family so that the strain of the day will not wear you out.

Confetti: The Kids' Make-It-Yourself, Do-It-Yourself Party Book
Phyllis Fiarotta and Noel Fiarotta
Workman Publishing
1978   224 pp. $5.95

This book contains over 150 easy-to-follow, imaginative crafts for more than 20 of the best bashes, from birthdays to the last day of school party: Fish kites, bing-banger noise-makers, ice cream castles, totem poles, lovebird mobiles, delicate Valentine hearts, handmade greeting cards, and of course, confetti.

George Washington, Christopher Columbus, and you have one thing in common, a yearly birthday celebration. That's right, your birthday is just as important as the other two. This year, circle your special day on the calendar and plan to have a rip-roaring, All-American carnival party. Scatter plenty of balloons around the party room. In the center of the table place a delicious carrousel cake and alongside it, a jester filled with party favors, one for each guest. Give everyone a clown mask as well as a pointed pompom hat. Ice cream, popcorn balls, candy apples, and hot chocolate with melted marshmallows are all-time favorites. This party might just turn out to be "The Greatest Show on Earth."

The Dynamite Party Book
Linda Williams Aber
Scholastic Book Services
1978   80 pp. $1.50

This book offers new and different party themes and ideas for children, from a Mystery Party with FBIce Treats and A Nose For Crime Game to a Hooray for Hollywood Party, which includes a Gossip Column Game and Hollywood Heroes sandwiches.

Strike up the band! Turn down the lights! And bring on the dancing ghouls! You're having a monster of a party and all your favorite friends are invited! It's going to be a glorious get-together with demonish decorations, ghoulish games, fantastic food and more fun than a barrel of bats.

Camps	Communication	Cultural Awareness
Child Care	Cooking with Kids	
Clothing	Creative Expression	

CAMPS

See also Away from Home.

Summer camp can be a very pleasant experience for children, especially after they have had some experience away from home, either at day camps or nursery schools. When you are looking for a camp, get recommendations from other families, finding out which camps are most popular, the programs they offer and their staff qualifications. Explore camps which offer special programs: diet, horseback riding, sailing, music, dance and the arts are some examples.

Before your child leaves for camp, make sure her health forms and other information are completed. Talk about the camp experience and the different activities and opportunities camp offers. Make sure your child knows how to make her own bed. Have her take a supply of stamped postcards addressed to home, and send along a minimum of clothing. Most camps will suggest what clothes to bring along. Plan for parent visiting days, a pleasant time for you to be with your child. While your child is at camp, you and your mate may want to enjoy a vacation or rest.

The Guide to Summer Camps and Summer Schools
Porter Sargent Publishers
1979-80   445 pp. $12.99/$9.00

This yearly publication offers comprehensive information on summer academic programs for children, summer camp listings and descriptions, as well as information on unusual opportunities such as the Outward Bound program and camps for the handicapped or maladjusted.

Organizations (See Appendix A)

American Alliance for Health, Physical Education and Recreation

American Camping Association

Boys' Clubs of America

Boy Scouts of America

Camp Fire Girls

Girls' Clubs of America

Girl Scouts of the United States of America

Local YMCA

Local YWCA

Religious groups also sponsor camps.

CHILD CARE

See also Away from Home; Baby-Sitting; Nursery and Preschool Care.

With millions of mothers working, child care is used by many families. It is needed by all families at some time, and thus it is important that parents work together to provide the best child care possible in their communites.

Child care is any service for children provided at home, in someone else's home or at a day-care center. Here we are specifically referring to care outside the home.

The checklists which follow will help you locate an adequate child-care center. Publications on child care are listed as well.

Follow the suggestions in the Away from Home section to be sure that you have prepared your child. Reassurance that you are coming back and know and trust the person that you leave him with can calm fears.

If you are fortunate, you may have a variety of types of care to choose from in your area. When child care is available, you may be able to return to school or work and feel assured that he is well cared for while you are away. It can also provide your child with new friends and opportunities.

It is good to develop a play group when your child is small, because it gives you the chance to get to know other parents as well as to have an opportunity to develop a baby-sitting exchange. If you are using a day-care center, check it out carefully. Find out the adult-to-child ratio, what activities are provided, whether there is sufficient indoor and outdoor space, the kinds of play equipment that are available and the schedule of activities. Children should not be overly organized and should not spend too much time sitting or napping. Be sure you visit the facility that you are considering and observe the way the children respond to the adults around them.

The following checklist gives you some ideas on what to look for in a possible nursery school or child-care program for your child. This list covers just part of the picture. You should also investigate the emotional climate, the learning environment and the social aspects of the program. Take the time to look to find the best possible program for you and your child.

Copies of the checklist and other ideas are found in *Choosing Child Care*, a guide for parents from parents. It may be purchased from the Institute for Childhood Resources, 1169 Howard St., San Francisco, CA 94103 for $3.50 per copy (make checks payable to Parents and Child Care Resources).

- Can the facilities be reached easily?

- Do the children and staff interact happily and communicate easily?
- Is each child respected as an individual?
- Are my needs for the caregiver to be dependable and to value me as a parent considered?
- Can I afford the fees at this facility?
- Is the facility suitable for my child and my situation?

Organizations (See Appendix A)

Administration for Children, Youth and Families
Child Welfare League of America
Day Care Council of America

Physical Facility Checklist

Look over the space for the safety features, well-planned and adequate space, the condition of play equipment inside and out, and overall attractiveness.

1. Does the space seem in good repair and safe? (Are light sockets covered or out of reach?)   Yes   No
2. Is there enough open space, and is it well planned for children?   Yes   No
3. Is the equipment inside and out varied, sturdy and appropriate for a child to use?   Yes   No
4. Is the place attractive and comfortable? (Are there plants, pets and special areas for activities?)   Yes   No
5. Can the children get inside and outside easily and safely?   Yes   No
6. Are the materials ample, in good condition and easily available? (Can children reach the variety of books, toys, art supplies?)   Yes   No
7. Are the bathroom facilities clean, easy for a child to use and in good repair? (Easy-to-reach faucets, toilets, toilet paper, toothbrushes and toothpaste, paper towels, etc.?)   Yes   No
8. Are meals nutritious, well balanced and varied? Is the food prepared and served attractively?   Yes   No
9. Do the children have a comfortable and quiet place for naps? Do they nap on cots or beds?   Yes   No
10. Does the facility have provision for an isolated place for an ill child?   Yes   No

Tally of observations on physical facility:

Total Number of Yes Answers _____

Total Number of No Answers _____

Words I would use to describe the place

How would my child feel about this place?

How do I feel about this place?

INTRODUCTION TO CO-OPS

C

Nursery school tuition can cost from $50 to $130 per month. Many funded schools are restricted by their funding to low-income families.

If you are one of the many families caught in this double-bind, you might consider the alternative of the cooperative nursery school. Tuition at cooperatives can be as reasonable as $19 per month. The explanation for this difference can be found in that key word "cooperative."

In a cooperative nursery, or day care center, parents provide many of the services for which a school would normally have to pay. For example, maintenance is provided by parents at "work parties" scheduled as tasks arise, or on a regularly assigned basis. A spring work party might consist of painting a classroom, repairing outdoor equipment, and replacing floor tile. Fences must be mended, bookcases painted, and the kitchen cleaned. Each family must usually contribute a certain number of hours during each year to these jobs.

Another area of parent responsibility is the conduct of business. There are tuition clerks, purchasers, membership chairpersons, treasurers, and so forth. These jobs are easily managed in a school of 15 to 30 children, but often need to be shared in schools which may have 50 or 75 children.

The third and most important area of parent participation is in the classroom itself. A parent is usually required to participate in the class one day per week for each child he or she has in the school. Father or mother may come to school on the assigned day, and some fathers with flexible schedules, such as students, seasonal workers, or those temporarily out of work, participate regularly. Each day there must be enough parents and trained teachers to meet regulations. Parents with particular skills or interests are encouraged to share them with the children. Thus a mother who plays the guitar or accordion will bring her instrument to school, play for the children, and let them try to pluck the strings or press the keys. A mother with special cooking skills will plan to assist the children with one of her recipes; children participate in making egg rolls, latkes (potato pancakes), and tea cakes, and learn about each other in this way. Cultural backgrounds and interests are shared, offering the children an opportunity to grow in their learning about and appreciation of the world and its diverse people.

Meetings are an integral part of cooperatives. Since parents work in the classroom, they are an important part of the teaching staff, and most cooperatives have at least one meeting per month—and some as often as one per week —to plan activities and discuss the emotional and physical development of the children, individually and as a group. If a family has had a crisis, such as a divorce, this is shared in the group, and parents discuss ways in which to help the child deal with this. Also, since parents cooperate on the same day each week, the Wednesday cooperator may never see the Friday cooperator, except at these meetings.

Structure of Cooperatives

Most cooperative nurseries and day care centers have a parent Board, elected by the membership. The Board may consist of President, two or three vice-presidents (in charge of, for example, human relations), secretary, and treasurer. In most co-ops, the Board is entitled to set up the budget, approve expenditures, and hire teachers. Teachers may or may not be considered members of the school community, with voting rights. Some cooperative day care centers are staffed by parents entirely, aided by students or volunteers, who meet collectively to make decisions about policy or program.

Forming a co-op—Small co-ops are often organized by young mothers looking for quality programming for their children, but unable to spend a great deal of money. Frequently a notice in supermarket or laundromat will bring a group together for this purpose. The Parent Cooperative Preschools International has published a manual which carefully details the procedure for setting up a co-op nursery, with specific instructions for licensing, hiring, health, equipment, etc. Many other books are available in this area.

Why choose a co-op? If you want a shared experience with your child and an opportunity to grow as a parent with a support system, co-ops may be for you. Co-ops are also a bargain today. In a morning nursery, a parent is committed to one morning a week, plus perhaps an average of two hours per month at maintenance, or an hour or two per week purchasing, as examples. A monthly meeting adds two more hours. These commitments may not be realistic for a family where both parents work.

C
A co-op can be an enriching experience in many ways. Parents and children learn together—to tie-dye, batik, or make egg rolls, projects which may then be carried out at home. Each parent is exposed to the parenting styles of the others, and learns new ways to cope with a tantrum or a fight, observes the teachers' techniques, and tucks those too away for future reference. For families new to a community or isolated from the extended family, the co-op is a place to make new friends, where people care about each other and the children. The group provides enormous support to families with problems, often assuming the role of the missing extended family.

And what does the child gain? Children and parents alike are bolstered by seeing the parent in a positive role of facilitating the child's growth, development, and education. A shy child feels better when his mother cooperates, and learns to feel at home more rapidly. The child's classmates are real to parents, so that stories of his school day are more meaningful. The parent gains a certain prestige in the school for work she may do. When mothers are at home most of the time, confined to being chief cook and bottlewasher, this can be a tremendous boost to the ego.

Who chooses co-ops? Because of the commitment to cooperate, private co-ops tend to be composed largely of middle-class, two-parent families. University students tend to choose co-ops for their children, as do faculty families. As previously mentioned, co-ops may create a hardship if both parents work. In recent years, though, employers have become more aware of the parent's obligations, and permit the employee to use the time he needs for this purpose, making it up at other times.

A cooperative experience can be one of the most enriching in a young family's life. The key to this experience is the amount of investment you are willing to make. If involvement in your child's education seems exciting to you, then the chances are that your family would be happy in a cooperative.

There is also a large body of knowledge which suggests that when parent training through meetings is an integral part of the program, the family and even the community will benefit. This was one of the reasons that much of the Project Headstart planning included parents. Leadership qualities developed through work in the group can translate effectively into the community, when previously disenfranchised people challenge public schools and other institutions. There are, in fact, a small group of people who consider co-ops a political statement, one step toward changing society.

Irene Cohn
Parent, Lawyer, Co-op Founder

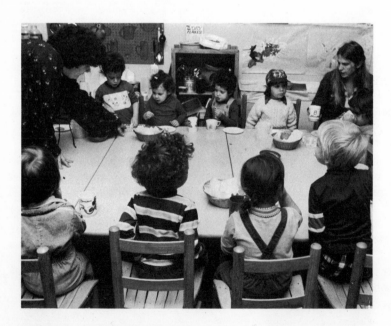

Sharing the Children
Nora Harlow
Harper & Row
1976   154 pp. $2.95

A funny, unorthodox account of small-town-type child care in the heart of New York City. Six mothers unable to pay for day care share care of their children, each taking one day a week. When more parents participate, the group encounters institutions and city bureaucracies in their effort to set up a storefront center.

Our center was going to be more humane, run by the community, and cozier, but essentially the same: set up to meet the needs of the business world.

Organizations (See Appendix A)

National:

Administration for Children, Youth and Families

Child Welfare League of America

Day Care Council of America

Education Development Center

U.S. Department of Health and Human Services

Local:

Bananas Child Care Information Service

Children's Council of San Francisco—Childcare Switchboard

Day Care Council of Nassau County

Maryland Committee for Children

Parents as Resources Project—Evanston, Ill

Magazines (See Appendix B)

Children Today
Day Care and Early Education
Handbook for Working Women
Voice for Children
Working Mother
Working Woman

CLOTHING

See also Part 1—Layette and Nursery Needs

Color-fast washable clothing that is simple to get on and off is the best day-to-day apparel for children. Versatility and comfort are the most important criteria. Shoes should be comfortable and roomy and worn with socks that will not slip into them. With a few shirts, sweaters, a bathing suit, several pair of play pants and a dress-up outfit, he or she will be sufficiently prepared for school, play and special outings. Since children grow so quickly in the first ten years, large wardrobes are expensive and impractical. Brothers and sisters can share clothing with each other, and clothing swaps are popular among many families.

Appendix D lists manufacturers and distributors of children's clothing. We have selected items from each company which are durable in construction and/or pleasing in design.

Golden Hands
Sewing Children's Clothes: A Pattern Book
Random House
1973   128 pp. $7.95

A good book for beginners, with easy-to-follow instructions for making collars, buttonholes and decorative touches. Includes sixty designs for making everything from pajamas to overalls and winter coats.

Any hem over four inches deep will only add weight to the garment and make it look shapeless. Bear in mind, too, that when a dress becomes too short for a growing child it affects not only the hem but also the length between shoulder and underarm and this, in turn, makes the sleeve too tight.

COMMUNICATION

See also Discipline; Emotional Development; Language and Speech

Through three levels of communication—verbal, tactile and visual—we express our love, disapproval, anger and encouragement to our children. A familiar complaint is that while we spend hours talking to our children, we are not really communicating with them. We are hearing words, but not responding to the emotion behind them. In this hectic world, conversation often becomes a mere transfer of facts and information, even between parent and child. The ability to empathize with one's children takes time, perception and a bit of work to achieve. But it can result in true communication and sharing of ideas and emotions, not just a verbal barrage which leads to misunderstandings and hurt feelings.

Familiarity with these three levels of communication will make you a more effective parent. Tone of voice is crucial in communication. While you may often want to express your anger, a well-modulated tone of voice is likely to be more effective than harsh tones, which can scare a child. We all lose our tempers from time to time, but remember that children often don't know why we are mad. Loud noises can frighten children.

C Touching and hugging are now known to be vital to the well-being of babies and children, stimulating their physical growth and emotional stability and happiness. A hug and a kiss to begin and end each day can say "I love you," and give your child the security that no matter what happens, he is safe with you.

Children are also perceptive to nuances of expression. Often you can discipline with a look and never say a word. Be aware of your expressions. You could be conveying a mood which has nothing to do with your child, but which he interprets as such.

If you make an effort to listen to your child's ideas, offer praise and support for his endeavors and remember the importance of physical affection, your communication with your child will be vastly improved.

RECLAIMING THE CHILD WITHIN THE CHILD

Have you caught yourself reacting to the demands of a child with irritation and frustration, perhaps uttering such phrases as:

> *"Can't you do anything for yourself? What's the matter with you anyway?"*
> *"Shut up, or I'll really give you something to cry about."*
> *"You're big enough to do that for yourself."*
> *"When your brother was your age, he could tie his own shoelaces. Why can't you?"*

As parents, we have all experienced some level of displeasure at having to tend to a new arrival in the early hours of the morning as the child's demanding cries intrude into our peaceful sleep. These kinds of responses from us are used by the child as an excuse to deny personal self-worth.

While it is true that an infant is less able to tend to the physiological needs of survival than we are, it is equally true that this being in a tiny body has a capacity for joy, a passion for life, an adventurous curiosity, and a level of creativity that we may not have known in years.

As I look around, I see hordes of adults afflicted with terminal normality suppressing their spirit to fit into the mold of the sector of the society they claim for peers. Recall even the dreary conformity of the nonconformist youths of the late 1960's.

The magical child in your life offers you an exquisite opportunity: the opportunity for you to heal your wounded spirit, rehabilitate your capacity for ecstasy, and to rediscover love. Love is the experience of knowing that another truly sees you and conveys to you that they will not harm you, that they accept and do not judge you, and that they celebrate and support the essence of your being.

While you offer the child the opportunity for physiological life, the child offers you the chance to regain emotional, mystical, and spiritual integrity and to heal the wounds of the past.

It is a relationship between two equals: a person called a parent and a person called a child. The parent-child relationship, when this opportunity is recognized, is a truly balanced, inspirational, loving and creatively productive adventure.

Stewart Emery
Founder, Actualizations

Body Language of Children
Suzanne Szasz
W. W. Norton
1978   159 pp. $10.95

This book explores physical clues to a child's posture and expression, giving universal meaning to elevated eyebrows, placing of a hand on the head, turning of the open palm upward, and so on.

The body language of children is the most reliable way of understanding their feelings and desires. . . . For example, parents have to learn to distinguish between a hunger cry, a lonely cry, or a bored cry by observing the infant's physical clues. A good parent-child relationship demands that parents quickly tune in to their children's nonverbal language and, at the same time, that children learn what their parents' body language is telling them.

Listen To Us!
Dorriet Kavanaugh
Workman Publishing
1978   255 pp. $5.95

This book contains collected opinions of children between the ages of six and thirteen on such topics as school, corporal punishment and sex education.

Karen, 9: Sometimes if I'm on the phone, my mother hollers at me and makes me get off the phone. She goes on hollering at me because she knows I'll be embarrassed. And the next day I go to school and somebody asks me why did I hang up the phone on them. So when I get home, I tell my mother all about it and she says, "I'm sorry." It happens again and again and again.

And everytime it happens again, she says, "Sorry," but it happens over and over anyway. I get mad at her for a long time—about a half an hour or an hour. Then she comes over and she hugs

me and squeezes me and embarrasses me. I always get mad at her and she says, "I made a mean child." I have my eyes all down, all squinched up.

How to Get Your Child to Listen
Thomas J. Banville
Condor Publishing
1978   211 pp. $2.50

Nearly all persistent, unacceptable behavior in children has its roots in poor listening, according to Banville. Chapters offer a step-by-step guide to help them develop proper listening habits. Included are appendices of auditory exercises and body-image activities.

It's always a good idea to begin the search for causes of poor listening with a thorough examination of your child's hearing. A child who doesn't seem to respond to directions may be unable to do so because he can't hear them. If your child hasn't had a hearing examination, have that done before you try to do any of the exercises with him.

Getting Along in Your Family
Phyllis Reynolds Naylor
Abingdon
1976   112 pp. $5.50

For youngsters, this book deals with problems of relating to brothers and sisters, understanding parents, sharing tasks, and the like. Also discussions of what it's like to be youngest, oldest and middle child are presented.

Happy families don't just happen, they are made—by lots of effort and patience. Just wishing won't do it.

Some of the ways of working at it are really very simple.

When someone in the family is in a bad mood, it makes sense to stay out of the way until he or she

feels better. People who are very upset or angry or tense are in no condition to listen to someone else. Instead, they want others to understand them, and at that moment they are not especially concerned about how others may feel.

COOKING WITH KIDS

See also Food and Nutrition

Children enjoy learning how to prepare food and should be allowed to experiment and master this skill. They also need to clean up after themselves, shop for food and prepare food properly. Taking the time to teach children these skills is worthwhile. Cookbooks written especially for children are enjoyable for them to use and have easier-to-follow directions.

A few references for these books are:

Crunchy Bananas and Other Great Recipes Kids Can Cook
Barbara Wilms
Sagamore Books/Peregrine Smith
1975   111 pp. $4.95

Kids in the Kitchen
Lois Levine
Macmillan
1973   192 pp. $1.25

Many Hands Cooking: An International Cookbook for Boys and Girls
Terry Touff Cooper and Marilyn Ratner
Thomas Y. Crowell (Harper & Row) in Cooperation with UNICEF
1974   50 pp. $4.95

Strawberry Shortcake Cooking Fun
Michael Smollin
Random House
1980   38 pp. $1.25

C

Skills List for Little Cooks

- mixing
- beating with an eggbeater
- stirring
- whipping
- mashing
- measuring
- leveling
- packing
- squeezing drops
- cutting
- slicing
- chopping
- spreading soft onto firm
- washing
- draining
- straining
- kneading
- squeezing
- rolling
- grating
- cracking
- peeling
- tossing
- shaking
- turning
- unscrewing
- pouring
- dipping
- scrubbing
- tearing, breaking, snapping
- juicing with a juicer
- grinding with a hand grinder
- wrapping

CREATIVE EXPRESSION

See also Games and Activities.

Children express themselves by their continuous and natural creativity—through singing, dancing, moving, playing and creating art and music. Children are creative in play with other children, when they are by themselves playing dolls or dress-up or creating their own dramas and puppet shows.

All too often we remember times when our parents stopped our creativity when we were in the midst of something that was important to us. Try to respect your child's needs to express himself as best he can and give him time to share his creativity with you. It is important that home and school nurture and support children's creative expression in art, music, dance and theater, so that children's personal expression can flourish. Creative expression is as important as other learning; maintaining a balance between intellectual and creative expression is important.

Imagination and Fantasy

Fantasy is a very important part of children's growth. They need to spend time in imaginative play to develop their creative ideas. They do that in a process of play by themselves, often making up imaginary friends as well as playing with other children. These fantasies are an important part of this process. It is important that you do not make fun of them or ridicule them or tease them about their imaginary playmates. Children work out feelings and ideas through working with their imagination.

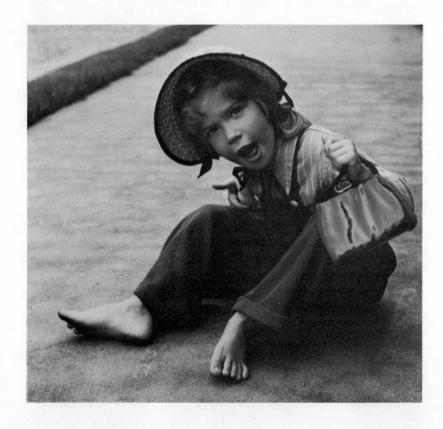

CREATIVITY FOR CHILDREN

C

By a creative life for children, we mean a creative life for all children—not only specially talented children or specially bright children or children with some gift for seeing and hearing differently from others, but *all* children. We mean the kind of creativity that is possible for every child in every kind of home in every kind of community. We mean a chance for every child, as he grows and comes to understand the world, to make new a part of the world he sees. It means giving children a chance to do in play, as they grow, the kind of thing that is done by poets and landscape architects, scientists and statesmen to such a superb degree.

This may seem to be contradictory. If only a few adults have such great creativity, how can all children be creative? This is partly because during the time they are growing, their whole being is involved with growing taller, stronger, and more mature, and growth itself is creative. Each day is a new day. The child makes it so because the child has grown. This is the day when, for the first time in the world, Jimmy or Betty can stand, or swim a hundred yards, or climb the tallest pine tree in the wood. As creativity is essentially making something new, all those who are busy growing are naturally creative.

Each time a piece of learning takes place, we realize anew the extraordinary quantity of knowledge that all young children are absorbing, even in a home where the parents are busy and harassed or are very little informed. The child is learning who he is and what he is, what the difference is between things that are alive and things that are not, between human beings and animals or insects, between the familiar and the unfamiliar, what is *up* and what is *down*, and what is *across*. When we talk about making a child's life creative, we are in a way talking about adding something new to this natural absorption of the world—about how to make the learning that will take place anyway be more meaningful and more alive.

One very important way is to provide the conditions within which the child himself can discover the complex things in the house, in the town, in the natural world, with just enough help to be sure the clues are right. Ants live in ant hills. If you follow them from the spilled sugar to the place where they are going in a straight line, each carrying a tiny crystal of sugar, you will find where they came from. What is honey? What is a bee? A few days later, a sting teaches all too well what a bee is. But what has honey to do with stings? It may take a trip to the country or a picture in a book and a honeycomb to provide the information the child needs—the facts of the hive, the bees coming and going looking for clover, the beeswax. Left all alone with wonder and questions and doubt about the connections between what happens at the same time or in the same place or with the same word used for two different things, the child is often lonely, frightened, in despair for fear he can *never make sense* of the world. "Mrs. Jones calls her little girl 'honey.' Is she a bee?" Children need the help of grownups to get a lot of these things straight.

Because the child, growing and learning, creates anew the experience of inventing a calendar or a telephone or of discovering the idea of transparency, people sometimes speak as if children were repeating the history of the human race. Long ago, mankind had to learn where honey comes from, how to make a calendar, how to make rope, how to weave, and many, many centuries later, Benjamin Franklin attracted electricity from the clouds, and, still later, the telephone was invented by Alexander Graham Bell. A child, as he learns something that adults already know, is repeating not the history of the human race but only the history of human children. Children in each generation have to re-create all the discoveries and creations of previous generations. Once upon a time, no one could count to six. But the child who is playing with the silver drawer or the kitchen utensils and who, discovering six knives and six forks and six teaspoons and six tablespoons, suddenly discovers *sixness*, is not making an original discovery of the same kind as the man who learned to count beyond five. The sixness is there in the half-dozen spoons and half-dozen forks, and it is expressed in all sorts of half-dozens as mother counts the laundry or orders rolls. Children discover for themselves the wonders that their parents and teachers already know. Those few who keep the freshness of a child's mind can go on to the other kind of creativity as adults.

Some people have also thought that a child has a more creative life if he lives very simply, perhaps on a small farm, and that things like candles are easier to understand than electric lights, wood fires than gas stoves. They think that because the child lives a simple life among things that are easier to understand, this will somehow make the child's understanding more creative. But this is not necessarily so. If a child's father is a farmer who knows a

C great deal about plants and animals and can understand what the child is wondering about and where his questions are leading, life on a farm can be very creative. And if a child's father is a skilled mechanic who understands about radio and TV and electric stoves and a.c. and d.c. current, then living in a city as the child of a skilled mechanic can be equally creative. What the child needs is someone wiser and more experienced than he is to whom he can go for an explanation when he is puzzled.

Margaret Mead
A Creative Life for Your Child
U.S. Children's Bureau
HEW, 1973

ART FOR CHILDREN

Some children are not consciously resistant, but are so inhibited or tight that they may need to first experience some safe activities that may help free their imaginative processes. I know that some children are quite fearful about letting go of themselves in some of the ways I suggest, and I may deal directly with the fear behind the resistance. Or I may just allow a child to decide for himself when he is ready to risk something that is difficult for him. He will become more open as his trust builds; he will begin to risk as his sense of self strengthens.

When the children begin to express themselves easily through the fantasy material and the varied types of expressive projections, I attempt to guide them back gently into the reality of their lives—by having them own or accept the parts of themselves they have exposed so that they can begin to feel a new sense of self-identity, responsibility, and self-support. This is difficult for many children. I continually attempt to guide the child from his symbolic expressions and fantasy material to reality and his own life experiences. I approach this task with much gentleness, though there are times when I am firm and other times when I find it best to give no guidance at all, and be patient.

One of the most effective techniques for helping children through their blocks is what has been termed modeling. In either a session with an individual child or a group, if *I* do what I ask the children to do, they will do it too. If a child cannot find a picture in his scribble after two or three attempts, I will do one of my own. The child is fascinated, now knows what I'm asking of him, and feels better about doing it once I do.

Violet Oaklander
Windows to Our Children
Real People Press
1978   335 pp. $8.00

Art

Children enjoy creating with their hands—shaping figures with clay or using plaster of paris, for example. They also love using tools such as crayons and paint brushes. Art is important to a child's development in that it helps develop muscles and motor control. Encourage your child to draw by making available crayons (nontoxic), paper, play dough and simple finger paints that are easy to prepare. Make sure your child has a specific place where she can be creative without making a mess or marking walls and floors. Spread newspaper out and give the child a specified area in which to work. Scribbles may not be recognizable to you, but they are expressions of a child's experiences, fantasies and special moments. Talk about the artwork by asking questions about the pictures she creates.

In nursery school, play groups and child-care centers, art is an important part of the day. Children's work is hung up on the walls, and children are very proud of their pictures. Be sure you notice your child's work at school.

Only three or four basic colors are necessary for painting. Jars of powdered poster colors are very inexpensive and can be mixed in a pie plate by sprinkling powdered color with water.

Children also enjoy cutting paper into objects and making collages, three-dimensional creations or masks. Older children are able to do more detailed and complicated art.

Other forms of artwork include needlework, mask-making and finger painting using powdered colors spread on pieces of wrapping paper. Blot pictures are fun: spread plain paste on a piece of paper and distribute paint or ink on one side of the paper. Fold the paper in half, and the surface is blotted. Open the paper for the finished art.

Children enjoy doing artwork alone or in groups. Have supplies available for the times when other children are visiting.

The selected activity books have many other creative ideas.

Metaphoric Mind
Bob Samples
Addison-Wesley
1976   209 pp. $5.95

This book presents an argument for teaching and developing our creative side to balance with our rational, analytical side.

The image of mental health that I favor is one in which both capacities, the rational and the metaphoric, are legitimate. It is an image of equal access to the functions of both cerebral hemispheres and to the mind functions celebrated by both. The joy of closure and convergent mind function is only matched by the joy of new metaphoric nonconvergent discovery. When both of these capacities are considered legitimate and celebrated fully, the synergic mind prevails. Synergy occurs when all things work together so that the sum of the energy in a system exceeds the total of the parts. There is a magic "catalyst" that makes things work better than they otherwise would.

Projects Using Inexpensive Materials

Stockpile some of the materials below for "what-can-I-do-now" projects. All are inexpensive. A few suggestions for each creative project are listed, but you and your children will think of many more.

Scrap Box—Try to secure discontinued wallpaper samples (check your local paint and wallpaper stores), yarn, spools, sandpaper, glitter, sequins, construction paper, old greeting cards, tissue paper, round cardboard tubes from paper towels, tiny boxes, and crepe paper. (Have a pair of scissors, paste, and Scotch tape available for use with these materials.) Let your child use the above listed items to create projects.

Music Box—Tack two bottle caps facing each other to the end of a tongue depressor. Repeat this process one inch above the first two bottle caps. Use like a rattle. Glue sandpaper to two small wooden blocks. Attach small handle of wood if desired. Use vertical movements of the hands, rubbing the two blocks together. (Used as rhythm instrument.) Buy ½ inch dowel rods. (Usually cheaper at the lumber yard.) Cut dowels into 8"–12" lengths. (Use as rhythm sticks.)

Pegboard—Use acoustical ceiling tile with pre-punched holes. Use golf tees of assorted colors to create pattern, make pictures or designs, and use as counting sticks.

Clothespins—to make into dolls or turn into butterflies with construction paper as wings and pipe cleaner antennae.

Alphabet Macaroni—to make into words or names. Glue on tongue depressors or Popsickle sticks to make place markers.

Odd Shaped Macaroni—to color with paint or crayon and string for jewelry. You can punch holes in shell macaroni with a heated ice pick, then string on elastic band for bracelet, or on yarn for necklace. (A small macaroni with a hole in it is now on the retail grocery shelf.)

Wooden Blocks—for building trains, tracks, skyscrapers. Giant dominoes (also for building) or just for playing dominoes.

Package of White Paper Plates—to decorate with crayons, turn into picture frames, make into clocks by adding numerals and hands, or edge with bells for a tambourine.

Flannelboard—Acquire ¼" plywood or masonite in one-foot-square piece. Make pillowcase style flannel covering for it (this makes washing easy). You will also need material like felt, Pellon, or flannel. Cut this material into shapes, figures, numerals, and letters. The felt or flannel adheres to the flannelboard and allows the child to create.

Housekeeping Kit—Acquire discarded forks, knives, spoons, utensils, eggbeater, dishes, play money, dish towels, napkins, and discarded sheeting for tablecloth, "dress-up" clothes. Your child will enjoy playing house. (This play activity applies to boys as well as girls.)

Assortment of Small, Multicolored Notepads—to make parking tickets, train tickets, paper money, or just to stimulate drawing.

Box of Assorted Buttons—to sort into families, string, use for soldiers, to populate block buildings, or for tiddledywinks.

Paper Lace Doilies—to color, make into placemats or bonnets, or use as clothes for clothespin dolls.

Balloons in Interesting Shapes—to paint with faces, use as balls, twist into animals, or for games.

Paper Clips—to string into necklaces and bracelets.

Peanut Shells—for finger puppets. Put half of an empty shell on each fintertip, make faces with paint, crayon, or ink.

Tin Cans in Assorted Sizes, Without Sharp Edges—for nested blocks, buildings, or telephones (two cans with hole in each bottom connected by string).

Large Sheet of White, Dull Finish Oilcloth—You can draw a rough map of your neighborhood's streets: let your preschooler construct the buildings he knows with small boxes, using blocks as trucks and cars.

C

---

*From Dr. D. Birchfield, *Handbook for Parents and Teachers*, 1970, 40 pp., out of print.

C *Old Sheeting*—to cut up for place-mats or doll house bedspreads and curtains. You can decorate it with crayons, then place color-side down on newspaper and press with hot iron and warm, wet cloth for added permanency.

Finger Paint—It's easy and inexpensive to make at home, using liquid laundry starch and food coloring. Paint on white shelf paper, dampened with a sponge.

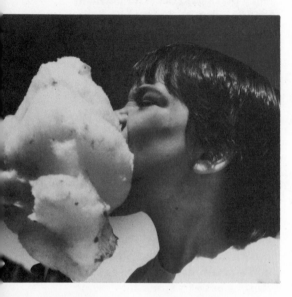

Save a Life Bank—Make a storage container from a one pound coffee can with a plastic top. Cut hole in plastic top about the size of a half dollar. Show the older children how to put all small objects, such as buttons and pins, into the container. The smaller children will also want to put things into the can. This teaches responsibility.

Simple Puzzles—Simple puzzles help the children to develop eye-hand control. Puzzles will also help children in learning to match shapes and forms. To make these simple puzzles, use cardboard box sections for back of puzzle pieces, then paste pictures from magazines upon the sections of cardboard, and cut into puzzle pieces.

Baby Reflection in a Mirror—A favorite toy to gain the baby's attention is a round or square non-breakable mirror. Hold the mirror so the baby can see himself, mother, and other members of the family. Discuss with the baby exactly what the reflection of the mirror projects.

Cradle Mobile—Obtain a piece of plastic covered clothes line or twine, long enough to tie across the crib. String such items as old jewelry, bright buttons, bells, and bright pieces of cloth. This will encourage the baby to watch the objects, recognize shapes, colors, and sizes.

Homemade Piggy Bank—Place open ends of two paper cups together. Seal both cups together with tape. Cut a slot for coins. Color the piggy. Attach paper ears, string tail, and cardboard legs.

Indoor Basketball Game—Fold a plastic potato sack over a rounded coat hanger. Run string through punched holes to secure the sack on hanger. Cut open the bottom end of bag, turn the hanger hook up and hang it over a doorknob or tightly secured hook on the door. Use small plastic or rubber ball to toss into basket.

Sound-Effects Box—Place 40 to 50 cooking style beans inside two large paper cups. Place open ends of cups together. Tape cups together. Shake the cups vigorously to produce sound of a steam train. Shake slowly for calypso rhythms, etc.

Harvest Puppets—Make puppets, using a different vegetable for each puppet's head. Add beans, raisins, radishes, and pepper slices for features. To hold the puppets up for viewing, insert tongue depressors or ice cream bar stick.

Paper-bag Puppets—Save large grocery shopping bags. Paint zoo, farm, or wild animal faces on bottom of bag. Cut holes for eyes, mouth, and nose. Children like to slip large bag down over their heads and do some playacting as a lion, monkey, or pig.

Drum—Hat boxes, abalone shells, wastebaskets, food cartons, bowls, barrels, hollow logs, cake boxes, or embroidery hoops make good drums. A drum may be short, long, thick or thin. The size of head as well as the size of the body influences the pitch and quality of the tone. The drum head may be made of any dried animal skin such as sheep, calf, suede, plastic, parchment, canvas, linen, and oil cloth.

Dance Rattle—Make an Indian dance rattle from an empty round cardboard box. Put metal noise-making objects, such as bottle caps, into the box. Tape lid down. Punch two holes opposite each other through the sides, push a sturdy stick through, and secure it with a string. Decorate rattle with poster paint or food coloring.

Gift or Toy Bucket—A large transparent plastic container can become a useful bucket. Burn holes at opposite sides of the container. Run heavy string or fancy lace through the holes and knot ends on the inside. Paint or paste colored paper to the lid.

Hand Glove Puppet—Tuck the two middle fingers of an old glove into the palm and sew up openings. Use dress snappers to make eyes, yarn to make whiskers and nose. Stuff ears and head with cotton or small pieces of newspaper. Pull thumb around neck and sew in place. Fit glove over hand and use middle finger to move puppet's head.

Paper Pay-Up Game—Cut pictures of attractive objects from old magazines and paste them to cards cut from cardboard such as cereal boxes. On the back of each card write a stunt, such as "Walk like a monkey." Place cards on a table with the picture side up. Each player picks up a card that appeals to him, then "pays-up" by doing what it says on back of card.

Mirrored Rag Doll—Cover a small round mirror with heavy clear plastic. Use the mirror for the face of an old-fashioned rag doll. Young children will enjoy holding their dollies and seeing themselves in the mirror.

Counting Rod—A counting rod which is entertaining as well as educational can be constructed by stringing ordinary metal nuts from a tool box on a wire clothes hanger that has been straightened. The sharp ends should be folded under and covered with heavy tape. Young children can add or subtract by manipulating the nuts. For older children, one might separate each group of 10 nuts with a butterfly nut. In this way, children can be helped to comprehend the place value of 10.

Photographs and Scrapbooks

Photographing your child from birth through different events over the years is a lot of fun. You don't need an expensive camera; something simple and easy to operate will do. You will enjoy having these pictures over the years to share and reflect on. As your children grow older they can take pictures of the whole family.

Simple scrapbooks can be made easily, and they will help keep the treasures in one place.

Add your child's art and drawings as they are produced. This is an activity well worth the time and energy. Through your children's artwork, you can see their development, how they see themselves and their world.

Recipes

Paste

- ½ cup water
- ½ cup flour

Mix the flour and water in a bowl with a spoon or your hands.

For a more lasting paste: put the flour in a saucepan and slowly stir in the water. Bring to a boil over a low heat; keeping this mixture stirred until thick and shiny. Store in a jar with a lid.

Finger Paint

- small amt. paste
- a few drops food coloring
- 1 or 2 spoonfuls soap flakes

Mix paste, coloring and soap flakes in a bowl. Let the children do their painting right on the kitchen table (the paint will wash off of everything except wood). First put a few drops of water down, then dab on paint mixture and watch the fun!

An old shirt for a smock and a handy sponge will be most helpful.

Play Dough

- 1 cup flour
- 1 cup water with food color added
- ½ cup salt
- 2 tsp. cream of tartar
- 1 tbsp. oil

Mix dry ingredients with colored water and oil. Pour gradually into saucepan. Cook 3 minutes or until mixture pulls away from sides of pan. Cool and knead. Store in airtight container.

Music

Home music activities can be quite varied. Music is more than just singing. Rhythms and movement are a part of music too. Here are some simple suggestions you and your child might enjoy:

- Ask your child to teach you a song. Encourage him to share those he has learned with you.

- Teach your child some of the songs you learned as a child. Sing them together.

- Clap out rhythms and let your child echo you by clapping them after you. Change places and you be the echo.

- Clap the rhythms to familiar songs and see if your child can guess the song you are clapping. Let your child clap them for you to guess.

- Listen for sound and rhythms around you—your heart, a dripping faucet, rain falling, a tree scraping against something in the wind, the sound of popcorn popping, the jingle of a dog's tag, etc.

- Play a singing echo game—sing phrases of songs you know and have your child sing them back to you.

- Encourage your child to move to music—moving the way the music makes him feel.

C

Homemade instruments are always fun. Old boxes and containers with pebbles inside make fun shaker noise-makers. An old can and a stick or pencil makes a drum. Two pencils can make rhythm sticks. You can think of many more. Try it!!

Your child would probably enjoy making up simple songs. These can be sung over and over. You might even sing them as rounds. Having fun and enjoying music is all that is important.

If you have a record player and some children's music, encourage your child to skip, run, jump, hop, swing and sway to the music. You can do it too, it's really great exercise.

Pointers for Parents,
Florida Dept. of Education

Creative Activities for Young Children
D. Keith Osborn and Dorothy Haupt
Merrill-Palmer Institute
1964   101 pp. $1.50

A collection of ideas to stimulate creativity in children. The activities include cooking, woodwork, clay, painting and paper work.

Paper work—For some children activity in this area may mean: "I'm really making something," "I'm doing real, hard work," to others it may offer a challenge in terms of the processes involved; for still others it may give a sense of self-sufficiency and an opportunity to share knowledge. Whatever the meaning for children, the demand for adult ingenuity and skill in guidance is great. Certainly this is most true when the children's goals exceed their current level of manual dexterity, or of eye-hand coordination, or their ability to follow verbal directions and complicated hand maneuvers of adults.

Children Drawing
Jacqueline Goodnow
Harvard University Press
1977   159 pp. $3.95

Provides parents, teachers and psychologists with clues to understanding children's drawings as aspects of development and skill, as well as descriptions of children's thoughts and methods of problem-solving.

Our interest is a direct response to children's drawings in their own right. Most of them have charm, novelty, simplicity, playfulness, and a fresh approach that is a source of pure pleasure. But we are also interested because drawings are indications of more general phenomena of human life.

Kiddie Kreations (Kit)
906 North Woodward
Royal Oak, Michigan 48067

With a Kiddie Kreations kit, your child can draw her favorite illustrations, write her message, or simply put her name on the outside of her very own mug, bowl or tumbler. Send $2.00 to Kiddie Kreations, and they will send you specially sized drawing paper on which your child will do her artwork. Return the artwork to Kiddie Kreations with $1.25 for each mug, bowl or tumbler, and in a few weeks your child receives her personally designed dishware in the mail. Perfect for a special event or birthday-party activity.

Make a Plate (Kit)
Makit Products
4659 Mint Way
Dallas, TX 75236
$5.00

In just two easy steps your child's original drawing done with either water-color pens or water color crayons can be made into a keepsake 10" Melamine plate which can be used as wall decorations, given as gifts or used for regular dinnerplates.

Write to them for a kit which contains paper mats, instruction sheet, return mailing label for plate order form, protective cardboard stiffener and pre-addressed return envelope ($5 includes whole set including plate).

Kites—Sculpting the Sky
Tsutomu Hiroi
Pantheon Books
1978   140 pp. $4.95

In this survey of kite history with step-by-step instructions for building kites, the emphasis is on calculating weight, wingspread and tips on successful launching. Includes photographs.

Kiting has been called the celestial art. To appreciate the aptness of the term, it is enough to see a kite climbing gracefully to the sky, reflecting the glitter of the sun's rays, its shape changing with every gust of wind.

Listen: And Help Tell the Story
Bernice Wells Carlson
Abingdon
1965   172 pp. $6.50

This collection of nursery rhymes and poems is designed to stimulate listening skills in children by challenging their imagination through sound, action and participation.

Before you read or recite one of the verses, get the child's undivided attention. If he is a very young child, or a child with a short attention span, remove from his reach any objects that might distract him. Tell him about the verse or story and explain what he is expected to do. Read in a rhythmic manner. Choose selections from one part of the book and then another, or let the child choose.

Encourage the child to join you in making the expected response, in making the action or in saying the sound or phrase, but if he fails to do so do not scold him or retard the flow of the story. Praise the child or the group who listens. Without preaching you will demonstrate that it is fun to listen.

Singing and Dancing Games for the Very Young
Esther L. Nelson
Sterling Publishing
1977 71 pp. $5.95

Music and movement come naturally to young children, and the author has included in this book games for children ages two to eight to teach ease and freedom of movement. Familiar songs such as "Who's That Tapping at the Window?" "Humpty Dumpty" and "A-Hunting We Will Go" are included with others like "Catch a Falling Star and Put It in Your Pocket" and "I Had a Little Sailboat."

Don't worry about how well the children do the dances or exercises, as long as they are focusing and trying. There is no need to judge them or compare one to another. Each child will do what he or she can; there's no rushing their physical development. Each time you repeat the same dance, however, they get better at it; their coordination improves, their body awareness heightens, they move more parts of their bodies, their sense of rhythm develops and their joy increases.

For Children

I Can Dance
Brian Bullard and David Charlsen
G. P. Putnam's Sons
1979 127 pp. $10.95

This beautiful book uses stroboscopic (freeze-action) photographs to demonstrate basic dance movements. The engaging photographs on every page of this book not only teach the skills to enjoy and appreciate the ballet, but encourage the reader to participate in the exercises and to learn to dance. Sets of elementary choreography are included so that these basic ballet steps may be turned into a small dance production.

This book would be excellent reading material for the budding dancer, and would be equally appropriate for teaching dance appreciation.

From the foreword by Melissa Hayden:

Dancing is an adventure, from the time you first learn the basic steps to the moment you put it all together and bring it to an audience. Just think how far you've come from the day you put one foot in front of the other and took your first step!

Learning to walk sets you free —learning to dance gives you the greatest freedom of all: to express with your whole self the person you are.

Creative Dramatics for All Children
Emily Gillies
International Association for Childhood Education
1972 64 pp. $3.25

Photographs and text explain basic principles of creative dramatics to enable children to express themselves freely, openly, with concentration and respect for one another.

The leader in creative drama must not only listen—she must learn unrelentingly to write down what she hears, for through the children's words she will begin to understand the meanings behind the voice of each child speaking, the whir of each mind thinking and working as no other mind has ever worked before.

Making Puppets and Puppet Theaters
Joan Moloney
Frederick Fell
1973 64 pp. $7.95

The author believes books for children should encourage them to make and do things, so this book includes working drawings for making glove puppets, marionettes and puppet theaters, with a complete list of materials and tools needed.

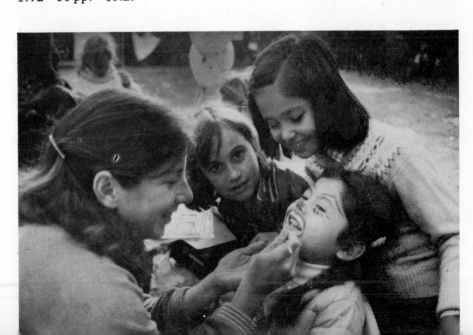

C

Normally shy children forget themselves and give their imagination to dressing puppets and seeing them live and move in their creations. An interest in, but lack of talent for any form of art, can find a satisfying creative outlet through shadow puppets which need not be elaborate figures but interesting movable shapes. Also, puppetry offers group-activity projects not always possible in other mediums. Each child contributes the talent he or she has—one to make the theater, another to carve or cut out the puppets, another to sew the clothes, and so on.

Mime—A Book of Silent Fantasy
Kay Hamblin
Doubleday (Dolphin Books)
1978   191 pp. $6.95

Photographs and text illustrate basic techniques of pantomime: movements, characterizations, illusion of objects and makeup.

See Appendix C for Films and Audio-Visual Aids

Rainbows—An Album for Kids
P.O. Box 118
220 Redwood Hwy.
Mill Valley, CA 94941
$7.00 (includes postage)

A tape of original joyful positive music by Joseph and Nathan Segal and friends with sound effects—"Songs are Magic in The Air," "Everyday People," "Rainbows, Would You Please Be My Friend;" "Singing Is Laughing." Perfect for children preschool to age 10.

CULTURAL AWARENESS

See also Literature for Children; Parenting; Religion.

Whatever your ethnic background and cultural experience, it is important to transmit it to your child. If you speak a foreign language, your child (up to age 5) will pick it up as a first language. He will learn English in time, as well. Once the child has become fluent in your language, it will be easier to learn a second or third.

Children love to go to ethnic fairs, museums and folk dances and dress in costumes from different cultures. If you eat special foods and celebrate special holidays, share the history of your rituals and the preparation of ethnic dishes. Stress that every child belongs to several different communities: the community of his parents and his own home, the parents' culture and the larger society.

Cultural Awareness: Resource Bibliography
Velma E. Schmidt and Earldene McNeill
National Association for Education of Young Children
1978   121 pp. $4.75

Provides annotated listings of posters, children's books, film strips, museums, records and newsletters to be used in planning experiences for children which increase awareness and understanding of diverse U.S. cultures. Also includes guidelines for choosing nonracist and nonsexist children's books and an address directory of over eight thousand suppliers.

While materials can help develop cultural awareness, especially for young children, real experiences in interacting with children and adults of other cultural groups—engaging together in ethnic dances, songs; having an adult from that culture explain artifacts, dance, sing or recite poetry; eating foods representative of a particular culture—are more meaningful. In

fact, real experiences often stimulate children to read books to find out more about a new interest. Adults can use the resources listed in this book to plan for real experiences and increase their own cultural awareness.

Children Are Children Are Children
Ann Cole, Carolyn Haas, Elizabeth Heller, Betty Weinberger
Little, Brown
1978   208 pp. $6.95

This book presents a series of activities based on customs of other countries to acquaint children with other cultures. Activities include creating a miniature Amazon rain forest to making a terrarium; playing the game Prince of Paris to learn counting in French, and making Iranian yogurt.

Children are children are children . . . whether they live in ancient Esfahan or modern Brasilia, there are many common threads running through their childhood years. Children everywhere enjoy jacks and jump rope; hopscotch and hide and seek; ice cream, candy and birthday candles. Games like "scissors, paper, stone"—"jan ken po," "les ciseaux, le papier, la pierre"—in whatever language, have been used by children for centuries; whether it is a French fête, a Brazilian festa, or a Japanese matsuri, everyone feels the excitement of fireworks, singing, dancing and colorful parades.

Organizations (See Appendix A)

Black Child Development Institute
Coalition for Children and Youth
National Conference of Christians and Jews
United Nations Children's Fund

D

DEATH

Losing a relative, friend or pet creates sad feelings and a sense of loss for all children. Encourage your child to express feelings and share the sadness. Don't pretend the death didn't happen.

One of the best books about coping with grieving and loss is *Learning To Say Good-Bye* by Eda LeShan, a book written for children. During the first stage of grief, people just cannot accept the fact that someone they love has really died. You hope for some magic to happen, wanting desperately to believe it is all a bad dream, but it is not.

Gradually the time comes when you begin really to understand that the person you love will never come back. This is usually months after his or her death. At first you may wonder why you are crying harder and more often now than right after it happened. It seems strange. Actually, it is very natural and makes good sense. You have had time to become stronger and more able to face the fact that never again will you be with that person.

We also include resources for parents who have lost a child and those whose children are faced with death.

Bereaved Parent
Harriet Sarnoff Schiff
Penguin Books
1978   146 pp. $2.95

For parents whose child has died, Schiff offers guidelines, practical suggestions for coping with grief, facing the funeral and rebuilding the marriage. Written by a mother whose son died at age ten.

Parents, unable to understand how it could be that their child died, take to lashing out at their spouses. Indeed, each sometimes blames the other for the death. This blaming over the cause of death may appear ludicrous—the spouse is after all making what is tantamount to an accusation of the murder of their child to a vulnerable, susceptible mother or father. Just the mere hint of such a thing to grieving mates could be enough to make them believe they were indeed responsible for the death of their child. If in the back of the mind there is the least shred of doubt about personal judgment or responsibility, a question could be planted that would not be undone in a lifetime.

Care of the Child Facing Death
Lindy Burton
Routledge and Kegan Paul
1974   217 pp. $14.95

Most families faced with supporting a potentially dying child are often at a loss to know where to turn for help. This book is concerned with pinpointing the problems which exist for parents and those involved in the care of sick children. The question of what and how much to say to a sick child about his or her illness is fully discussed, as well as how to deal with an exacting treatment regime.

Parental attitude is therefore essential for optimal physical functioning, and is also of immense significance in terms of the child's overall development. If he is to remain happy and positive he must be challenged to maximum achievement within the limitations of his illness state. This is not an easy task for parents—it involves rethinking their objectives and expectations for the child, inevitably relinquishing some of the fantasies and goals which were attached to him when he was healthy.

Should the Children Know?
Marguerita Rudolph
Schocken Books
1980   128 pp. $5.95

This book introduces ways to help prepare children for coping with death. It helps children recognize and express fears and feelings of loss at death of family member or friend.

D   *In the course of living with children, while teaching parenting, working with, or simply befriending them at various ages and levels, we are bound to encounter death. The death may be regarded as unreconcilable tragedy or resented as an act of intrusion in the activities of the living, or it may cause feelings of helplessness and fear in adults as well as children. However, taking into account children's understanding and feelings appropriate to their ages, adults can help children (and themselves) by clarifying experiences of separation, by offering religious or spiritual explanations and by using artistic means for expression or release of ideas and feelings about death. Thus, through death one may acquire a deeper knowledge of life and of living.*

Talking About Death—A Dialogue Between Parent and Child
Earl A. Grollman
Beacon Press
1976   98 pp. $9.95

Grollman suggests that a parent must tell a child about death immediately after one occurs in the family. The approach must be warm, sympathetic and kind. Included is a listing of professional services, films, agencies and other books for further information.

While you will not deny a youngster the opportunity to weep, neither should you urge the child to display unfelt feelings. Youngsters should not be subjected to emotional blackmail in which they are urged to behave in some particular manner, such as remaining still when they need to run and jump. . . . There are other outlets for emotion besides tears. Allow them to express those feelings appropriate to their needs.

There Is a Rainbow Behind Every Dark Cloud
Gerald Jampolsky
Center for Attitudinal Healing
1978   96 pp. $5.95

A book about children by children who have had to face life-and-death situations because of serious illness. The presentation is simple and direct, and the children deal with problems such as going to the hospital and talking about death. Imaginative, heartwarming drawings by children enhance the text.

We all found it helpful to talk about death. It seemed easier to talk about being afraid of dying with other kids than to talk about it with adults. Lots of times adults get nervous, change the subject, and tell us that we shouldn't think of things like that.

Drawing pictures about what we thought death was like and talking about the pictures with each other made it less scary to talk about.

For Children

About Dying
Sarah Bonnett Stein
Walker and Co.
1974   47 pp. $5.95

This black-and-white photo essay about acceptance and understanding of death is for both parent and child. The narrative for adults gives comforting guidelines, while the children's text expresses a child's feelings about the death of a loved one.

It is best to say what's wrong and not make dying a lonely child's guessing game. You can explain that the person is very seriously sick. You can say that a person could die of that sickness. And if you can, help your child visit like this child is visiting his grandfather. It is the beginning of saying goodbye for both of them.

This was Grandpa, who gave the children Snow; who drew pictures with them, and smiled; who took them to the park. Until he got sick. Then the grown-ups said, "Be quiet. Grandpa is sick."

Learning to Say Good-Bye
Eda LeShan
Avon
1978   117 pp. $2.95

A frank, easy-to-read book about the feelings children experience when a parent dies, it is designed to be read aloud. This book encourages discussion and a sharing of feelings. The author discusses the different ways people share grief and the different ways people recover from grief.

Your mother or father was different from anyone else in all the world. There never was anyone like him or her—and there never will be. What a remarkable idea that is! If we were all the same, it wouldn't matter so much when one person died. The loss of someone is so painful because of that uniqueness. We can find other people to love, but each love is special and different.

DENTAL CARE

Visiting the dentist with your child is extremely important, and the child should have his first dental examination when he is two and a half years old. Children should visit the dentist at least once a year to detect any serious complications early enough to take preventive measures.

Feeling comfortable at the dentist's office is important, and your dentist should do everything to make your child feel at ease. Some dentists specialize in the treatment of children; these dentists are especially competent at quieting the fears or anxieties of children. Your local dental association or dental school can provide you with names of good dentists. Your friends or neighbors might also be able to recommend a dentist they have used and felt comfortable with. You might want to visit and talk with several dentists before you select one. It is often a good idea to stay with your child for several visits, until you are certain she is comfortable.

Ask your dentist to instruct your child in daily dental hygiene —brushing and flossing—and give an explanation of how food particles cause cavities. After your child's permanent teeth come in, your dentist might recommend orthodontia to correct a defective bite. Orthodontia is extremely expensive, so you would be wise to shop around for the best orthodontist you can find whose services you can afford.

Your Child's Teeth—A Parent's Guide to Making and Keeping Them Perfect
Stephen J. Moss
Houghton Mifflin
1979   143 pp. $3.95

For Children

My Friend the Dentist
Jane Watson
Golden Press
1972   31 pp. $2.95

My Dentist
Harlow Rockwell
William Morrow/Greenwillow
1975   32 pp. $7.50

For free pamphlets such as *A Visit to the Dentist* and *Cleaning Your Teeth and Gums* you may write to:

American Society of Dentistry for Children
American Dental Association
211 E. Chicago Ave.
Chicago, Ill. 60611

DISABILITIES

See also Health and Hospitals; Eyesight; Language and Speech; Mental Health; Sensory Development.

You can usually do a great deal for your child if the handicap is discovered early enough and you get sufficient help. Your physician will be of some help in getting information for you. In addition, we have included resources from major organizations involved in specific areas of developmental disability. Other parents who share the same problem can offer help. Your child's needs for love and attention are more complex than those of a completely healthy youngster. Confronting your feelings will be an important challenge. You should share these feelings with your mate. We have included a variety of books for a variety of problems, as well as other resources you can turn to in seeking help with these problems.

Finding help for the child with a developmentally disabling condition can involve a lot of time and research. Services are available for specific problems, which can considerably lessen their severity. Be sure you discuss the situation fully with your pediatrician and find out what services are available in your own community. The organizations listed in the Appendix section will help you find assistance with specific problems. Explore services designed to help parents cope with the problem.

Use the resources listed in this book for assistance in learning more about specific problems. In your community, there are teachers and other professionals experienced in working with special children who will be able to help you. Do not be discouraged, and do not let your child feel discouraged. Miracles have happened with children who might have been given up. Blindness, deafness or other physical or learning disabilities are not impossible problems to cope with. Your child will achieve to the extent to which he or she is capable—with your love and support.

Physical Disabilities

Depending on the nature of his delayed development, the child may look normal and be completely independent in daily activities or may be somewhat behind in his toilet training, feeding patterns, or socialization abilities. The behavioral difficulties he may present, such as hyperactivity or impulsiveness, may be manifestations of his abnormal development and do not necessarily imply emotional disturbance or problems at home. Any emotional disturbances he does manifest may be organically based or may be wholly emotional.

D Possible Problems

- Has trouble with fine motor co-ordination such as in coloring or eating.
- Is clumsy in gross motor activities such as running and playing outdoors.
- Receptive difficulties—has trouble understanding what others are saying.
- Expressive difficulties—has trouble saying exactly what he means.
- Displays articulation errors or stutters.
- Exhibits gross fluctuations of behavior with periods of being especially "bad."
- Has a low frustration level; is very impulsive and shows a lack of judgment.
- Can be "set off" by any activity that is not routine, i.e. free periods, music, field trips.
- May be hyperactive with a short attention span.
- May have a short attention span but not be hyperactive.
- Hyperactivity (super-active): never sits still.

Sometimes children are born with physical and/or mental conditions which hinder normal growth and development. Occasionally a child will acquire a handicap or abnormality from an accident.

Fortunately, many of these conditions can be changed and sometimes be completely corrected if they are spotted early in the child's life and something is done quickly. Failure to recognize and deal with these abnormal situations or behaviors can result in an unnecessary lifelong problem.

Early Warning Signs Checklist

Take a few moments and read this Early Warning Signs Checklist. If for any reason you suspect that your child may have special needs, seek help at once. *Don't wait until your child begins school!* It might be too late.

Vision Checklist

Get Help If Your Child . . .

- has difficulty picking up or locating small objects which have been dropped.
- rubs eyes frequently or complains that eyes hurt.
- has red or watering eyes. Eyelids are encrusted.
- holds head awkwardly, or tilts head to either side, or moves head backward or forward when looking at a particular object or person.
- has frequent crossing of eyes.

Playing Checklist

Get Help If Your Child . . .

- by age 1 . . . does not wave bye-bye, play patty-cake or peek-a-boo.
- by age 2 . . . does not mimic the family members doing household chores.
- by age 3 . . . does not seem to enjoy playing alone with toys, pots and pans, in a sandbox, etc.
- by age 4 . . . does not participate in simple games with other children about the same age.
- by age 5 . . . will not share or take turns.

Talking Checklist

Get Help If Your Child . . .

- by age 1 . . . does not say "Mamma" or "Dadda."
- by age 2 . . . cannot say names of close relatives/family members and identify toys.
- by age 3 . . . is unable to recite TV jingles or common rhymes.
- by age 4 . . . is not talking in short sentences.
- by age 5 . . . is not understood by persons outside family circle.

Activity Checklist

Get Help If Your Child . . .

- by age 1 . . . is not able to sit up without support.
- by age 2 . . . is unable to walk without assistance.
- by age 3 . . . cannot walk up and down steps.
- by age 4 . . . cannot balance on one foot for a short period.
- by age 5 . . . cannot throw a ball overhand or catch a large ball which is rolled or bounced.

Hearing Checklist

Get Help If Your Child . . .

- does not turn toward the source of sounds or voices by six months of age.
- has runny ears or earaches.
- talks unusually loudly.
- does not respond when called from another room.
- turns same ear toward a sound he/she wishes to hear.

Thinking Checklist

Get Help If Your Child . . .

- by age 1 . . . does not react to his/her name.

- by age 2 . . . is unable to identify eyes, ears, nose, mouth, and hair by pointing to them.

- by age 3 . . . fails to understand simple stories which are read or told.

- by age 4 . . . cannot give reasonable answers to questions such as: "What do you do when hungry?" or "What do you do when you are sleepy?"

- by age 5 . . . cannot seem to understand the meaning of the words: "today," "tomorrow," "yesterday."

Try to work with your child in the areas of concern. Often a child will not have experienced a particular occurrence. Children learn from watching and then participating . . . often over and over and over again.

If an unusual behavior persists, *take action!!* Seek help at once. REMEMBER: the earlier you notice a problem . . . and the sooner you get help . . . the better the chances of preventing complications.

Prepared by the State of Utah Office of Child Development
250 East Fifth South
Salt Lake City, Utah 84111

Let's Play to Grow (Kit)
Joseph P. Kennedy, Jr., Foundation
1701 K Street N.W.
Washington, DC 20006
$2.50

A useful play kit, this includes games and simple activities designed to improve the capability and self-confidence of handicapped and retarded children.

About Handicaps
Sarah Bonnett Stein
Walker
1974   47 pp. $6.95

Part of a collection called Open Family Books designed to help children cope with fears and hurts, this edition discusses a boy's concerns when he meets another child, handicapped by cerebral palsy. Large print and photographs stimulate children's discussion, while smaller-print text provides adults with insight into the specific problems encountered.

Matthew doesn't like Joe's crooked legs. He copies the way Joe walks. Whenever Joe comes to play, Matthew jumps and runs around very fast. He makes sure his own legs work right. He is afraid they could get like Joe's. (child's text)

Most of us can remember back to times when we scrutinized our own bodies with the sharper eyes of childhood—when the conformation of our bellybutton was as mapped as the location of each mole or wart or the pattern of our palms. No doubt each person, searching so diligently for both uniqueness and perfection, has found some small imperfection too. Ears that seem too long, a bulgy navel, a nose tipped at a fashion we wish it weren't. (adult text)

Are You Ready To Mainstream?
Samuel J. Brawn and Miriam G. Lasher
Charles E. Merrill
1978   148 pp. $4.95

This book presents a brief history of the development of educational programs for children with special needs with suggestions for creating healthy learning environments.

Negativism, tantrums, refusal to try tasks, overdependence on an adult, aggressiveness, and excessive activity level are all familiar to any adult who works with "emotionally disturbed" children. Sometimes adults are too quick to conclude that a problem is interpersonal in nature; therefore, they are too ready to address themselves exclusively to feelings and family dynamics. However, these same behavior problems frequently conceal an underlying deficit in the child's learning abilities.

Bernard—Bringing Up Our Mongol Son
John and Eileen Wilks
Routledge and Kegan Paul
1974   157 pp. $6.50

An account of John and Eileen Wilks's demanding and often painful task of bringing up a mentally handicapped child. For anyone involved with a mongoloid child, this book offers a chance to compare notes and to gain strength from a couple who used a tragedy as an opportunity to enrich family relationships. The authors describe their difficulties teaching their son to talk, to eat properly and to behave in public situations.

From the beginning it was fairly clear to us that a mongol could make life difficult for his brothers and sisters. If we had had any doubts on this point, they were certainly removed by the number of times we were advised not to let the other children suffer. However, to begin with, there was not much we could do, but wait to see how things turned out. . . .

D

Birth Defects—The Tragedy and the Hope
March of Dimes Birth Defects
Foundation

This pamphlet gives the parent important information on birth defects—their causes, treatments, how they are diagnosed and how they can be prevented.

Caring for Your Disabled Child
Benjamin Spock and Marion O. Lerrigo
Macmillan
1965   359 pp. $4.95

This reference book for parents of mentally, physically or emotionally handicapped children covers medical care, rehabilitation, education, and vocational future. Chapters focus on play activities and methods of helping children to develop sexually and socially. One important section deals with tools and techniques, such as artificial limbs, hearing aids and wheelchairs.

It's very helpful for a father to chat often with his son about the kind of work the boy thinks he wants to do, to evaluate his plans, and to encourage him, if this is justified. Yet a father may fail his handicapped child in this way, because of uncertainty about what he can advise. He needs to keep in close touch with the vocational guidance his child is receiving. A mother may fail to teach her handicapped daughter the elements of homemaking because she doubts that the girl will ever have her own home. The handicapped child, who longs to be treated like other children, interprets these omissions as evidence of his parents' lack of confidence in his future.

Deaf Like Me
Thomas S. Spradley and James P. Spradley
Random House
1978   280 pp. $8.95

A moving story, this book records the moments of discouragement and frustration and finally the joyful triumphs of a family with a deaf child. More than 22 million Americans have some degree of hearing loss, and thousands of deaf children are born each year. This story points out the barriers of silence separating the deaf from the world around them.

By denying Lynn's deafness and treating her as if she were normal, we actually made her feel different. Even in the most ordinary family activities, by talking as if she could hear when she could not, we created for her the profound feeling that she was on the outside, a stranger to what was going on. Only after we began to sign regularly did we realize how the pretense of normality had appeared to Lynn. For the first time in her life she did not merely sit at the table watching our mysterious lips, seeing us laugh and smile for unknown reasons. She began to share the day's activities.

Handling the Young Cerebral Palsied Child at Home
Nancie R. Finnie
E. P. Dutton
1975   330 pp. $5.95

For therapists as well as teachers and parents, this book focuses on the importance of parental and home management in total treatment programs of children with cerebral palsy. Included are chapters on special problems of toilet training, bathing, dressing and feeding, plus a guide to community resources and suppliers of accessories and equipment.

It is . . . very important . . . not to stand still in your mutual development with your handicapped child, so that you both remain locked firmly in the earliest infant-parent relationship, with no changes occurring. Behavior such as scratching your face with his fingers, and pulling your hair, may be attractive in an infant. Its encouragement at first by parental smiling and gentle vocal response is appropriate for the development of the social bond between parent and child, and essential for the acquisition of movement skills and for the learning of body awareness. At a later stage, however, the child should learn to be gentle as he grows in strength, because he needs to become aware of others' feelings, and he should be moving on to exploration of toys, objects, and his physical environment.

Help Them Grow!
Jane Blumenfeld, Pearl E. Thompson, Beverly S. Vogel
Abingdon
1971   64 pp. $2.75

This pictorial handbook for parents of handicapped children provides suggestions for teaching in the home, developing basic skills which enable children to grow as individuals.

Give practice in use of utensils by giving every opportunity for child to use them, such as at snack time and extra practice time.

Use finger foods, such as celery, carrots, small cuts of meat, hot dogs, crackers, toast, and bread sticks.

Brightly colored foods on spoon or fork may encourage use of utensil.

Make a game of bringing spoon to mouth.

Put food on spoon or fork that will stick to it and that the child really likes.

D

Helping the Mentally Retarded Acquire Play Skills
Paul Whelan
Charles C. Thomas
1977   210 pp. $12.50

This how-to book describes ways to train play skills in mentally retarded children, who do not play spontaneously but need guidelines, with teaching procedures and techniques to develop play behavior.

During winter season, playing in the snow or making a snowman are skills which the severely handicapped individual should be given an opportunity to learn. Tree climbing, hiking, piling up leaves, and playing in a river or lake are other possible illustrations of learning to play in the natural environment. In addition to being an excellent means of learning the environment and different seasons, this is also more consistent with fostering normalization and integration with nonretarded peers in the community.

Helping Children With Learning Disabilities
Ruth Dinkins Rowan
Abingdon
1977   128 pp. $5.95

Information on how to help children with learning problems is contained in this book, with subjects ranging from symptoms to the need for proper nutrition and the value of the parent/teacher working relationship. Case studies demonstrate why these children fail and how different behavior patterns set them apart from other children.

Learning disabilities are so diverse, taking a different course in each individual child, that consideration of some definitive characteristics may prove helpful. No child exhibits all these traits, and conversely, the presence of only a

few of these is not indicative of a learning disorder.

- *Very good in some skills, very low in others; good reader, poor in math; great conversationalist, can't write; good at sports, can't read.*
- *Performs differently from day to day.*
- *Doesn't play well with other children.*
- *Doesn't respond to jokes.*

How to Create Interiors for the Disabled
Jane Randolph Cary
Pantheon Books
1978   124 pp. $5.95

Suggestions to make the home environments safe and free of frustration for the physically handicapped are in this book. Also discussed: life for the disabled in the community; traveling and information on consumer groups for the handicapped.

Reach. Grasp. Twist. Pull. Back up. Turn. Go around. Repeat all over again. That's getting a door open and closed. No wonder the physically handicapped declare doors are energy-sapping, frustrating barriers they'd gladly do without. Some are necessary for privacy and safety, such as privacy and entry doors and those at bathroom and bedroom. Basement stairways and other dangerous openings in a home should be blocked also. But in general, regard every door as an expendable barrier that you should either remove or at least make easier to operate.

Side-hinged swing-out doors are the most difficult for the disabled to handle. Almost all doors inside the house will be of this kind. Either prop them open permanently or take them off their hinges and store them—under beds and behind a sofa if need be.

Why Your Child Is Hyperactive
Ben F. Feingold
Random House
1975   211 pp. $7.95

Feingold presents case histories of hyperkinetic children who, through experimentation with a synthetic-free diet, become calmer and more able to cope. He tells how to apply a synthetic-free diet and gives suggestions for menus plus recipes for specific dishes.

Frustrated easily, he would flare out against others or turn wrath inward by biting himself. Punishment means nothing. He was on the verge of being "unmanageable," according to his immediate supervisor. Fifty milligrams of Thorazine had been prescribed as a control.

Yet hyperkinesis is not usually associated with PKU. The supervisor, searching for a method of added control, learned of the elimination diet and wondered if certain foods might not be stirring up the patient. The boy ate the same institutional foods as the other children, but experimentally, the staff member eliminated all natural salicylates from his diet. Within three weeks, most of the hyperkinetic symptoms had disappeared.

Improving Your Child's Behavior Chemistry
Lendon H. Smith
Pocket Books
1978   256 pp. $2.25

Poor diet and body chemistry may be the cause of such problems in children as nightmares, bedwetting, allergies and even hyperactivity, according to the author. The author shows how with diet and vitamin therapy along with counseling, dozens of common behavior problems can be effectively overcome.

Parent as Teacher
D. H. Scott
Fearon Pitman
1972   136 pp. $3.95

D This is a guide for parents who wish to teach their learning-disabled children, stressing home care for those unable to locate special-education consultants and/or psychologists. Learning games and materials are suggested.

. . . If your son or daughter is a lazy reader, what will really count is the interest you show. This may need endless patience, without nagging or bullying. Go to some trouble to find out the right level of reading material both in difficulty and what interests him. Show him how he can follow sports better or learn more about his hobby by being able to read. In consultation with him, you should buy the right kind of book or magazine. Don't object if he prefers comics which appeal to his more primitive instincts. What matters is the habit of reading—even sitting down quietly reading nothing but the captions of comic strips. Try to insist that there should be a regular reading hour each evening.

Raising The Young Blind Child: A Guide for Parents and Educators
Shulamith Kastein, Isabelle Spaulding and Battia Scharf
Human Sciences Press
1979   224 pp. $14.95

In this sensitively illustrated book, parents are guided through the day-to-day situations involved in caring for and educating a blind child. As specialists in the education of the blind, the authors reveal that blind children can grow up to be productive, independent and self-fulfilled individuals when they have lived in an environment that provides enriching human relationships and emotional and in-tellectual growth. Throughout this work, emphasis is placed on the role of language in the child's emotional and cognitive development.

Seizures, Epilepsy, and Your Child
Jorge C. Lagos
Harper & Row
1974   223 pp. $9.95

Nature, origins, diagnosis, treatment and management of epilepsy are discussed here, with clear, realistic answers to questions such as: What is the prognosis for such a child, and is there a relationship between epilepsy and mental retardation?

It is little known by the general public that a large number of young children, usually between the ages of six months and two years, may have convulsions in association with febrile illnesses (illnesses accompanied by high fever) such as a viral infection, an ear infection, a strep throat, or some of the other common illnesses of childhood. These so-called febrile seizures are always of the major type (grand mal), with loss of consciousness, stiffening of the body, and jerking of the four limbs.

Some Mothers I Know
Tom Wakefield
Routledge and Kegan Paul
1978   93 pp. $9.00

In a subjective account of four mothers, each of whom has a handicapped child, the mothers tell their own stories about the strains and the rewards of raising handicapped children, discussing such things as the great expense involved and the anxiety connected with assessing their children's future.

I had a vague notion what epilepsy was and I had seen one or two people have what I knew was a fit, but I never thought it could happen to my family. We were only a small family anyway. 'Oh,' was all I could say to my sister. I thought, 'Why should this happen to me?' Yet it had happened and after this he was transferred to Queen Elizabeth Hospital. He was sent home again, but every ten weeks the attacks came back regular as clockwork. I had got used to the procedure by now and I even held the oxygen mask for him in the ambulance. This went on for another four years before I realized, without thinking about it too much, that I was having to live with my son's illness in much the same way as he was having to grow in spite of it.

Something's Wrong With My Child
Milton Brutten, Sylvia O. Richardson and Charles Mangel
Harcourt Brace Jovanovich
1979   219 pp. $3.95

The focus here is not on mentally retarded children but on children who have all the mental potential for learning and growing and yet, due to some physical impairment, fail to learn. The authors assure the parents of such children that most have potential to lead productive lives if they are treated properly. Parents are warned that rearing such children is more time-consuming and arduous than raising normal children. Case histories are presented to demonstrate the proper care and treatment of these children.

The learning-disabled child may find school hard from the very first day. He can't cut with scissors, can't color inside lines, has difficulty matching shapes and sizes. He may have trouble grasping abstract concepts (are jets and buses both means of transportation?) or relating what he has learned in one context to another.

Special Child Handbook
Joan McNamara and Bernard McNamara
Dutton
1978   330 pp. $12.50

This practical, compassionate, nontechnical manual helps parents and professionals understand and fulfill the special requirements of handicapped children.

When you work with your child, you need to keep in mind the differences in individuals and their methods of dealing with life. Some children are natural "go-getters" who will try anything once, while others tend to be cautious about new situations. If you set up a model of the way in which your child should handle himself, you are bound to be disappointed. This is especially true if you base your expectations on what you have seen in late-night TV movies and novels. The classic stereotype of the martyr, a polite, modest person with a handicap who knows his place, is reminiscent of attitudes toward other minorities who have been expected to stay out of the mainstream of life and all its opportunities. Another stereotype, the hero or the brave gutsy person with a handicap who overcomes it to become a celebrity, is perhaps an ideal that parents hold up in efforts to force their child into achievements that can bring them pride at whatever price. Parents may try to fit themselves into these roles as well.

The Special Children
Nancy C. Schumacher
Vantage Press
1977   90 pp. $5.95

Written by the mother of a learning-disabled child, this book provides an overview of learning-disability symptoms, testing and diagnostic procedures, as well as

teaching methods in classroom and school.

There are a lot of different sides to special education. I think the prime ingredient is patience and a teacher who will take the time to get along with her children.

Teaching Parents to Teach
David L. Lillie and Pascal L. Trohanis
Walker
1976   205 pp. $11.95

Full involvement of parents in early education is increasingly recognized as a critical factor in the successful teaching of handicapped children. Therefore the authors have pooled suggestions from psychologists and educators on seeking more meaningful ways in which parents can participate in the lives of their offspring.

The family with a handicapped, deviant, or chronically ill child has special problems which set the stage for unique pitfalls. Pediatricians are all too familiar with families of children who have serious chronic or life-threatening illnesses. The devotion of economic resources, emotional and physical energy, as well as time itself, to one member of the family may produce a situation in which others suffer needlessly. Such a danger exists even when parents are truly involved in trying to aid any child in the family who has a problem.

Visually Handicapped Children and Young People
Elizabeth K. Chapman
Routledge and Kegan Paul
1978   150 pp. $15.50

A child cannot make out numbers on a bus or recognize the face of a friend across the street. How

much should be done for this child in terms of education for the visually handicapped? This easy-to-read book focuses on the education of such children from preschool through high school. In early chapters, the reader learns the causes of sight defects, while other chapters deal with counseling and educational aids.

A diminished visual field may be evident as apparent clumsiness and seemingly poor eye-hand coordination; difficulties in seeing clearly may present themselves in the unusual position or movements that a child shows while working, such as tilting his head forward, whilst facial grimaces such as frowning or squinting can in some cases indicate sight problems. Actions indicating discomfort such as rubbing the eyes, or excessive blinking and complaints of dizziness, headache and nausea, covering one eye with the hand, and poking the corner of it with the finger are all signs indicating the possible presence of visual dysfunction.

Organizations (See Appendix A)

National:

American Academy of Pediatrics

American Association of Ophthalmology

American Dietetic Association

American Foundation for the Blind

American Medical Association

American Podiatry Association

American Speech and Hearing Association

Appalachian Regional Commission

D

Association for Children and Adults with Learning Disabilities

Children in Hospitals

Council for Exceptional Children

Epilepsy Foundation of America

Fight for Sight

March of Dimes Birth Defects Foundation

Muscular Dystrophy Association

National Association for Retarded Children

National Institute of Child Health and Human Development

National Society for Autistic Children

U.S. Department of Health and Human Services

Local:

Devereux Foundation

Erikson Institute for Early Education

See Appendix C for Films and Audio-Visual Aids.

DISCIPLINE

See also Abuse of Children; Communication; Rights of Children.

Disciplining children is, of course, a matter of individual judgment. You may choose to be either strict or permissive, depending upon your personality and the needs of your child.

I advise that you set limits before a child undertakes an activity, rather than afterward, when he may have unknowingly gone beyond the acceptable bounds.

Allow your child to make mistakes. If an accident occurs, such as breaking your favorite vase, try to be understanding and lenient. Child-proofing your house is probably the best way to avoid unnecessary discipline. While children move and need space, they also need to know what your restrictions are. Your discipline should be fair and consistent.

Don't let punishment go on for long periods of time, as that is abusive. The purpose of discipline is for the child to learn or relearn acceptable behavior and to learn that you have set safe limits for their protection. It is not an outlet for parental hostility or an opportunity to frighten a child. If your children understand that you have a healthy viewpoint on discipline, they will probably need less correcting and will not confuse their impressions of your feelings about them. Effective discipline depends upon how you view yourself and your child, and how you use available parent-training resources.

DIVORCE

See also Single Parents.

Breaking up a family through divorce is never easy at best, and at worst it can engender pain and blame far beyond that which caused the split between the parents. A child's need for love and support from both parents is especially crucial through a divorce.

Both parents should spend time with their children and attempt to reduce the trauma by providing an atmosphere of security and love. Beware of using your children as weapons against your former spouse; it can only hurt all of you.

Before you consider divorce you should explore the alternatives; counseling, discussion with friends you trust and a short separation are some. Try to recapture some of the feeling you had when you were first married. Probe the underlying reasons behind your problems. Often children cause a strain in a relationship because of the new demands they make on adults who are unprepared to cope with children. Talk over your mutual needs and try to find paths of compromise.

If divorce is inevitable, you can ease the trauma by casting as few aspersions on your former partner as possible. Excessive daily upsets caused by discussions of each detail of the divorce will cause your child's sense of security to crumble, and his relationships with other children may suffer, as may his schoolwork. Children may lose their sense of financial security as well if the primary breadwinner (usually the father) moves out and the remaining parent can't afford to maintain their former life-style.

Above all, be sure that your child knows that he is not responsible for the divorce. Reassurance that the other parent will love him, even when they aren't living as a family, is vital.

IDEAS FOR SEPARATED OR DIVORCED MOMS AND DADS ON VISITS WITH CHILDREN

D

- Allow yourself and your children time for readjustment.

- Remember and share the best parts of your marriage with your children honestly.

- Assure your children that they are not to blame for the breakup, nor will they be abandoned or rejected.

- Continuing anger or bitterness toward your former partner is far more injurious to your children than the marital breakup itself.

- Refrain from criticizing the other parent; foster respect by your children of both parents.

- Do not force or encourage your children to take sides.

- Try not to upset a child's routine too abruptly.

- Be frank about financial pressures.

- Be honest in telling children what is happening and why, in a way children can understand and digest.

- You may need to retell the story about your divorce or separation after the children get older and consider life more maturely.

- Don't let your negative feelings (guilt, anger, depression) interfere with consistent disciplining of your children.

- Don't pity your children. Your expectation that they can handle difficult situations will encourage them.

Parents Without Partners, Inc.

Co-Parenting—Sharing Your Child Equally
Miriam Galper
Running Press
1978   158 pp. $4.95

An alternative to traditional forms of custody arrangements, co-custody, or co-parenting, is a system in which the child spends equal amounts of time with each parent, and parents share equal responsibility for the child's care. This arrangement allows parents to maintain pleasurable, ongoing, intimate relationships with their children and to play a major part in their development.

After separation takes place, differences seem clearer to the child. He learns what the expectations are for his behavior when he is with one parent or the other. Some rules belong in mother's house but not in father's. Father is strict about some things that mother doesn't care about. When a child is with his father, he understands that he can behave in ways which might be unacceptable to his mother.

See also *The Disposable Parent: The Case for Joint Custody.* Mel Roman and William Haddad, Penguin Books. 1978   197 pp. $3.95
Excellent new book.

Fathers and Custody
Ira Victor and Win Ann Winkler
Hawthorn Books
1977   181 pp. $8.95

In this book to help fathers win the custody battle, the authors present a case for divorced fathers and their children by showing through interviews and case histories fathers who are coping successfully in a one-parent household.

They explore problems such as joint custody, remarriage and attitudes about the divorced parent, and an appendix lists divorced fathers' groups, single-parent and child-help groups, as well as legal-advice-referral agencies.

More fathers are fighting for full custody. More are fighting for joint or split custody (one or more children to each parent, depending upon the individual situation). Many more are fighting to have their visitation rights enforced. They want something more than a surreptitious phone call every year and a half. Others are fighting because they feel that their visitation rights, when carried out according to the letter of the law, can destroy a father-child relationship far more effectively than a court order forbidding a father to have anything to do with his children.

D

Marital Separation
Robert S. Weiss
Basic Books
1975   326 pp. $4.95

This book contains practical suggestions for adults designed to ease the transition of separation and aid in organization of a new single life. Topics include erosion of love, identity change, legal matters, single parenting.

Separation is an incident in the relationship of spouses rather than an ending of that relationship. It is a critically important incident, to be sure; an incident that ushers in fundamental changes in the relationship. But it is not an ending. Months after the individual has moved to a hotel room, furnished flat, friend's apartment, or back to the parental home, the spouse is likely to remain the most important figure in his or her world.

Parents' Book About Divorce
Richard Q. Gardner
Bantam Books
1979   300 pp. $2.95

A positive book to help divorced parents maintain loving, supportive relationships with their children. Problems covered include: when and how to tell children of approaching divorce, how to settle custody and visitation rights, how to alleviate anger and fear of abandonment and how to determine whether professional help is needed.

Many problems may arise for parents with regard to the question of what to reveal to the children when an extramarital sexual involvement has been the precipitating cause of the separation. When such involvements have been a central cause of the separation the children do best if they are told. In the situation where both parents consider infidelity to be a symptom of more basic difficulties in their relationship, difficulties that they have been unable to resolve, they do well to present to the children the fundamental contributions of each and describe the affair as a common outcome of such problems. To withhold the information may make the parent more comfortable, but the children will be impeded in their abilities to deal optimally with the trauma of separation.

Talking About Divorce
Earl A. Grollman
Beacon Press
1975   87 pp. $2.95

Grollman helps parents face reality and the consequences of a family breakup. The first section, for children, is an illustrated read-along, treating divorce in a straightforward, honest, compassionate manner. The second section is a parents' guide for these dialogues, encouraging sharing of the child's real feelings of anger, resentment, hostility, and perhaps relief that the unhappy family is separating.

"You are not the reason for us wanting to live away from each other . . . You are not to blame for the divorce . . . Do you think you are?"
. . . Say again and again that you are unhappy with each other but not with him. The reason for the divorce is not because the child was bad. As long as he believes that he has caused the separation, he can conjure up the illusion that he has the power to bring you all back together.

When Parents Divorce
Bernard Steinzor
Pocket Books
1969   339 pp. $1.25

Steinzor maintains that divorce is healthier than an unhappy marriage; the turbulent period of adjustment prior to and immediately after separation can be a time of growth, fulfillment, and liberation for parents and child. Topics discussed include custody and visitation rights, property and support payments, and coping realistically with the former partner.

Divorce, then, may be a way of increasing the child's capacity for the growth of love, which means a readiness to be open and clear with another as a person and not as a means to an end.

For Children

Divorce Is a Grown Up Problem
Janet Sinberg
Avon
1978   100 pp. $2.95

This is a book designed to help children understand what has happened to their family when a divorce occurs and to be read aloud by a parent—hopefully by both parents at different times. The author warns that during and immediately after a divorce, a child needs to talk, to cry, to feel angry and sad but most of all to find her way through the confusion.

Your child is still a child. It won't help him or her to be told "Now you're the man of the house" or "you're Daddy's little woman now." A child needs to know that adults are still in charge of his world and will continue to be so.

Boys' and Girls' Book About Divorce
Richard Gardner
Bantam Books
1971   158 pp. $2.50

This guide for children of divorced parents addresses such topics as: "Who's To Blame?" or "How To Get Along Better With Your Stepmother and Stepfather."

Many children of divorced parents wish their mothers would marry again. Most of them wish it would be to their father, and if not to him then to another man. These children keep asking their mothers over and over when they're going to get married again. This usually upsets the mother and makes her feel bad about the divorce. It would be a great mistake if such a mother were to marry a man she did not love just because she thought this would make her child happier.

What's Going to Happen to Me?
Eda LeShan
Four Winds Press
1978   132 pp. $6.95

One in every sixth child lives in a one-parent family. Divorce has become so common in the lives of so many children that when one little boy wrote a fairy tale for school he ended it: "and so they lived happily together for quite some time." The author talks to children in this book, striving to help them understand how they feel and how their parents feel and encouraging them to get in touch with their feelings.

Right now it is probably hard for you to get through one day at a time. All you can think about is how angry or confused or scared you are, yet it seems as if most people expect you to go on living as if nothing was happening. Your

teacher gets upset if you aren't listening; your grandmother gets angry if you yell at her; your father doesn't understand why you won't talk to him anymore; your mother thinks you are much too old to be wetting your bed at night or needing a night light. You may feel like it's the end of the world, but all these things are natural and normal things that can happen to a child when parents are getting a divorce.

Organizations (See Appendix A)

American Association of Marriage and Family Counselors

Jewish Board of Family and Children's Services

National Council on Family Relations

Parents Without Partners

Contact also local family service agency or church clergyman for additional support and referrals for counseling or legal assistance.

DRAMA. SEE CREATIVE EXPRESSION.

DREAMS

Dreams are a natural and a necessary part of sleep. When your child has nightmares or upsetting dreams, reassure her and encourage her to share her dreams with you. Frequent nightmares may indicate that your child is suffering some stress or upset during the day. Explore the possible causes

with your child (and perhaps her teachers) to eliminate the source.

For Children

D

A Child's Library of Dreams
Sheri Clyde
Celestial Arts
1978   69 pp. $3.95

Containing dream stories emphasizing sharing of dreams to stimulate imagination and creativity and to overcome the frightening experience of a "bad" dream, this collection of children's dreams and the author's own conception of them is geared to children ages six to twelve, but is very acceptable bedtime reading material for younger children as well.

You are galloping on a black horse, through a thick green forest at midnight, bright with silvery moonlight. The wind is blowing your hair, and the moonlight is shining gently on your face and arms. Your arms are tightly wrapped around the neck of the magnificent beast. Faster, faster the magic black horse races the wind. You bury your head and face in his wild mane, peeking out just enough to see the pines and oaks and rocks and bushes and silver streams fade dizzily as you and your strong animal friend rush on and on and on through the night.

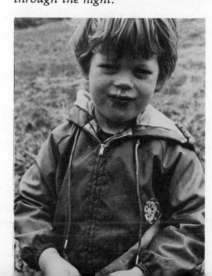

CHILDREN'S DREAMS AND NIGHTMARES

D The best thing a parent can do to help children tap the immense resources of insight and creativity available through their dreams is to act as an eager listener. The worst thing a parent can do is to act as a pushy dream interpreter.

Parents should take the time to ask children about their dreams in the morning, showing consistent interest in the detail of the events and feelings of the dreams by asking questions like, "Do you remember a dream from last night? I'd love to hear all about it." If the parents will also share with their children a few of their own dream sagas the rewards can be great. First, of course, the children will love the attention lavished upon their nightly masterpieces and they will be less motivated to produce or overemphasize nightmares in order to get that extra attention. Second, by validating the children's dream life, parents encourage their children's creative, synthetic, problem-solving abilities, which are at their best in the sleep state. Third, by regularly sharing dreams at breakfast, a family can find itself communicating in very open, humorous and meaningful ways. If the family agrees not to try to interpret each other's dreams, or to judge them, but to listen appreciatively to each member's dream-stories, a great deal of trust can be built up.

Indeed, there is very much to be gained from the skillful interpretation of children's dreams. However, this skill requires study and tact in its application and is described in *Living Your Dreams* for those interested in learning how to interpret and direct dreams. The techniques presented therein are easily taught to young people.

When children have nightmares, encourage them to describe in detail the whole drama. Suggest that the children look at the dreams as if they were scary movies. Assure them that no dream-movie monster can ever *really* hurt them. Then rehearse with them their plan of action for any frightening dreams they might have in the future. While awake, the children should tell themselves that the very next time a monster or threatening animal or person chases them in a dream, they will not run but turn and face the pursuer and ask, "What do you want, and why are you in my dream?" With a little practice, children will find that they automatically follow this strategy while asleep and that whenever a frightful dream-enemy is confronted, it will reveal itself as a friend in disguise who only wanted to tell the dreamer something about himself. The ability to confront and understand a dream-enemy gives children a new sense of mastery and self-confidence as well as valuable insights into the parts of their personalities they need to better understand.

One of the most important and fortunately, one of the easiest ways to tap into the practical problem-solving abilities of the sleep state is through dream incubation. This is the process of going to sleep with a specific problem on your mind and awakening in the morning with a dream that helps you to understand or solve the problem. Suppose a child has a difficult decision to make, or perhaps she needs a good idea for a school project, or perhaps she needs help in adjusting to the parents' separation. Before she goes to sleep, if she writes on a piece of paper her one-line request for understanding or a good idea, places the paper by her bed, and then repeats the incubation request over and over in her mind as she falls asleep, she will likely awaken with a dream answer to her request. Since incubated dreams are often easier to understand than spontaneous ones, they offer a good starting point for beginners in dream study. They also help children and adults to solve big and little problems more quickly and with much less pain than usual. After one's first successfully incubated dream, one realizes beyond any doubt that a dream is a terrible thing to waste.

Gayle Delaney
Living Your Dreams
Harper and Row
1979   232 pp. $8.95

DRUG ABUSE.
SEE HEALTH AND
HOSPITALS.

E

Ecology
Education

Emotional Development
Environments for Children

Exercise and Sports
Eyesight

ECOLOGY

Our nation and the world are facing a crisis in terms of the use of natural resources and the availability of undeveloped land. You can teach your child about the environment and ecology at home through animals, flower and vegetable gardens, nature walks, visits to woods, and with books on animals and plants. Teach your child to protect the environment and to conserve energy and other resources at home, school and in the community.

As a child grows, his world expands. His small playpen universe enlarges to include his yard, the park, his neighborhood and the outdoors. Children are fascinated by the plants and creatures of this new world, and teaching your child about his environment is not only a way to help him develop an awareness of and concern for living things, but it is also great fun!

We have included some books and magazines that will provide interesting information and ideas for you to share with your child, records that you can listen to together and coloring books that instruct as they entertain. We encourage you to investigate these natural history "teaching aids" and to consider making the study of nature part of your regular activities with your child. Not only will you learn a great deal, but you will be instilling an appreciation of our

environment that is becoming increasingly necessary in our current ecological crisis.

Mrs. Terwilliger's Coloring Book
Write for information to:
P.O. Box 668
Tiburon, CA 94920
$3.00 (includes postage)

This fascinating coloring book teaches natural history to your children while they are developing art skills. Based on the teaching of Elizabeth C. Terwilliger, a naturalist and wildlife specialist who teaches children and adults, each drawing features an informative caption.

Look for the little red cap on the back of the Acorn Woodpecker's head, and his black chin and yellow throat. He stores acorns in the bark of trees.

My Garden Companion
Jamie Jobb
Charles Scribner's Sons (Sierra Club Books)
1977   336 pp. $4.95

Gardeners are special people, says the author of this volume of useful information. This sourcebook includes: locating a plot, what to grow, when to plant, how to dig and prepare soil and how to pinch and prune.

You will save yourself a lot of trouble and disappointment if you find out which types and varieties of common garden plants grow

best in your area. This is especially true for a food or flower garden.

Anywhere you live you can have a garden: in a house, apartment, trailer, treehouse, or even on a sailboat. All you need is fresh water, soil, sunlight, and permission. You can have a garden that is very little and quiet, or very big and busy, or very in-between.

North American Wildflowers Coloring Album
Troubador Press
$2.50

This coloring book offers highly detailed drawings of North American wildflowers in a large ($8\frac{1}{2} \times 11$) full-page format suitable for framing after coloring. On the facing page of each drawing is a clear, concise description of the flowers found in the drawing, with complete botanical information on the characteristics of the plants.

Sierra
Sierra Club
530 Bush Street
San Francisco, CA 94108
Nonmembers—$8/year
Subscription & membership—
$20/year
Single issue—$1.50

This bimonthly magazine features environmental awareness/protection articles and also includes outdoor product information, outdoor activity articles and book reviews.

Sierra Club Summer Book
Linda Allison
Charles Scribner's Sons (Sierra Club Books)
1977   160 pp. $4.95

E   This book celebrates the earth in summer through numerous activities, toys and games for children. Creative projects include constructing a gum wrapper thermometer, high noon portraits, potato gargoyles and an outdoor West African game (Yote) played with sticks and stones.

Whenever there is strong sunlight, the conditions are right for high noon portraits. Grab a friend, a pen, a paper; hold still and get traced. Write a letter on the back and send it to grandma. She'll love it.

Smithsonian
Smithsonian Associates
900 Jefferson Drive
Washington, D.C. 20560
U.S. and possessions—$12/year
Elsewhere—$15.50/year
Single issue—$1.25

This monthly publication includes a variety of natural-history articles, information on Smithsonian exhibits, geographic articles and more.

Terra
Natural History Museum of Los Angeles County
Exposition Park
Los Angeles, CA 90007
Family—$25/year
Student—$15/year

This quarterly magazine is devoted to articles on natural history. Includes such topics as "From the Gold Rush to the Hollywood Rushes: Butterfly Farming in California."

Tripping with Terwilliger
Write for information to:
P.O. Box 668
Tiburon, CA 94920
$5.75 (includes postage)

A recording of Elizabeth Terwilliger teaching natural history

to children. Selections include: "Mighty Sea," "Grasshopper," "Sierra," "Sights and Sounds of the Seasons" and many more. (Songbook included.)

View from the Oak
Judith and Herbert Kohl
Charles Scribner's Sons (Sierra Club Books)
1977   110 pp. $4.95

This book introduces children to the world of animals and insects by exploring the ways they experience space, sense and time and communicate with others of their kind. It includes activities, experiments and illustrations to help young readers enter different worlds through an understanding of the senses of animals.

All dirt might smell and feel and look alike to us. But for the mole each part of its territory has a particular density, smells of all the creatures that do or have lived there, and has its own texture. To understand how a mole knows its territory, the next time you go to a beach, pick up a pinch of sand and take it home. Then look at the individual grains of sand under a power magnifier. Are there any two grains alike? What is the range of colors? of shapes? of densities? Imagine being just a bit larger than the grains of sand. A pinch of sand would be as varied and complex as the dirt around the mole's tunnel is for the mole.

Organizations

Appalachian Regional Commission

Friends of the Earth

Greenpeace

National Geographic Society

Sierra Club

EDUCATION— GENERAL

See also Alternative Schools, Child Care, Nursery and Preschools.

The Teacher and You

Your part as a parent in preparing your child for his first play or group experience away from home is to make sure your child understands the basics about the class, teacher, travel to and from and as much as you can explain before the first day of school. Hopefully you will be satisfied with the teacher your child has. If not, talk to the teacher before the end of the first week about any changes you feel are necessary in the best interests of the child.

Teachers have various degrees of training and ability. They are overworked and often underpaid for the work they do and the responsibility they have. They educate and care for anywhere from ten to thirty or more children a day and are responsible for all aspects of their learning and social development.

If your child's teacher does not assist him to your satisfaction, first have a conference with the teacher to find out why. The problem may be with your child, and it is necessary to hear how the teacher feels. If this approach does not work, if possible, request a change of class by discussing the situation with the director or principal of the school. A talk with a counselor or a psychologist may be helpful if your child is having a problem that moving into a new situation will not help.

Certain kinds of behavior are disruptive to everyone in the classroom. A counselor can help you explore the causes. The first steps to finding the source of behavioral problems include: a physical checkup, a controlled diet (free of additives and sugar) and discussions of the problem of respect for the rights of others with your child. The important point is that your child be in a school situation in which she feels totally comfortable and can function to her greatest potential.

Some Ways of Distinguishing a Good School or Center for Young Children

- Is there space for running about freely for active play and still other space where quiet play may go on undisturbed, both indoors and out?

- Is there sufficient space for a cot for each child during rest periods and a two-foot aisle between the beds?

- Is there a place where children may be isolated if needed, for instance, in case of a sudden "runny nose"?

- Is there approved fire protection and does every member of the staff understand what to do in a fire emergency?

- Are heating facilities adequate and officially approved? Is there sufficient ventilation?

- Is there protection against drafts, dampness? Check for unbroken flights of stairs, unprotected stairwells, uncovered radiators, and any other possible dangers to children.

- Does the center carry liability insurance?

- Are the rooms well-lighted, without glare? Are they well ventilated? Are they kept clean?

- Are toilets and washbasins sanitary and sufficient in number? (At least one to every 15 children.)

- Are provisions made for medical examinations at least once a year, and preferably more often, with a parent present? Is the center given a full written report by a private physician, health clinic, or other community agency, before the child is admitted? Is there a supervising pediatrician for the school? (on call)

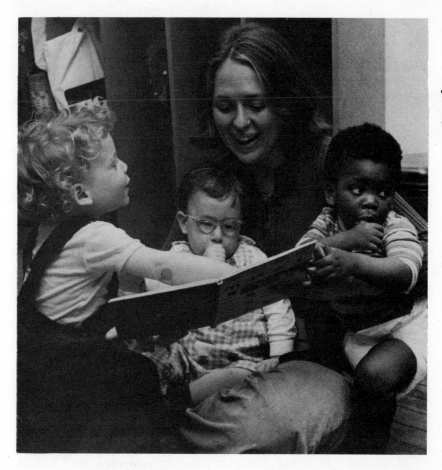

E

- Is a person trained in first aid always available? Are there adequate first aid supplies safely stored, out of reach of the children, yet readily available to the adults? Is there close observation at the beginning of the day and during the course of the day by a responsible person to prevent the spread of communicable diseases common among young children?

Single copy furnished free upon receipt of self-addressed stamped #10 envelope.
National Association for the Education of Young Children
1834 Connecticut Ave., N.W.
Washington, D.C., 20009

Parent Involvement

One of the greatest problems of the school today is that it tells children they should think, and then refuses to acknowledge or tolerate any new ideas. Basically, it's trying to mold children to function within the system—not to work to make needed changes.

Parents must learn that the schools should be established to serve the community and the community's opinion must be respected; they must question the arbitrary rules of traditional education, they must know and believe that they can make changes that they feel are necessary.

Many teachers just can't measure up—they've done nothing for so many years that it is impossible to start to move now. What about those teachers who can move and recognize a real need in providing for your children a learning environment which stimulates growth and development in a meaningful way?

Before you can answer this, you need to ask yourself questions which will aid you in gaining insight into your own feelings:

- Am I in awe of the teacher because I think she knows so much more than I?

- Did unpleasant memories of a bad experience with the teacher of my older child influence my feelings with this teacher?

- Do I have a feeling the teacher really isn't interested in my child because she has so many others?

- My child is so difficult to deal with, shall I avoid talking to the teacher about him?

- Am I blaming the teacher and the school too much for all my child's unfortunate behavior lately?

- Do I disagree with the school's philosophy at times? What have I done about changing that philosophy?

What the Kindergarten Teacher Should be Doing for Your Child

The kindergarten teacher should create an environment that is stimulating, not overwhelming or confusing, and supplied with equipment and material. Children require quiet places to play, sufficient materials, balanced opportunities to paint, draw and use different media. A balance of activities allows for opportunities in science, math, language. The teacher should talk with children so that they understand and can feel her confidence in them. Her attitude should be enthusiastic and positive. The classroom should have moveable materials with opportunities to sort, classify, compare and allow for many different sensory experiences. Materials should be available to allow children to create, measure, work with plant life and learn the differences between big and little. They need to have opportunities to play in different media.

What Can Parents Do?

IN THE HOME

Parents can encourage and provide learning activities at home that will help to create a home-school climate conducive to a child's total learning and development. The following suggestions are just a few of the things parents can do at home to help.

Read daily to your children, especially your pre-school ones.

Listen to your child read or pretend to read.

Take time to talk with your child as opposed to talking to him.

Talk with your child about "what happened in school today?" or what happened while he was out playing.

Provide a quiet time in the home each day for reading and study free from interruptions by the radio, television, and telephone.

Reinforce activities that originated in school. (Parents can play word games with their children such as asking the child to "Tell me all of the words you know that begin like baby, or like dog," etc. Or, "Tell me a word that rhymes with toy, or cake," etc.)

Take children on weekend outings, holiday trips, and vacations. Then talk with your child about what he saw, the order in which he saw it, and how he felt about what he saw.

Help your child create a story by letting him tell it to you so that you can write it down.

Help your child draw a picture about an experience you have had together. Then talk about the picture together.

There are many other things you can do—ask your friends and neighbors to help you think up others.

Pointers for Parents
Florida Dept. of Education
Tallahassee, Florida

Education by Choice: The Case for Family Control
John E. Coons and Stephen D. Sugarman
University of California Press
1978   223 pp. $10.95

In this examination of the concept of family choice in education, the authors present theories and arguments suggesting that the best authority over a child's education should be the family, supported by professionals. Alternatives to our present system of education such as vouchers, entitlements and education stamps are presented. The authors maintain that via such alternatives the ideological strains can be reduced in society. Chapters deal with ideological pluralism, racial integration and the nature of subsidy for education.

What effect would the liberty to attend a school chosen by themselves and their family have on children who are potential academic failures? In our opinion a significant proportion among the dropout and truant cadres would today be engaged in some organized pursuit of learning had they not been effectively expelled from that pursuit by compulsory assignment to a school experience they plainly despised.

Getting Ready
Lois Mark Stalvey
William Morrow
1974   313 pp. $7.95

This book deals with one of the most tragic and dangerous problems in American society: the mental and spiritual crippling of minority children in urban schools. The author writes about the experiences of her daughter and sons in Philadelphia's predominantly black public schools, and tells how the problems at her children's school led her to the conclusion that schools are often not living up to the challenge of educating students.

Parents Organizing to Improve Schools
Happy Fernandez
National Committee for Citizens in Education
1976   53 pp. $1.50

This pamphlet is directed to parents concerned about children's educational environments, who want to organize parents' groups to make positive contributions toward improving schools.

The primary goal of a parent group should be recognition by other parents that it is an effective organization working to benefit the children at your school. Recognition by school officials should be a secondary question, and it will come only after or as a result of being known as a voice for parent and student concerns. The best way to establish your identity is to take action that improves the quality of education at your children's schools.

Parent Power
Martin Buskin
Cornerstone Library
1977   173 pp. $1.95

In this handbook for dealing with your child's school, discussion of suburban schools dominates most chapters. Suggestions are offered for coping with and improving the daily reality of classroom life.

One important question to ask about class size—and school administrators have to be watched here for their tricky use of statistics—is what the average class size is in the specific school your child is attending. The average class size for a district may sound wonderful, but if your school happens to be the district's one overcrowded school, the overall district's statistics won't mean a thing.

Who Controls The Schools?
Carl Marburger
National Committee for Citizens in Education
1978   76 pp. $2.00

A handbook for parents answering such questions as: who makes the decisions about what happens to children in public schools, what is the role of parents and citizens in that process and who should make decisions.

[The] inability of citizens to affect their educational institutions is a major problem. Some of the difficulty lies with the parents/citizens themselves. Frequently, parent groups cannot agree on what they want the schools to do and so cannot exert any united influence. Moreover, parents and citizens are still quite confused about how

schools operate, both in theory and in practice. Despite decades of talk about community relations from schools and administrators, the public is quite uninformed about school affairs.

E

Organizations (See Appendix A)

National:

Administration for Children, Youth and Families

American Association of Elementary-Kindergarten-Nursery School Educators

American Association of Sex Educators and Counselors

American Montessori Society

Appalachian Regional Commission

Association for Childhood Education International

Black Child Development Institute

Children's Defense Fund

Education Development Center

National Association for the Education of Young Children

National Education Association

National Forum of Catholic Parent Organizations

National Society for Hebrew Day Schools

P.E.E.R.S.

United Synagogue of America

Magazines (See Appendix B)

Children Today
Day Care and Early Education
Early Years

E EMOTIONAL DEVELOPMENT

See also Communication; Disabilities; Mental Health.

Emotions are what we feel and experience every day. They are reflections of love, friendship, success, failure, daily stresses and strains. Children need to be allowed to express their emotions freely, as long as they do not become hurtful to anyone else. Unfortunately, we have been taught to be embarrassed by emotions and to stifle them. The more expressive you are, the more open your child will learn to be. If you are uncertain about your feelings or your child's feelings, do not hesitate to turn to people who can help you clarify and understand them better—a psychologist, a social worker, a helpful teacher or a sympathetic friend.

The emotional social side of children's development is as important as the intellectual cognitive development. Ideally, children should have the opportunity to keep both aspects of themselves in balance, and thus will be able to achieve and do well both in their personal and school activities.

Be prepared to deal with a range of emotions. Anger is common. If your child is furious and demanding, he may say, "I hate you." Usually this is because you have asked for something he doesn't want to do or doesn't perceive as reasonable. Often a child is right, and it is important to examine your own demands and question your own responses.

Here are some additional points to remember: Do not have your child focus his attention on you all the time. Do not confine children for long periods of time.

Do not ignore your child when he needs to throw a tantrum. Do not worry if you say no. Do not be overprotective. Do not overpower your child.

Assert Yourself
Merna Dee Galassi; John P. Galassi
Human Sciences Press
1977   237 pp. $7.95

Presents a variety of discussions and exercises with the goal of increased self-expression and assertion for a "variety of users." Maintaining that "learning to behave assertively does not come overnight and that it takes time and hard work," this book offers a strong hand to guide one through the arduous course. There is an overview for the self-help user and an overview for those who wish to develop their own training programs.

You have the right to say no to requests that are unreasonable and to requests which, although reasonable, you do not care to grant. Being able to say no when you mean no is important for a variety of reasons. First, it helps you to avoid becoming involved in situations which you think you will regret being involved in at a later time. It also helps to prevent the development of circumstances in which you will feel as though you have been taken advantage of, abused, or manipulated into doing something which you did not care to do. Finally, it allows you, rather than the other person, to make your decisions and to direct your life in that situation.

Family Communication
Sven Wahlroos
Macmillan
1976   328 pp. $1.95

In terms of prevention, it is important to reiterate that the in-ner security on which nondefensiveness rests is a direct result of the love a person has experienced as an infant and child. The younger the human being, the more important this love seems to be for future development. The love does not need to be communicated in words: The love must be communicated through tenderness, bodily contact, a clearly communicated wish to be with the child, and a clearly communicated attitude that the child is important, not only as a human being but as a very special human being. The love must also be communicated through firmness and through clearly showing the child that you will help him control his impulses when he is not able or willing to do so himself. This control must be exercised with reasonableness and fairness, however, and the object must be the gradual abandonment of external control and its replacement by the development of inner discipline.

Feeling Child
Arthur Janov
Simon and Schuster/Touchstone
1975   286 pp. $4.95

Excessive daydreaming, fear of the dark, emotional problems in school—these are all problems parents often have to deal with in bringing up their offspring. This guidebook for parents who want to rear emotionally healthy children discusses these problems as well as the common failures of most parents in family living.

What I am saying is that the seeds of neurosis may well begin before birth, and that experience by the fetus in the womb may be as important, if not more so, than subsequent social events.

Feeling Good Cards
507 Palma Way
Mill Valley, CA 94941
$7.00 (includes postage)

Playing cards that ask energizing questions for clear non-threatening communication for children and adults to play with and talk about together.

Help for the Lonely Child
Ernest, Rita and Paul Siegal
E. P. Dutton
1978   187 pp. $9.95

This is a book for parents and educators of lonely children. The authors discuss how inept nonverbal communication skills make a child feel frustrated, often hostile and plagued by feelings of self-doubt and self-reproach, which in the end produce a lonely child.

The authors provide workable techniques to improve a child's social perceptions and help her relate to others in a meaningful, satisfying way.

While making sure that the child gets experience at games is essential, it is even more important to provide him with the company of children his own age. At the beginning, he may not be capable of "playing" with them. Your job then is twofold. First, make certain that those children chosen as companions find the experience an enjoyable one. Unsatisfactory experiences can use up the supply of willing companions very quickly! Second, plan and structure the social experiences so that they build in two ways: (1) toward independent play, and (2) toward suitable time blocks.

How It Feels to Be a Child
Carole Klein
Harper & Row
1977   165 pp. $3.50

Klein dispels the myth of the happy child and emphasizes the importance of acknowledging children's right to experience painful feelings, since such feelings are natural in the process of growth and development.

Andy has been taught it is wrong to be seriously angry with his brother and to express that anger physically or verbally. The conflict over what he feels and what he's supposed to feel is obvious in his quick assurance that he loves his brother after that instinctive upper-casing of his resentment. But as Andy denies his spontaneous feelings, his isolation deepens. For he gets further and further away from his instinctual self. And a conviction grows, whispers bleakly in his ear, that if people knew what he was really like, they would not, could not, love him.

Teaching Your Child To Cope With Crisis
Suzanne Ramos
David McKay
1975   229 pp. $9.95

Guidelines on how to help children cope with divorce, death, surgery, alcoholic parents, extended separations and the like. One chapter deals with what happens to a child when a parent faces imprisonment.

In spite of the frequency of divorce, a child may not like it that one of his parents has been married to someone else. For this reason, he should find out about it from you. But again, try to bring it up in the context of a normal discussion. If your child says, "Hey, Dad, did you know that Billy's mother was married once to a different man and they got divorced?" you can say, "No, I didn't know that, but you know, Jim, I was married once to someone else. It only lasted a short time and we decided that we weren't right for each other and we got a divorce. A few years later I met your mother and we've been very happy together."

Self-Esteem: The Key to Your Child's Well-being
Harris Clemes and Reynold Bean
G. P. Putnam's Sons
1980   350 pp. $12.95

Two renowned therapists outline a unique program that shows parents and teachers how to give children the greatest gift of all—self-esteem. Experts agree that a child's feelings of selfhood are the key to well-being and to development into a mature and productive adult. The authors explore and discuss specific personal characteristics and psychological patterns, which, if properly nurtured, contribute to a child's confidence, the "Four Conditions of Self-Esteem."

Your child will have a good sense of self-esteem when these four crucial conditions are present:

- *Connectiveness—how children relate to other people;*

- *Uniqueness—how children express and feel their differences as individuals;*

- *Power—how effectively children influence the circumstances of their own lives;*

- *Models—how children clarify and manifest their goals and purposes.*

What Do You Do With Them Now That You've Got Them?
Muriel James
Addison-Wesley
1974   143 pp. $5.95

James uses transactional analysis to turn unpleasant feelings into pleasant ones. Each chapter starts with a typical family situation, demonstrating how to deal with feelings and behaviors that arise.

Your Child's Self-Esteem
Dorothy Corkille Briggs
Doubleday (Dolphin)
1975   341 pp. $2.95

This book promotes the concept of self-esteem as a child's most important characteristic, since her feelings about who she is will affect her development throughout her life.

We sometimes have less faith in our children's sprouting capacities than we do in our plants'. By pushing and urging and forbidding we try to force growth. When progress bogs down, we focus on them, rather than on the climate around them.

For Children

Feelings—Inside You and Outward Too
Barbara Kay Polland
Celestial Arts
1975   54 pp. $4.95

This book, which helps young children understand why they feel as they do and how they can express these emotions to others, is also excellent for parents seeking a bridge between their own and their children's feelings. It demonstrates ways to exchange inner feelings and reflections in a sharing, caring, growing atmosphere. Contains large black and white photographs.

PAIN—It can be awfully painful inside when feelings get hurt. What is the meanest of mean things anyone has ever said to you? Pretend you are telling that person OUTLOUD how these mean words made you feel inside.

Liking Myself
Pat Palmer
Impact Publishers
1977   80 pp. $3.95

This is a fun book for young children to read themselves or

have read to them, offering exercises and questions designed to help them feel okay about themselves.

Liking yourself and being your own good friend helps you to like other people and be a good friend to them. It is fun to give other people a treat, such as . . . scratching their backs . . . (the way you like it, too!) . . . sharing your favorite cookie . . . telling them nice things you like about them . . . giving them turns on your bike . . . Share the good parts of you with others!

Meditation for Children
Deborah Rozman
Celestial Arts
1976   151 pp. $4.95

This book offers advice for initiating and continuing meditation periods within the family or school, with chapters on yoga and evolutionary awareness exercises included. Written in gentle yet concise language, it is also suitable for adults.

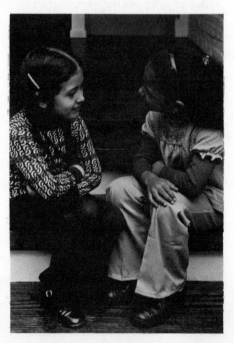

A child who meditates correctly every day keeps some contact with the Real Self inside that is never conditioned by what happens, that is always pure. He is not as influenced. This does not mean that he is insensitive or closed to other people; it means that he doesn't have to look outside himself so much for authority, security and confirmation. He has his own direct contact with inspiration and bliss and does not need to depend so much on all the external stimulation that bombards children.

Mouse, The Monster And Me
Pat Palmer
Impact Publishers
1977   78 pp. $3.95

Assertiveness training for children is presented in this book, including a "Strengths Game," where friends sit in a circle, fold paper in half, list good qualities in themselves, then pass paper to person on right, who in turn lists good qualities he or she sees in the other child on the other half of the paper. The game allows a child to discover his self-perceptions and compare them with ways in which others see him. The "Saying No Game" helps a child learn to say no firmly but without hurting others' feelings.

Mice can be nice. And people who act like our friend mouse are sometimes so nice that they allow themselves to be walked on by other people. . . .

Monsters, on the other hand (actually you probably prefer not to have a monster on either hand!) are seldom friendly or thoughtful or nice. . . .

Of course, all people are not mice or monsters. Most are just themselves. Friendly. Honest. Thoughtful. Fun to be with. You probably are too, but we can all learn to like ourselves more.

New TA For Kids
Alvyn and Margaret Freed
Jalmar Press
1977   101 pp. $4.95

This book uses simple words and phrases to explain the concepts of transactional analysis to children. Chapter I illustrates how each individual is three personas (Parent, Adult, Child); following chapters deal with how personas function; the final chapter tells how to be an "OK" person.

What we want to talk about now is how to make use of TA so that you can become skilled at helping other people feel OK and, in turn, to feel OK yourself. The first job then is to tell ourselves every day, "I'm OK—You're OK." Put a bumper sticker on your mirror and read it out loud every morning. This means that other people are worthwhile, adequate, and important and so am I.

It's Scary Sometimes
"I and Others" Writers Collective
Human Sciences Press
1978   29 pp. $6.96

Designed to help young people understand and cope with fear, this book explores the psychology of fear, including information on how adults can help children overcome and minimize fright. The pictures and words of the children are invaluable, each quote highlighting a child's scary experience.

When I turn on the T.V. at home and hear music and then I turn it off and I hear only silence, I'm afraid because I hear the silence, so I stamp my feet to hear a noise and that way it seems like there's someone there.

Stories About the Real World
Richard A. Gardner
Avon
1972   137 pp. $1.50

Excessive involvement with fantasy may make it difficult for a child to deal with reality. The author offers stories for children to tip the scale more toward reality. Stories are designed to present real-life situations and offer satisfying real-life solutions.

Oliver also started to look at what he was doing with his friends. He didn't like to hear that he was selfish, that he always wanted to go first and that he wouldn't let other children play with his toys. But he realized—for the first time—that loneliness was even worse. So Oliver thought about how he acted with the other children. It made him feel bad but he knew that thinking about his problems would help him change them.

It was hard, at first, to let other children play with his toys.

It was more fun to be first in a game than to wait his turn . . . but he knew that if he wanted to have friends he would have to feel bad at times and let them go ahead of him.

ENVIRONMENTS FOR CHILDREN

See also Disabilities; Playgrounds.

The world your child lives in every day consists of both a physical environment and an emotional environment. A home may be beautifully decorated and perfect, but living within that environment is what is important—how parents talk to each other and to their children and the degree of warmth and responsiveness people show to one another. Your environment should reflect your values and the way you feel about your family.

Children need a space to call their own. A private room is ideal, but even if it is a bed, a dresser and half a closet, let your child know that the space is for her alone. You have the right to set limits about cleanliness and neatness of that space. Sometimes your child will need help attaining those standards.

Children enjoy the opportunity to design their own storage and shelf spaces. Closets, storage space, toys and books—as well as kitchen and bathroom items—should be within easy access. Pillows, soft lights, desks, a record player, a table, extra chairs and an easel are all items that make your child's room more pleasant. You also might wish to add some plants or a small pet; children enjoy taking care of living things.

Once you and your child have set up the physical environment, the emotional climate grows out of your experiences together each day—how much you enjoy and share together, and how you handle any problems that arise. Each day it is up to you, as a parent, to create an environment of love for yourself and your family.

Wherever children are is an environment for children. We can help make that environment a stimulating, meaningful place. By now everyone knows about low furniture and "mini" mops and brooms. How much else can be or has been "mini"-mized for the children? (Not that reduced size is the whole answer to the question.) Perhaps the information provided by the references in this section will help parents, and educators, expand their concept of suitable childhood environments.

From their first days on earth, too many children are mishandled in hospital nurseries, where harsh

E

E and inhuman fluorescent lights shimmer, and at home they are often confined to cribs and play-pens without enough opportunity to move. We must be more aware of their basic needs and make vital adaptations to these needs.

There is another important category, which must exert profound influence—the special nature of the needs of children. Among them: rest, play, quiet, noise, privacy, social contact, adult love, adult models, safety, growth, cleanliness and development—at home and in school.

For help in designing a room for your child, send for The Children's Design Center catalogue. It provides information on children's furniture and other equipment which is highly functional and often transformable. Recognizing that apartment dwellers often have limited space, the Design Center offers, through mail-order, such things as high chairs that can later be used as standard-sized chairs, and cradles that convert to desks. You can call the Center's toll-free line (within the continental U.S. (800) 833-4755, within New York State (800) 342-4774). The Center makes a special effort to locate products for handicapped children. For catalogue ordering information see the Toys section, page 246.

Checklists for Spaces, Furniture and Outdoor Equipment

Design Considerations for Children's Activities

- size
- durability
- flexibility
- quality
- safety
- attractiveness

- usefulness
- adaptability
- cost
- easy maintenance
- warmth
- rest
- quiet
- visual stimulation
- verbal stimulation
- physical movement
- sensorial experiences
- freedom
- security
- opportunities for spontaneous activity

A Child's Place
Alexandra Stoddard
Doubleday/Dolphin
1978   164 pp. $5.95

Stoddard approaches a child's room from his scale and view, with an eye toward creating challenges, fun and stimulation as the child grows.

As behavior patterns change, so should the environment. A revolving room design can be changed as often as you would change a bulletin board. The display shelves that once housed miniature horses and Beatrix Potter rabbits might later display knitting or a rock collection.

Child in the City
Colin Ward
Pantheon Books
1978   211 pp. $12.95/$6.95

Through photographs and text, this book explores relationships between children aged five to sixteen and their urban environment. It explores their ingenuity in exploiting what a city has to offer, and demands that cities be made more accessible, negotiable and useful to children.

Every generation assumes that the street games of its youth have been destroyed by the modern city. Yet they survive, changing their form in innumerable adaptations to exploit environmental changes. The lifts of the tower block, the trolleys from the supermarket, are incorporated into the repertoire of playthings, often to the great discomfort of the adult world. The very outrageousness some of the forms these adaptations take surely suggests that children are demanding their share of the city and knocking for admission into this adult world which monopolizes the city's toys and forgets that the most precious gift we can give to the young is social space: the necessary space—or privacy—in which to become human beings.

Sunset Ideas for Children's Rooms & Play Yards
Lane Publishing
1980   96 pp. $3.95

This book contains ideas and suggestions on how to create your children's rooms to be much more to them than just places to sleep. You can devise for your children a friendly, cozy and safe environment in furnishings and arrangements that make a big difference. This book also helps with problems that occur if kids' rooms are undersized and shows diverse and imaginative solutions to other typical children's room problems.

Children's outdoor play varies endlessly and the book gives good ideas for increasing the potential of backyard and playground fun in ways that parents can manage better than can kids, left to their own devices. It includes safety tips and first-aid techniques.

EXERCISE AND SPORTS

See also After School Activities; Games and Activities; Playgrounds; Playing.

Developing your children's interest in regular exercise and sports is a gift you can give them for the rest of their lives. Everything from playing ball with them to running to teaching them to swim or play tennis adds to your child's balance, enjoyment and ability to be with other children, and is essential to keep your child in good physical condition. Actually, many parents rediscover their own love for exercise and sports when they share these activities with their children. Doing yoga together or exercising, riding bicycles or engaging in other sports could be a great deal of fun for your family.

Your child should have regular exercise every day out-of-doors; walking and bike riding are excellent. Dancing to music in the house is also fun, and regular sport activities are something to be encouraged.

Overcompetitiveness in some team sports is not necessarily advantageous for children, particularly if too much stress is placed on winning. The most important part of a child's development is learning how to play the game and playing it. Winning is important, of course, but it is not the end in itself; the process is what is important. Children should enjoy their activities and be able to know that they are loved even if their team does not win the game.

Public Information
Travelers Insurance
Hartford, CT

For Children

Girl Sports
Karen Folger Jacobs
Bantam Books
1978   180 pp. $1.50

The author interviews fifteen female athletes who have been successful in sports events long considered "for boys only." The females, who have excelled in sports from wrestling to judo, discuss how they came to be involved in their sport and how it has affected their life-styles.

They talk about training, competing, winning and losing.

"I love competition: I want to be the greatest. I want to be like Mohammed Ali and Bruce Jenner. They are the greatest! If you're the greatest, everyone looks up to you, and you get in the papers. My picture was on the cover of Runner's World two times."

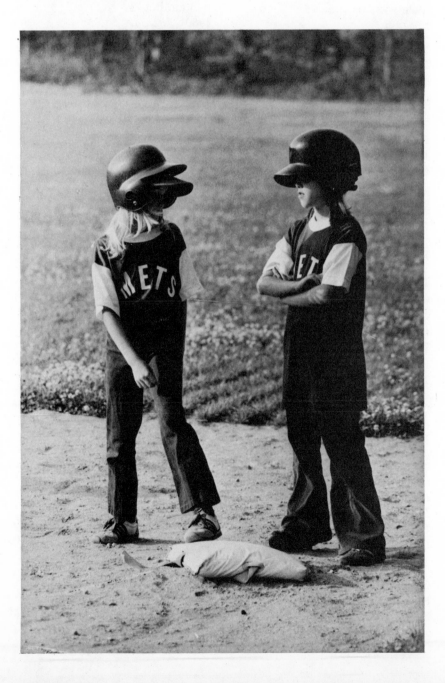

E

E

Play Ball with Roger the Dodger
Al Campanis
G. P. Putnam's Sons
1980   80 pp. $7.95/$3.95

Aspiring Little Leaguers will find valuable tips on how to play baseball in this lively, fun book. In clear, funny, cartoon-style art, Roger the Dodger demonstrates each aspect of the game, from batting and running to pitching, catching, and fielding. This how-to-book provides basic advice that will help young players improve their game.

Bunting is when you hit the ball lightly without taking a swing at it. Bunting is used under certain conditions. A good bunt can make the difference between winning or losing a game.

Yoga for Young People
Michaeline Kiss
Bobbs-Merrill
1980   92 pp. $5.95

This book teaches children the basic principles and techniques of yoga, to develop a healthy body and mind through coordination and concentration.

The Yogic Deep Breath is a complete breath. It uses three areas of the body: the lower abdomen, the rib·cage, and the chest.

Here is how it works: As you breathe in, you expand, or push out, first the abdomen, then the rib cage, then the chest. As you breathe out, you contract, or pull in, first the abdomen, then the rib cage, then the chest.

All breathing should be done through the nostrils. They are filters that purify the air for us.

More Books on Sports, Games, Keeping Fit and Healthy

In addition to the books listed here, see detailed descriptions in the Creative Expression, Ecology, Games and Activities, Playing, and Toys sections.

Any Child Can Swim
Jeanelle Ankeney
Contemporary Books
1976   123 pp. $6.95

Playbook
Steven Caney
Workman Publishing
1975   240 pp. $5.95

See & Be:
Yoga and Creative Movement for Children
Rachel Carr
Spectrum (Prentice Hall)
1980   114 pp. $6.95

Your Own Horse: A Beginner's Guide to Horse Care
Patrice Clay
G. P. Putnam's Sons
1977   127 pp. $7.95

Games of the World: How to Make Them; How to Play Them; How They Came to Be
Frederic Grunfeld
Ballantine
1975   280 pp. $7.95

Games Babies Play: A Handbook of Games to Play With Infants
Julie Hagstrom and Joan Morrill
A & W
1979   84 pp. $4.95

Perfect Balance—The Story of An Elite Gymnast
Lynn Haney and Bruce Curtis
G. P. Putnam's Sons
1979   60 pp. $8.95

Concise Encyclopedia of Sports
Keith Jennison
Franklin Watts
1979   218 pp. $8.95

The Great Game of Soccer
Howard Liss
G. P. Putnam's Sons
1979   64 pp. $8.95

Yoga for Your Children
Lyn Marshall
Schocken Books
1976   64 pp. $4.95

Kids Book of Games for Cars, Trains & Planes
Rudi McToots and Drednaught
Bantam Books
1980   162 pp. $4.95

Street Games
Alan Milberg
McGraw Hill
1976   302 pp. $7.95

Best Rainy Day Book Ever: More Than 500 Things to Color & Make
Richard Scarrys
Random House
1979   Unpaged $4.95

Everybody's A Winner—A Kids' Guide to Sports
Tom Schneider
Little, Brown
1976   139 pp. $7.95/$4.95

Sports Superstitions
George Sullivan
Coward, McCann & Geoghegan
1978   71 pp. $7.50

How to Teach Your Baby to Swim
Claire Timmermans
Stein & Day
1975   159 pp. $8.95

Organizations (See Appendix A)

American Alliance for Health, Physical Education and Recreation

EYESIGHT

See also Disabilities; Sensory Development.

Watch for These Signs of Eye Trouble in Children

Behavior

- Rubs eyes excessively.
- Shuts or covers one eye, tilts head or thrusts head forward.
- Has difficulty in reading or in other work requiring close use of the eyes.
- Blinks more than usual or is irritable when doing close work.
- Stumbles over small objects.
- Holds books close to eyes.
- Is unable to see distant things clearly.
- Squints eyelids together or frowns.

Appearance

- Crossed eyes.
- Red-rimmed, encrusted, or swollen eyelids.
- Inflamed or watery eyes.
- Recurring styes.

Complaints

- Eyes itch, burn or feel scratchy.
- Cannot see well.
- Dizziness, headaches, or nausea following close eye work.
- Blurred or double vision.

If your child has any of these signs, a professional eye examination is advised.

Facing the Problem

It is estimated that one in every 20 preschool age children in the U.S. has a vision problem which, if uncorrected, can seriously interfere with his development and schooling. For some of these children, those with "lazy eye," discovery and treatment before school age is especially important.

A child thinks that everyone sees the way that he does. If he doesn't see well, he probably won't complain—he doesn't know he has a "vision problem."

It's up to you to see if your child has normal vision. This Home Eye Test is a good start; but in no way takes the place of a professional eye examination.

Testing the Child

First, explain to the child that you are going to play a "pointing game" with him. (Avoid coaxing or insisting. If the child doesn't want to, choose another time.)

Create and cut out a big "E" and teach him to point like it "points" when held in the four different directions (up, down, right, and left). Say to him, "point like this." Show him if he needs help. Continue until he can point in the four directions without help. Praise him each time he responds.

Write for your copy of the above to:
National Society for the Prevention of Blindness
79 Madison Ave.
New York, N.Y. 10016

Total Vision
Richard S. Kavner and Lorraine Dusky
A & W
1978   251 pp. $8.95

In this practical guidebook to help preserve, protect and improve the quality of eyesight, the authors have included exercises and games that families can perform at home to help achieve heightened perception, keener memory, stronger powers of concentration and overall better vision. Chapters explain how stress, emotional trauma and even faulty posture can cause distortion of images and eye ailments.

You may do remarkably well reading those letters on the chart, but good vision includes all those other skills, and more. Vision is tied up with how a person moves, thinks, comes to a decision; visual problems can give us clues to what kinds of stresses the person operates under. Distortions of the eye are considered to be problems in reaching a decision, reflections of behavioral style, and indications of some form of stress, whether it be physiological, cultural or environmental. It just might be something as simple as the fact that you didn't have proper lighting on the bedside table all those nights you stayed up until three o'clock and secretly read while your parents thought you were sleeping.

Organizations (See Appendix A)

American Association of Ophthalmology

American Foundation for the Blind

Fight for Sight

F

FAMILY

See also Fathering; Marriage and Shared Roles; Mothering; Parenting; Section I—Preparing for Parenting; Single Parents.

The child first learns about life within the family group—from parents, grandparents, cousins and friends or anyone who is a part of the extended family or support system. Most families in America consist of either two parents or a single parent raising children. In many families, grandparents or relatives and friends are also responsible for the child. Other familial arrangements are a possible part of the child's immediate family. Sometimes due to special family circumstances a child must be relocated in a new family, through foster care or adoption.

A foster family consists of people who care enough about children to want to provide them with temporary homes. In many cases, the foster care comes at a time when a child is vulnerable and needs particularly loving support. An adoptive family is one which provides a loving home to the child when there is no parent who can be responsible.

All families go through many changes by the time the child reaches adulthood. The family establishes its own customs, traditions and life-style.

A great deal of attention has been given to families over the past years. Many books have been written to describe different family situations, but no one knows or understands a family better than its participants—each member has his or her own perspective, needs and experiences.

Each family is unique, based on the value systems and the ideas of its own individual members.

Family Council

A regular family council meeting can be very important. Everyone in the family should have an opportunity to participate. Everyone should have an equal say in the activities. Any voting that takes place should avoid struggles between parents and children by mutual agreement. If decisions cannot be reached, they can be put off until the next meeting.

It takes time to get everyone to talk together and feel satisfied, so do not get discouraged. Sometimes people don't believe that this can be an effective way of participating in the family, but in fact, everyone enjoys the opportunity of these special meetings. Find a convenient time when everyone can sit down together and work out problems. Anyone in the family should be able to initiate an emergency meeting, if necessary.

Family Council
Rudolf Dreikurs, Shirley Gould and Raymond J. Corsini
Henry Regnery Co./Contemporary Books
1974   128 pp. $3.95

The family should operate in an orderly manner with a minimum of conflict and with all family members contributing, according to the authors, who offer a step-by-step guide for setting up and maintaining a family council. The authors stress ways to handle conflict and methods of teaching responsibility and fostering equality.

In any conflict, it is necessary to discover and pinpoint the issue. The real issue is never what people are arguing about. The real issue is the disturbed relationship. . . .

Creative Family Activities
Valerie Sloane
Abingdon
1976   128 pp. $4.95

This book contains suggestions for creatively motivating children through such family activities as backyard carnivals, cooking together, shopping expeditions and amusements for the sick child.

A divorced father who spent Sundays with his twelve-year-old daughter encountered a problem trying to simulate a normal family situation in his bachelor apartment. He could sense that a visit to a movie, restaurant, or other commercial attraction was no basis for building a father-daughter relationship. He knew the girl didn't particularly enjoy spending a day at his place, and he felt them drifting apart.

One day she said to him, "I'm sorry, Dad, but it's boring at your apartment. I'd rather stay in my own room and read magazines and listen to records."

Capitalizing on the girl's interest in country and western music, her dad suggested that they build a gutbucket. Together father and daughter began a search for the materials needed to build this simple percussion instrument.

How to Strengthen Your Marriage and Family
G. Hugh Allred
Brigham Young University Press
1976   388 pp. $7.95

Using case histories, the author suggests how to create harmony, happiness and meaningful productivity in marriage and family, as well as how to improve communication among family members.

F

FUNCTIONS OF THE FAMILY

What is a family? What does it do? Presumably—and we can't really go beyond speculation here—families came into existence because of the need to formalize child rearing. Divisions of labor notwithstanding, it was that little creature who clearly belonged to the woman in the den but whose relationship to the hunter was probably less clearly understood, who across the centuries helped establish a pattern of bonding which held people together into family units. We sometimes think of the family as a female invention, but the complicated social patterns of regulating family life which gradually evolved offer in many ways greater protection to men.

Prior to full understanding of the process of procreation, paternity was not easily demonstrated. It had to be established by regulation of the ambience of women and then advertised and preserved by such customs as patronymic designation and a genealogy formalized through the father. Many of the important antecedents of our complicated legal system are rooted in the family, such as the concept of legitimacy, patterns of determining inheritance, etc. All of these bear witness to the fact that family law historically protected the male of the species and enhanced his security just as much as that of the female.

The biological definition of family involves no sentimentality. It describes a classification and nothing more. However, the connotative and social definition of family carries with it a broad array of expectations. That the individual family has perhaps not always provided these highly desirable characteristics is implied in the following sardonic but hopefully tongue-in-cheek definition of a family offered by Sussman: "The family is a group of people somewhat haphazardly assembled (at least initially), related by blood or by marriage, and ruled by its sickest member."

In some respects, the question of what a family actually is can be as difficult to specify as what a family should be.

Maybe it would help to re-define *family*. A family is a group of people living together with trust, having clear relationships, and who aid in each other's growth. So divorced or not, a family is what you make of it. If everyone loves and is willing to let others in the family be, then everything will be great. But if there are expectations of what someone should do, then everything gets messed up. Constructive criticism is fine, but must be stated as that. It cannot sound like screaming; it has to be done calmly.

Also if the constructive criticism is not accepted, then one must have enough trust in the other person to solve his problem for himself.

Trust is the key word. Once you get away from trust you start coming upon hate, guilt, lies and other things that destroy a relationship. Trust is important, but clarity is also important. When someone does something that you do not like, react to it, find out why that person did or said that particular thing. If you do not then you start to have mad bubbles building up inside you. These bubbles lead to anger. Pop the bubbles before they pop you!

Bettye M. Caldwell
Child Development Specialist

F

Secrets in the Family
Lily Pincus and Christopher Dare
Pantheon Books
1978   44 pp. $8.95

The authors explore the social myths of birth, copulation and death and their impact on the family. Drawing on therapeutic case histories, they show how these mysteries can become the common domain of the whole family and have creative as well as detrimental effects.

Sensuality in the family has three components. There is the sex life of the parents; the children's developing sensual longing; and the parents' tendency to re-experience their own childhood sensuality in the relationship with their children. *It is therefore inevitable that incestuous fantasies are part of the secret life of every family. For children to develop into healthy, loving and sexual adults, these fantasies are necessary, but their overt expression has to be controlled by the parents.*

Your Family History
Allan J. Lichtman
Vintage Books
1978   200 pp. $3.95

The author believes strongly that family history can be exciting and can bring you closer to your parents, grandparents, children and other kin. He offers practical approaches to researching your roots, from informal chats with family members to collecting heirlooms or beginning an autobiography.

Don't be satisfied during an interview with vaguely phrased responses. Try to get a family member to translate such responses into concrete ideas and actual behavior that can be checked against information from other sources. For example, your grandmother might tell you that she came from a large family. Ask her how many brothers and sisters she had.

Organizations
(See Appendix A)

Administration for Children, Youth and Families

American Association of Marriage and Family Counselors

American Home Economics Association

Black Child Development Institute

Jewish Board of Family and Children's Services

National Council on Family Relations

U.S. Department of Health and Human Services

United Synagogue of America

Magazines
(See Appendix B)

Family Circle
Marriage and Family Living
Parents' Magazine
Redbook

FATHERING

See also Marriage and Shared Roles; Parenting; Single Parents; Part I—Sharing Roles.

Fathers, like mothers, love their children and have a strong investment in their future. Fathering is as much an art as mothering, and becoming a successful father requires a skill all its own. Children look to their fathers for many supports, both social and emotional, and like all family members, fathers need attention, care and understanding from both their spouses and their children. At first, men are no more prepared to be fathers than women are to be mothers; perhaps in time, schools will offer classes in parenting for both boys and girls.

F

The American Father
William Reynolds
Pocket Books
1980   224 pp. $2.50

A sharp and entertaining exposé of American family life, this book is designed to make the reader question current assumptions about parenting and fathering and the roles of mother and father.

Fathering, in fact, is a secondary interest to Father who is primarily occupied with the torments and rewards of being Mother's lover first and foremost. His children are seldom the center of his life and many of his dealings with them are influenced more by his feelings at the moment about Mother than anything in particular the children may be doing.

Fathering
Maureen Green
McGraw-Hill
1976   218 pp. $3.50

Deeply sympathetic to the father's plight in our changing social system, this book emphasizes the need for a strong father's role in the development of secure and happy children. Early chapters trace the father's transformation from patriarch to buddy; later chapters discuss fathering within the nuclear family.

Father's part after the infant years in teaching the children to become fully human obviously starts by just being there, giving them enough time to seize on the fact that men exist as well as women, that interesting and helpful, satisfying and violent feelings can exist between father and mother, as well as father and son, mother and son, father and daughter and mother and daughter. To be introduced to the rich emotional possibilities of life, a growing child

needs to see some of it in action. Most of all, children of both sexes get a chance to see how men and women get along together as adults.

How to Father
Fitzhugh Dodson
New American Library
1975   488 pp. $2.95

Dodson describes how a father can guide his child at each stage of psychological development, and urges fathers to become involved with a child from infancy rather than waiting for adolescence to develop close emotional and physical contact. A useful survival kit appears in the appendix, as well as a guide to toys a father can make, a list of children's books and so on.

It is important for you as a father to be firm in setting wise limits and boundaries for your child's actions at each behavioral stage. Limits and boundaries should be reasonable and based on what can normally be expected for his age. Then be firm in enforcing these limits and boundaries. By doing this you are helping his own inner controls of his antisocial impulses. If you are not firm in enforcing limits, you are making it that much harder for him to establish this inner control system; and a child who does not firmly establish an inner control in early life is going to become an adolescent who will have great difficulty saying "no" to drugs or other antisocial behavior during his difficult teen-age years.

The Liberated Man
Warren Farrell
Bantam Books
1975   384 pp. $2.95

An incisive exploration of sex-role myths, this handbook is for men who want to move beyond

the theoretical psychological view of masculinity. It discusses women's liberation, the movement's effect on men, the concept of fatherhood, and the like.

When a discussion of men's and women's liberation starts questioning one stereotype after another, men usually get frustrated: "Won't there be any differences left? Is everyone going to be alike —unisex, uni-everything?" The answer is exactly the opposite: people will develop as individuals rather than mold themselves into a sexual stereotype. Men still ask, "What will happen to the chemistry between the sexes?" The potential for chemistry among individuals whose attitudes and behavior cannot be predicted is much greater than it is between two persons who are largely two stereotypes. There is no chemistry in confinement. The person searching for a stereotyped self is escaping from the freedom to develop a true self.

Who Will Raise the Children?
James A. Levine
Bantam Books
1977   187 pp. $1.95

This is about men and child care, the social implications of men sharing care with mothers or being single fathers and the advantages of househusbands for children as well as to parents and society.

Our whole society operates, for the most part, on two interlocking assumptions: that it is the natural role of men to be, first and foremost, breadwinner, and that it is the natural role of women to take care of children. Even as the latter premise is challenged—as more and more women work outside the home—it highlights just how little the former is even questioned.

See Appendix C for Films and Audio-Visual Aids.

F FIRST AID AND SAFETY

We have included first-aid information so that you know what to do first in an emergency. The next step is to get prompt medical help. Know where the nearest emergency hospital is, as well as other emergency facilities, including burn and trauma centers if your community has them.

Emergency Care

How you handle yourself in a medical emergency situation is extremely important. Knowing the basics of first aid can give you an added feeling of confidence as a parent. Your local Red Cross chapter provides training classes. For information, consult your local telephone directory. Training may include mouth-to-mouth resuscitation, first aid for wounds, poison control and other emergencies.

Be sure to have the telephone numbers of your doctor, fire department, police department and ambulance service near your telephone at all times. Being prepared for an emergency includes developing a useful first-aid kit, which contains items you are familiar with. Your doctor or pharmacist may be good resources in choosing the contents of your kit, which should include Ipecac (an emetic) as well as other items.

Fill in the appropriate numbers and post this list next to your telephone:

Doctor _____
Fire Department _____
Police Department _____
Poison Control _____
Ambulance _____
Neighbor _____

Relative _____
Parent Work Phone _____
Allergies or Special Problems _____
_____

A PHYSICIAN SHOULD BE CALLED IMMEDIATELY FOR ALL SERIOUS INJURIES OR SUSPECTED POISONING.

DO NOT GIVE FOOD OR DRINK TO ANY SEVERELY INJURED PATIENT.

Bruises

Rest injured part. Apply cold compresses for half hour (no ice next to skin). If skin is broken, treat as a cut. For other injuries always consult physician without delay.

Scrapes

Use wet gauze or cotton to sponge off gently with clean water and soap. Apply sterile dressing, preferably nonadhesive or "film" type.

Cuts*

Small—Wash with clean water and soap. Hold under running water. Apply sterile gauze dressing.
Large—Apply dressing. Press firmly and elevate to stop bleeding—use tourniquet only if necessary. Bandage. Secure medical care.
Note: Do not use iodine or other antiseptics before the physician arrives.

Puncture Wounds*

Consult physician.

Slivers

Wash with clean water and soap. Remove with tweezers or forceps. Wash again. If large or deep, consult physician.

Bites or Stings

Insect

Scrape out stinger, if present, with a scraping motion of the finger nail. Do not pull out. Apply cold compresses. Consult physician promptly if there is any reaction, such as hives, generalized rash, pallor, weakness, nausea, vomiting, "tightness" in chest, nose, or throat, or collapse.

Animal

Wash with clean water and soap. Hold under running water for two or three minutes if not bleeding profusely. Apply sterile dressing. Consult physician.
Note: If possible, catch or retain the animal and maintain alive for observation regarding rabies. Notify police or health officer.

Snake

Non-poisonous—Treat as a cut.
Poisonous—(Keep calm—work fast.) Complete rest. Apply constricting band above the bite (not too tight). Get victim to physician or hospital as soon as possible.

Burns and Scalds*

Burns of Limited Extent

If caused by heat: Minor burns of extremities may be immersed in cold water and ice bag or cold wet packs applied to areas on the trunk or face. Cooling must be constant until pain disappears. Nonadhesive dressing should be used if available. Plastic household wrap makes an excellent nonadhesive emergency covering. Consult physician. Do not break the blisters.

If caused by chemicals: Wash burned area thoroughly with water. Consult physician.

---

* Protection against tetanus should be considered whenever the skin is broken or for burns even if skin appears intact.

Extensive Burns

Keep patient in flat position. Remove clothing from burned area—if adherent, leave alone. Cover with clean cloth. Keep patient warm. Take patient to hospital or to a physician at once.
Note: Do not use ointments, greases, powder, etc. Electric burns with shock may require artificial respiration. Pull the victim away with nonconductive material, such as cloth. Do not use bare hands.

Fractures

Any deformity of injured part usually means a fracture. Do not move person if fracture of leg, neck, or back is suspected. Summon physician at once. If person must be moved, immobilize with adequate splints.

Sprains

Elevate injured part. Apply cold compresses for half hour. If swelling is unusual, do not use injured part until seen by physician.

Eyes

To remove foreign bodies, use a moist cotton swab. Don't overdo it. Pain in eye from foreign bodies, scrapes, scratches, cuts, etc., can be alleviated by bandaging the lids shut until doctor's aid can be obtained. Immediate and abundant flushing out with plain water is procedure for chemicals splashed in eyes. Do not use drops or ointment.

Poisoning

Call the nearest hospital emergency room or poison control center at once. As soon as possible induce vomiting.
Exceptions: Vomiting should *not* be induced if the child has swallowed kerosene or other petroleum products, furniture polish, paint thinner, or a strong corrosive such as lye or acids. Vomiting should not be induced if the child is unconscious or convulsing.

To Induce Vomiting: Give one tablespoon (one-half ounce) of Syrup of Ipecac for a child of one year of age or older plus at least one cup of water. Keep child with face down and head lower than hips to avoid choking while vomiting. If no vomiting occurs in 20 minutes, dose may be repeated *once* only. Do not waste time waiting but contact the patient's physician, hospital emergency room, or poison control center at once for instructions as to the need for further treatment. If unable to obtain this advice, transport patient immediately to the nearest emergency medical facility. Bring package or container with intact label. If vomiting occurs, and advice is that the patient should receive further medical treatment, save some of the vomitus and bring with him to the treatment facility.

Choking

If the child chokes and is not breathing, turn him head and face down over your knees and forcefully hit his back between shoulder blades in an effort to propel the object from the windpipe. If he can breathe, do not attempt this maneuver.

Artificial Respiration

To be used for drowning, smoke inhalation, and electric shock. Continue artificial respiration until seen by a physician.

Mouth-to-nose or mouth-to-mouth rescue breathing is the method of choice.

Rescue Breathing Technique

1. Clear the throat—wipe out any fluid, vomitus, mucus or foreign body with fingers.
2. Place victim on his back.
3. Tilt the head straight back—extend the neck as far as possible. (This will automatically keep the tongue out of airway.)
4. Blow—with victim's lips closed, breathe into nose with a smooth steady action until the chest is seen to rise.
5. Remove mouth—allow lungs to empty.
6. Repeat—continue with relatively shallow breaths, appropriate for size, at rate of about 20 per minute. For infants only shallow puffs should be used.

Note: If you are not getting air exchange, quickly recheck position of head, turn victim on his side and give several sharp blows between the shoulder blades to jar foreign matter free. Sweep fingers through victim's mouth to remove foreign matter.
Do Not Stop. If one can observe the chest to rise and fall, all within reason is being done.

Prepared by Committee on Accident Prevention and Subcommittee on Accidental Poisoning—American Society of Pediatrics. Published with permission of the American Academy of Pediatrics.

Nosebleeds

F In sitting position blow out from the nose all clot and blood. Into the bleeding nostril insert a wedge of cotton moistened with any of the common nose drops. (If no nose drops are available, cold water or hydrogen peroxide may be used to moisten the pack.) With finger against the outside of that nostril apply firm pressure for five minutes. If bleeding stops, leave packing in place and check with your doctor. If bleeding persists, secure medical care.

Fainting and Unconsciousness

Keep in flat position. Loosen clothing around neck. Summon physician. Keep patient warm. Keep mouth clear. Give nothing to swallow. Do not splash water on the face.

Convulsions

Consult physician. Lay on side with head lower than hips. Apply cold cloths to head. Sponge with cool water. Give nothing by mouth.

Head Injuries

Complete rest. Consult physician.

Notify the doctor if:

1. There is loss of consciousness at the time of the injury or at anytime thereafter.

2. You are unable to arouse the child from sleep. You may allow the child to sleep after the injury but check frequently to see whether the child can be aroused. Check at least every one or two hours during the day, and two to three times during the night.

3. There is persistent vomiting. Many children vomit immediately from fright, but the vomiting does not persist.

4. Inability to move a limb.

5. Oozing of blood or watery fluid from the ears or nose.

6. Persistent headache lasting over one hour. The headache will be severe enough to interfere with activity and normal sleep.

7. Persistent dizziness for one hour after the injury.

8. Unequal pupils. Be sure the light is not shining in one eye or that pupil will normally be constricted and smaller.

9. Pallid color that does not return to normal in a short time.

Safety Pointers

In automobiles, be sure that your child is fastened in securely with a seat belt, that the doors are locked and that your children know not to stand up while you are driving.

Walking on the street, be sure that children know the safety rules and stop at the curb, looking both ways for cars. Be sure your child understands the traffic light signals. If she is not old enough, be sure a responsible person is with her.

Bicycle safety—Children enjoy bicycles with training wheels, three-wheel tricycles and two-wheelers. Be sure the bicycle is the right size for your child. Be sure the bicycle has safety equipment, reflectors and warning devices such as a bell or a horn. Apply light-reflecting materials to make the bicycle more visible. Be sure that all the hardware on bicycle is in place, the tires properly inflated and the chain cleaned and oiled.

Child-proof your house. Make sure children have areas to play in that are free of dangers. Make certain all dangerous items are out of reach. If your house has a swimming pool, be sure there is a locked gate with no access for your child without an adult. As early as possible, your child should learn the basic skill of blowing bubbles under water and should feel comfortable around water, particularly if you live around water. Be careful of chemicals and poisons. Be sure you know what they are and that they are on shelves the children cannot reach, in a locked cabinet.

Your child should know his name, address and phone number if you are going to be somewhere where there is a possibility of your child being separated from you for any reason. Be sure the information is attached to the child. Make sure your child knows what to do in an emergency.

Put safety latches on your cabinets or drawers. Some that are recommended are Kindergard Latch, Chris-Brooke, Safe-T-Loc, Child Guard and Safe-T-Latch. Watch for electrical cords, sharp edges, toys that have small button eyes that can be removed and anything painted which can be toxic as well as items in disrepair.

To "Poison-Proof" Your Home . . .

1. Keep household products and medicines out of reach and out of sight of children, preferably in a locked cabinet or closet.

F

Even if you must leave the room for only an instant, remove the container to a safe spot.

2. Store medicines separately from other household products and keep these items in their original containers—never in cups or soft-drink bottles.

3. Be sure that all products are properly labelled, and read the label before using.

4. Always turn the light on when giving or taking medicine.

5. Since children tend to imitate adults—avoid taking medications in their presence.

6. Refer to medicines by their proper names. They are not candies.

7. Clean out your medicine cabinet periodically. Get rid of old medicines by flushing them down the drain, rinsing the container in water, and then discarding it.

8. Ask for and use household substances which are available in child resistant packaging. Insist on safety packaging for prescription medicines. Resecure safety feature carefully after using. Safety packaging gives extra protection to your children.

To Prevent Suffocation and Choking

- Keep plastic bags, such as those placed on drycleaning, away from babies and children. One safe plan is to tear them into small pieces before throwing them away. It is not safe to use

Source: Your Child from 1 to 6, US Department of Health and Human Services, 1972 97 pp. $.20

thin plastic to cover a mattress. It clings to the nostrils and can cause smothering.

- Be sure that gas fixtures don't leak. Use rigid metal connections instead of rubber tubing which may wear and crack.

- Remove small bones from fish or chicken for children under 3.

- Blow up balloons before giving them to the baby to play with. And do not let him play with a collapsed balloon. The child too young to know how to blow may suck the balloon into his throat and choke on it.

- Keep small objects such as beads, coins, pins, and buttons picked up and out of reach. The baby is sure to put anything he finds into his mouth, and is apt to swallow or choke on small items.

- No toy should be smaller than the baby's mouth or have small removable parts.

- Don't force the baby to take any oily medicine. Oily particles, if inhaled from choking, can cause damage to the lungs.

- Place his crib away from venetian blind cords.

- Do not feed the baby nuts, popcorn, small candies or leave them within his reach.

- Avoid clothing with a drawstring about the neck.

- If the baby vomits, lift his hips slightly to permit the liquid to flow out of his mouth. Do not pick him up at such a time.

To Prevent Water Accidents

- Do not leave a child under 3 alone in the bathtub even for an instant. Empty or securely cover wading pools when not

in use. It takes only enough water to cover nose and mouth to cause drowning.

- Keep your eye on a child who can crawl or walk every minute you are at the beach, or near a pool or lake.

- Be sure all cesspools and wells are securely covered.

- Drain pools and puddles around the outside of the house.

- Do not leave bathtub filled or tubs of water around where a baby may fall into them.

- Turn handles of cooking utensils away from front of stove.

- Avoid tablecloths that hang over the table edge. The baby is sure to grasp the dangling corner to pull up by, and can pull off hot foods or a pot of scalding coffee along with the tablecloth.

- Use safety covers on electric outlets to keep out the baby's fingers and toys or other objects.

- Replace electric cords and equipment when they show wear.

- Keep steam kettle or vaporizer and portable heater out of the baby's reach, and do not place such items close to the child or bedclothes.

- Keep the electric coffee pot or the iron, hot or cold, and its cord well out of the baby's reach.

- Guard against overexposure to sun. A few minutes a day, at first, is enough. Keep the baby's head covered and eyes shaded against any continued exposure to direct sun.

F

To Prevent Falls

- Keep the stairs free of objects which can cause you to fall while carrying the baby. Keep one hand free to grasp the handrail.
- Place a guard across stairs. A folding gate is useful at doorways to confine the baby to a safe part of the house.
- Keep a harness or safety strap on an active baby in the carriage or stroller, and never leave an active baby alone in the carriage.
- Never leave a baby alone on a bed, couch, or dressing table for even a moment without a barrier to keep him from rolling off. The baby who cannot roll over one day may be able to do so the next. Babies sometimes can pitch backwards before they can creep forward.
- Buy a high chair with broad space between the legs so it will not tip over, or select a low table-type variety.
- Keep scissors, knives, and other pointed objects out of reach.

To Prevent Poisoning

- Follow the doctor's directions exactly in giving medicine. Be sure that all products are properly labeled. Read the label twice before giving medicine. Measure the dosage carefully. Never refer to medicine as candy. Do not permit another child to give medicine to the baby unless under strict supervision.
- Never store liquids which are not meant to be swallowed in food or soft drink containers, or leave them in unmarked jars about the kitchen. Cleaning materials, paint thinner, hair waving lotions, boric acid solution, and other clear liquids may be mistaken for water or sampled by the baby as he's learning to drink without a nipple.
- In order to avoid the possibility of lead poisoning from chewing or sucking on painted furniture, toys, or window ledges, use paint marked "for indoor use" or "Conforms to American Standard Z66.1—1955. For use on surfaces which might be chewed by children."
- Keep medicines and cleaning materials in a locked cabinet or closet.

WAYS TO KEEP OUR CHILDREN SAFE

Did you know that infants can learn to swim at a very early age—if carefully taught by experts? That's one new aspect of safety, as well as joy in life, that all parents and teachers can and should explore. Then, we can put a stop to many unnecessary drownings.

There are ways to prevent the many other hazards that threaten and kill little children. How? First, as parents, we can learn what to expect of our children in their development and their natural curiosity to explore. Secondly, we can help them to use their own inner resources while teaching them how to protect themselves in a positive way.

Today, accidents loom as the nation's Number One threat to all children and a very serious menace to infants. Each year, about 14,000 boys and girls under age 15 die, and about 23,000,000 under age 16 are seriously injured in accidents.

Choking, suffocation, automobile accidents, fires and falls cause a great many infant deaths. Children from 1 to 4 are menaced by motor vehicle accidents, fires and drowning. They are also frequent poisoning victims, especially at age one. School-age youngsters are threatened by automobile and bicycle accidents, drowning, fires and firearms.

Although not all childhood accidents can be prevented, complete prevention must be our ultimate goal. Yet, who would want to raise children so timid, so lacking in daring that they would *never* risk getting hurt? No, that's not what parents or teachers are after. Minor mishaps—bumps and bruises, scratches and scrapes—are part of the growing and learning process. It is impossible to teach a child caution without causing some fear. And it is difficult to discover a middle ground between over- and under-protection. The teaching process, however, can be carried out successfully.

Most serious accidents *can* be prevented. Studies show that certain types of accidents are more likely to occur at one stage of a child's development than at another. No two children grow and develop at just the same rate or in just the same way. Every child is a person with a temperament of his or her own. Nevertheless, knowing something about the general growth and developmental patterns of all children will enable many parents to foresee potential accident situations, and take necessary precautions.

A basic ingredient in childhood safety is an understanding of the young child's need to touch, to feel and to investigate. Youngsters get into trouble if left alone to find out the why of things. Patience and empathetic supervision will teach a child what he wants to know within the limits of safety.

Be on the Watch

There's no substitute for keeping an eye on the baby. In fact, that's just what you must do for the first few years of a child's life. Newborns are obviously quite helpless. They can't roll over and don't move around much. But you have to check them from time to time to make sure they are all right. See that the baby's face is free of covers, clothing or anything else that might interfere with breathing. It's best not to use a pillow in bassinet, crib or carriage.

As babies grow older and more active, you can give them something to play with in the same room in which you are working. You may get less done this way, but you will have more peace of mind when keeping an eye on the child.

If you have older children, they may be able to take over the watching for a short period, or at least you can call on them to check what the baby is doing from time to time. But it is seldom wise to count on an older child to watch a young baby for very long.

Keeping an eye on the growing child is one of the most difficult things to do. After all, so many of us live in small families without any help. Frequently lacking are community centers, day care or nursery groups where young children can go for quality care, play, learning and creative expression. Help from outside the family could (and one day will) help to keep our children safer and happier.

Look Ahead

Besides keeping an eye on the baby, you can prevent many accidents by anticipating what the growing baby and child can do. For example, your baby may be highly active—waving arms and kicking legs a lot. If so, you can expect the baby to wiggle and scoot before learning to roll over. So, it's wise to always stay with your infant when he or she is on a bed, dressing table or anyplace from which the baby might fall.

You also need to inspect playthings for tiny, sharp, detachable parts—pins, eyes, buttons, beads—and anything the baby might swallow and choke on.

Baby-Safe House

Before your child graduates from the playpen, be sure to "baby-safe" your home—or that part where you allow the baby to roam. According to one study, the most dangerous rooms for babies and toddlers are: (1) kitchen, (2) bedroom, (3) bathroom, in that order. Hazards come in the form of poisonous household substances, medicines, cosmetics, sharp objects and scalding hot foods and liquids.

You can give your child safe space for action and exercise by clearing away or locking up all harmful objects. Give the baby toys too big to put into the mouth. A variety of plastic or wooden kitchen materials—spoons, cups, pans and the like—can often be as interesting as the many toys available in stores.

It's wise to know what to do in an emergency, since accidents still do happen. Keep important telephone numbers near your phone. For example: physician, hospital, poison control center (if one is near you), police and fire departments, pharmacy, ambulance, taxi.

For more information on accident prevention as well as emergency medical care, write for Metropolitan's catalog, *Health and Safety Educational Materials:* Health and Safety Education Division, Metropolitan Life Insurance Company, One Madison Avenue, New York, N.Y. 10010. Or you may pick up a copy at a local Metropolitan office.

Joan W. Parks
Health Education Consultant

F Children and Cars

Auto Safety and Your Child
U.S. Government Printing Office
Washington, D.C. 20402

This pamphlet explains how deaths and injuries to infants and children can be greatly reduced simply by buckling them into crash-tested car restraints, and lists the different kinds of restraints and how they are properly used. It lists resources and groups that provide information on auto safety.

General Services Division (NAD-42)/The National Highway Traffic Safety Administration
400 7th St., SW
Washington, D.C. 20590

This federally-funded organization created by the Highway Safety Act of 1966 sets safety standards for motor vehicles under 10,000 lbs. and recalls cars not meeting the safety standards. They also award Traffic Safety Grants to states. They will provide free pamphlets entitled "Child Restraint Systems for Your Automobile" (DOT-HS-805-174) as well as loan out informative films on child passenger safety. For further information on child passenger safety associations contact your State Office of Traffic Safety.

Physicians for Automotive Safety
Communications Dept.
P.O. Box 208
Rye, New York 10580

"Don't Risk Your Child's Life"

Send a self-addressed, stamped, legal size envelope with 35¢ to obtain a copy of this booklet.

More Safety Resources

Among the many other safety materials you can obtain are:

A Sigh of Relief: The First-Aid Handbook for Childhood Emergencies
Martin I. Green
Bantam Books
1977   199 pp. $6.95

An accessible and clear first-aid handbook. The first half deals with the prevention of accidents and the creation of safe home, school, playground, car, camping and water environments. The second section provides fast, simple guidance on how to handle almost any medical emergency a child may encounter.

Preschool Children in Traffic: A Parents' Guide
Local American Automobile Associations (free)

Your Child and Household Safety
Dr. Jay M. Arena
Chemical Specialties Manufacturers' Association, Suite 1120, 1001 Connecticut Avenue, N.W., Washington, D.C. 20036 (50¢)

Panic or Plan?
Your Child's Safety
Metropolitan Life Insurance Company, One Madison Avenue, New York, New York 10010 (free)

The Children's Hospital Accident Handbook
Department of Health Education
The Children's Hospital Medical Center, 300 Longwood Avenue, Boston, MA 02115 (35¢)

Young Children and Accidents in the Home
U.S. Department of Health and Human Services
Order from:
Consumer Information Center, Pueblo, CO 81009 (65¢)

Tuffy Talks about Medicine
Aetna Life and Casualty
Order from:
Film Librarian, Public Relations & Advertising Department, Aetna Life and Casualty, 151 Farmington Avenue, Hartford, CT 06115 (free)

A Guide for Teaching Poison Prevention in Kindergartens and Primary Grades
U.S. Department of Health and Human Services
Order from:
Consumer Information Center, Pueblo, CO 81009 ($1.00)

Organizations (See Appendix A)

American Academy of Pediatrics

American Automobile Association

American Medical Association

American National Red Cross

Jewish Board of Family and Children's Services

National Institute of Child Health and Human Development

U.S. Department of Health and Human Services

See Appendix C for Films and Audio-Visual Aids

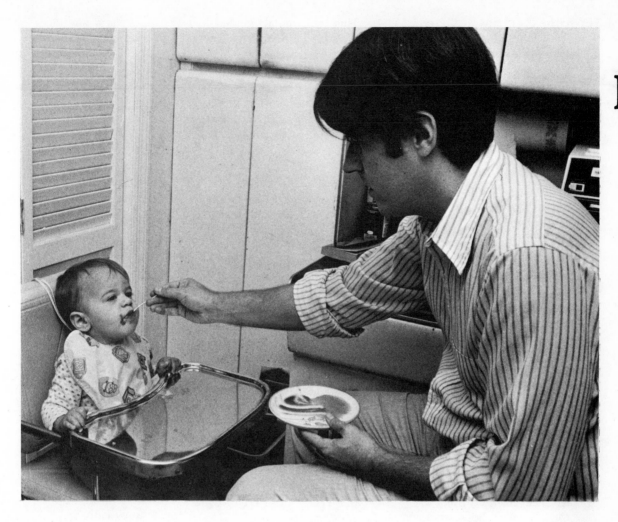

F

FOOD AND NUTRITION

See also Cooking with Kids; Part I: Feeding and Nutrition

What you feed your child is important. Be cautious about giving your child anything with sugar or overfeeding your child. A good balanced diet for you and your child is best. Give many choices of fruits, vegetables, meat, cereals, grains, chicken and eggs.

Children develop preferences for certain foods and dislikes for others. One good suggestion to encourage wider food selection: "Try a little bit of everything to know what it is, and then finish what you can." Parents often don't realize that children do self-select foods and they do enjoy variety. Children also enjoy food shopping, helping set the table, cleaning dishes and cooking simple foods. Cookbooks for children will give them new ideas.

Children watch their parents' responses to food, and they imi-tate. They follow your habits. If you never liked spinach or avoid it now, you may find that your child does also. A new way to prepare it may be as a salad with bacon bits and chopped egg. Use your imagination and enjoy the variety of new possibilities.

Mealtime is a good time for the family to get together to talk and share. Try new dishes for the family to enjoy. When your child prepares a dish, say positive things about the results or the cook will be discouraged from trying again.

Sample Recipes

Crunchy Home-made Cereal

F Use cereal for a three o'clock snack for the children. Be sure to add milk. This tastes better than anything you can buy in a cereal box.

> 4 cups quick-cooking rolled oats
> 1 cup wheat germ
> 1 cup finely chopped nuts
> ½ cup chopped coconut
> ¼ cup honey

Mix all together well and spread out on a cookie sheet or any flat pan. Bake for ½ hour at very low heat (250 degrees F.). Stir once or twice while baking. Store in plastic bag or empty coffee can. Add raisins when you serve it.

To Add Vitamin C: Fruit Kabobs and Popsicles

Slip onto a toothpick pieces of fruit such as banana slices, pineapple chunks, grapes, strawberries, melon cubes, prune halves, apple cubes and cheese cubes (dip apple and banana pieces in lemon juice to keep them from browning).

Or . . . make ice cubes or popsicles from orange juice or grape juice. Many hardware stores carry plastic popsicle molds.

Snacks to Limit:

candies, rich desserts, cakes, doughnuts, soft drinks, potato chips, commercially prepared cookies. It is difficult, but if you can make some rules about how often the children eat these non-foods, your reward will be better teeth, better appetites at the table and a much smaller grocery bill. All of these snack foods cost a lot of money!

Food Is More Than Just Something To Eat
U.S. Department of Agriculture
U.S. Government Printing Office
1969   32 pp.   Free

This nutritional guide discusses major nutrients and where to find them as well as the importance of nutrition during pregnancy, infancy and the school years. It also explains nutritional labeling on packaged foods and provides a daily food guide. Full-color illustrations.

Food is what you eat, nutrition is how your body uses food. And if you aren't eating foods to meet your body needs, you may be suffering from poor nutrition. Some of the damages caused by severe malnutrition may be irreversible.

What a young girl eats today may have an effect on the kind of pregnancy she will have years from now. What a pregnant mother eats may have an effect on her child's growth and development. What a child eats affects the way he grows and develops. What a person eats—as an infant, a child, or an adult—can affect the length and quality of his life.

Nature's Children—A Guide to Organic Foods and Herbal Remedies for Children
Juliette de Bairacli-Levy
Schocken Books
1978   148 pp. $2.95

Contained within this book are advice and recipes for natural living and healing, as well as herbal remedies for fever and cuts.

The simple rule to use when choosing foods, is to take only natural things. Cereals, with the exception of sweet-corn and barley and wheat, have to be prepared before they can be digested by man. Corn, cut fresh, can be eaten raw, and needs only to be soaked in a shallow covering of water from twenty-four to forty-eight hours to be palatable and digestible. Sprouted wheat can be eaten raw. All other vegetarian or dairy foods can be eaten natural and raw, direct from wild countryside, gar-den, orchard and dairy—or from the greengrocer's shop!

More on Food and Nutrition

How to Convert the Kids From What They Eat to What They Oughta
Polly Greenberg
Ballantine
1980   218 pp. $2.50

Feed Me! I'm Yours
Vicki Lansky
Bantam Books
1974   153 pp. $1.95

Diet For A Small Planet
Frances Moore Lappé
Ballantine
1975   410 pp. $2.50

Recipes for A Small Planet
Frances Moore Lappé
Ballantine
1973   366 pp. $2.50

Feed Your Kids Right
Lendon Smith
McGraw-Hill
1976   251 pp. $9.95

Making Your Own Baby Food
Mary Turner and James Turner
Bantam Books
1976   146 pp. $1.75

Organizations (See Appendix A)

American Academy of Pediatrics

American Dietetic Association

American Home Economics Association

American Medical Association

National Institute of Child Health and Human Development

U.S. Department of Agriculture

U.S. Department of Health and Human Services

GAMES AND ACTIVITIES

See also: After-school Activities; Creative Expression; Playing; Playgrounds; Sports

Activities to Do with Your Children

We have listed many different activities for you to do with your children. There are ideas throughout the book for art, music and all the different activities that are on the list. It is important to create a balance between activities that you enjoy and activities specifically for your children. Don't be surprised if at certain times, children are not interested in the activities that you recommend. Keep these in mind:

- cooking
- cutting pictures
- dancing
- drawing pictures
- games
- gardening
- laughing and jokes
- making and watching home movies
- photography
- playing games and puzzles
- preparing something (recipes, crafts)
- reading
- roller skating
- sports
- storytelling
- swimming
- talking
- trips to libraries, stores, zoos, museums, other homes, places of interest
- walking
- writing letters/stories

  Create your own Fun!

Tips to Assist Your Child to Beat Summer or After-school Boredom

- Sort school papers. Make a scrapbook of the best/favorite ones for math, reading, art, etc.
- Visit the library. Ask about the summer programs available. Check out some books for recreational reading.
- Write a letter to a relative in another state.
- Visit the park nearest your home. Relax and do some "people-watching."
- Do a good deed for someone in your family.
- Plan an indoor picnic for the next rainy day—food, fun, and friends.
- Save the seeds from a piece of watermelon. Plant them in a flowerpot and put it on a sunny windowsill. Don't forget to water them.
- Keep a daily record of what you see.
- Ask some friends to help you bake cupcakes. Decorate them with icing and candy to create funny faces.
- Say thanks to your parents for something. Write them a note.
- Write a poem about the Fourth of July.
- Make a drawing of a sunset.
- Write and read a short story to a small child.
- Put on a play about monsters.
- Write a "Dear Abby" question.
- Make your mother's or father's lunch.
- Take a hike with a friend.
- Write a 20-second commercial for your favorite gum.
- Review the multiplication tables or do other arithmetic games with someone.
- Make a dessert for dinner. Ask mom to help you select an easy recipe.
- Read good books.
- Count the cars that drive past your home for one hour.
- Spend fifteen minutes in quiet thought.
- Collect objects that are one-half, one-third, one-fourth, one-fifth and one-sixth of a total set of objects.
- Find some way to earn $2.
- Deposit the $2 in a bank account. Open a savings account if you do not have one already.

G

Paint and decorate a hard-boiled egg. Give it to someone.

Write a letter to a friend away at camp or elsewhere.

Make a sheet of math problems for mom or dad to do. Check the answers.

- Create and draw a comic strip.
- Do a good deed for a senior citizen.
- Clean your room and have a garage sale. Add the profits to your bank account.
- Make a greeting card for a sick relative or friend.
- List the letters of the alphabet. Cut out a word from the newspaper for each letter. Paste them on a piece of colored paper.
- Find an odd-shaped rock. Decorate it with scrap materials.
- Make up ten different, interesting math problems with the answer 12.
- Write new lyrics (words) for your favorite song.
- Name twenty nice things that happened to you this summer.
- Make a checklist of the things you need for school.
- Help mom or dad with one of the activities planned for the day.
- Go shopping for your school supplies.
- List the things you would like to· accomplish for the next school year.
- Go to bed early so you'll be rested and ready for the first full day of school tomorrow.

Pointers for Parents, Florida Dept. of Education, Tallahassee, Florida

Tips on Improving Perceptual Motor Activities

- Use an old paper sack. Put several pieces of crumpled newspaper in the sack. Tape or tie the sack closed. This makes an inexpensive "ball" for a young child to throw, kick, catch or bat with his hands.
- Coat hangers and old nylon stockings make interesting "tennis racquets." Squeeze the end of the hook toward the joint of the hanger for the handle. Hold the hanger opposite the handle in one hand and hold the handle in the other. Bend the hanger into an oblong or diamond shape. Put the hanger into the stocking as far as it will go. Tie the leftover stocking tightly with string. Balloons, small paper "balls" or yarn balls can be hit with this kind of racquet.
- Street curbs are good places to practice balancing. Walk, staying on the curb, placing one foot in front of the other. Cracks in the sidewalk or pavement can be used in the same way.
- Lines and dots designs. Make seven different-colored dots on a large piece of paper, spreading them out evenly. Have the child draw a circle around each dot until the circles meet each other. Use various colors and numbers of dots. Also, different shapes could be used—as squares around each dot or triangles, etc.
- Play the "What's Missing?" game. Place a group of things (such as a button, a spool of thread, a toy, a crayon, etc.) in front of the child and ask him to name the things and tell something about each that will help him remember it, as "The crayon is the only green thing, the button is shiny," etc. Now have child close eyes and you remove one thing. When he opens his eyes, ask what is missing. Vary the game by using more or fewer things, different things, or using a time limit.
- Bean bags for throwing and catching are easy to make. You can use old socks with the holes patched, scraps of cloth or whatever is available for the "bag." The insides can be beans, rice, etc. These are fun to catch and throw and to throw into containers or at targets.
- An old bleach container or plastic milk container can be used for a fun ball game. All you need to do is cut the bottom of the container off, leaving a scoop-like catching basket with a handle. Two children can play the game—one throws the ball and the other tries to catch it in his basket—or one can play alone, throwing the ball up in the air and catching it as it comes down.

Games

Children play games by themselves and with other children. There are many games that children play both verbally and physically. It is important that children develop a whole range of games that they can enjoy, especially activities that they can do alone when they need quiet time. Children invent their own games and enjoy many of the same favorites that every child has played for many years.

G

Who's Sitting on the Button?

You need a button.

- The child who is "it" leaves the room.

- Everyone else sits down and one child sits on the button.

- The seated children sing a song or clap their hands.

- "It" comes back and tries to find who is sitting on the button.

- The closer he comes to the button, the louder the singing; as he moves farther away, the singing gets softer.

- When the button is found, the child sitting on it becomes "it" for the next time.

I See Something Red— A Game Using Colors

- Parent looks around and sees an object . . . a book, a pencil, an apple, a bicycle, a fire hydrant.

- She says, "I see something red."

- The child tries to guess what it is . . . Is it a chair? Is it Susie's ribbon? Is it an apple?

- The answer is no until someone guesses right.

- The child who guesses right gets to choose the next object.

- She says, "I see something green . . . or yellow . . . or blue . . ."

Opposites—A Word Game

- Parent thinks of a word
- The child tells its opposite
- Parent says, "in"
- Child says, "out"
- Parent says, "up,"
- Child says, "down."

Look Around for Other Words:

light	dark
brother	sister
hard	soft
hot	cold
stop	go

The Cooperative Sports and Games Book
Terry Orlick
Pantheon Books
1978   123 pp. $3.95

In this book of games to teach children cooperation and sharing, the games are designed to maximize cooperation and participation and allow everybody to win. The activities highlighted by the author eliminate fear of failure and reaffirm a child's confidence in herself.

The findings of studies such as these emphasize the need to develop individual games and whole sports programs in which all participants can be accepted and experience at least a moderate degree of success. If children think they have won, there is no need for them to feel threatened or anxious, and every reason to feel happy with themselves and satisfied with the experience.

The Dynamite Year-Round Catalog of Hot Stuff
Fran Claro
Scholastic Book Services
1978   94 pp. $3.95

A collection of games, activities, ideas and projects assembled from *Dynamite*, a popular children's magazine. Designed in a catalog format, the book offers page upon page of crafts, recipes, jokes and games for children to use all year round.

Ringo-Levio is a free-for-all. Everyone gets a chance to run like crazy. Divide up into two teams about the same size. Pick one area to be the jail. Team One's members run in every direction while Team Two tries to catch Team One and bring them all back to jail. Once you get tagged, you are caught and must return to jail, but a player that has not been captured can run into jail and yell "free-all" and everyone in jail can escape. Or, if a jailor from Team Two comes too near the jail, the prisoners can pull him or her in and everyone in jail goes free. That means Team Two has to try and catch Team One all over again. When everyone on Team One is captured and in jail, the game is over. Then Team Two gets a chance to give the other team a run for its money!

The Family Guide to Amusement Centers
Susan Hunter
Walker
1975   183 pp. $9.95/$5.95

This illustrated guide to family amusement centers in America covers such things as accommodations, availability of nurseries, admission rates, food facilities and even suggestions on when the weather is best to visit each one.

It describes oceanariums and wild animal habitats—not just zoos—where the natural environment is recreated and where fish or animal and visitor get the greatest benefit. *The Family Guide to Amusement Centers* mentions those places where guides demonstrate scenes and tasks from America's past, and where early towns, such as Sturbridge or Williamsburg, are reconstructed.

Free Stuff for Kids
Pat Blakely, Barbara Haislet and
Judith Hentges
Meadowbrook Press
1980   128 pp. $2.95

This is a comprehensive, delightful collection of items that kids from six to twelve can send away for free or up to $1.00. It contains over 250 items, including games, maps, stamps, comics, posters, toys, coins and crafts.

The book is designed and written for children's use with complete, illustrated instructions for writing letters and post cards, addressing envelopes and handling postage. It's a learning tool in disguise.

Kids' America
Steven Caney
Workman Publishing
1978   414 pp. $6.95

This book contains activities, projects, tales and legends about America's history, spirit and lifestyles, including tap dancing, magic, weather forecasting, panning for gold and hobo sign language.

The early houses were not designed by architects, not built by contractors! Everything—including planning, clearing the land, cutting the lumber, gathering the stones, and construction itself— was done by the owner-to-be with help from his neighbors. American climate and materials were often unlike those of the settlers' homeland, and tools were hard to come by. Settlers really had to start from scratch.

New Games Book
Andrew Fluegelman
Doubleday (Dolphin)
1976   193 pp. $4.95

This sourcebook for games draws from a variety of cultures to foster imagination, honesty and body-mind involvement. History of the New Games movement, player-referee's nonrulebook and list of nonessential equipment are included.

AURA: Here's a one-on-one contest that's highly cooperative. You can't get it alone, but you can get it together. Stand facing your partner at arms' length. Touch palms and close your eyes. Now feel the energy you are creating together. Keeping your eyes closed, drop your hands and both turn around in place three times. Without opening your eyes, try to relocate your energy bodies by touching palms again. This game always makes it as a spectator sport and it is wildly contagious besides. Try playing it with your neighbor at the bus stop.

The 1980 New Games Resource Catalog: A Playful Guide to Literature, Games Equipment and Materials
New Games Foundation
P.O. Box 7901
San Francisco, CA 94120
Subscription price is $5.00/year

As kids spontaneously change games around all the time, it is helpful for parents to know something about the millions of games already in existence, ideas written down about games and playing, and options in equipment. The reason for this catalog is that resources are sometimes hard to find. The New Games Foundation community put together this catalog, having used all the items and found them worthy. This community sells the items, as well as lists them and has an on-going effort to find and make available literature, play equipment, and materials related to the freer style of play they advocate.

In addition, they publish a New Games News/Letter which is a quarterly journal about play available through membership in Friends of New Games or by subscription.

Magic Wanda's Dynamite Magic Book
Chip Lovitt
Scholastic Book Services
1978   80 pp. $1.50

This collection of magic tricks from *Dynamite* magazine includes vanishing rope, card tricks and mind reading games.

Doing a trick can be easy. But making a magic performance work while the audience's eyes are glued to your every move is a different story. It takes many things to make a magic show work!

Official Dynamite Club Handbook
Linda Williams Aber
Scholastic Book Services
1978   96 pp. $3.95

This handbook is to give ideas for a kid's club from *Dynamite*, a children's magazine. Contains club rules, official song, handshake, games, activities such as Sneaker Decorating Day, Creepy-Crawly Crab Race and starting a club newspaper.

When you meet another Dynamite Club Member, don't just settle for an ordinary "hi." Greet each other with this official Hi Sign —a sign that says right away that you're no ordinary kid, you're an extraordinary Dynamite Kid!

1. Make a fist with your right hand.

2. Bring it up about as high as your chest.

3. Make your right pointer finger point up to the sky. (That stands for one.)

4. Keeping your finger in that position, make two complete clockwise circles in the air with your whole hand. (That stands for two zeroes.)

Put it all together and you've got 100, which stands for—you guessed it—100% Dynamite, which you are, of course.

One Potato, Two Potato . . . The Secret Education of American Children
Mary and Herbert Knapp
W. W. Norton
1976   270 pp. $9.95

Explaining that traditional games, riddles and jump-rope rhymes are the first opportunities for exploring and exploiting sex differences that children have, the authors show how traditional lore

is used by children to cope with the stresses of their lives.

. . . If the function of games is to "prepare children for life" in modern, competitive society, then it seems to us that folk games, which involve verbal competition and individual judgment, are a more useful map of the territory ahead than organized sports, which emphasize physical competition and submission to authority.

Pumpkin In A Pear Tree
Ann Cole, Carolyn Haas, Elizabeth Heller and Betty Weinberger
Little, Brown
1976   112 pp. $4.95

This parents' and teachers' activity book covers all the holidays from Halloween to Hanukkah. Creative ideas include a March on Washington game for Martin Luther King Day and an experiment with flour and yeast to show what matzo's all about.

Make a Valentine Train by stringing together boxes of various sizes and shapes. Shoeboxes and milk and oatmeal cartons work well. Cover them with construction paper, adding a cardboard tube smokestack, paper windows and doors, and buttons, spool or jar lid wheels. Label each "car" with someone's name for "incoming" valentines or use the train to sort your "outgoing" valentines according to their destination: For School, For Home, For the Neighborhood, For the Post Office.

What Can I Do Today?
Joan Fincher Klimo
Pantheon Books
1974   58 pp. $2.50

Containing easy-to-follow instructions for projects to keep children busy, this book utilizes sculpting, printing, pasting and stitching skills. A list of supplies

needed to make party decorations, masks and collages is included.

Make the things you like and save them to give as Christmas and birthday gifts to your family and special friends. Once you choose a project, stay with it until you are happy with the results. Be sure to try them all, and when you are done, go on and create your own projects. Most important, do not feel limited to do the things shown here. Your creations can be just as good as those in this book—perhaps even better!

G

GAYS AS PARENTS

With the new freedom gays are beginning to enjoy, and with the examination of gay legal rights that has accompanied this, battles for gay rights are taking place in spheres that would have been unheard of a few years ago. One of these is the rights of gay parents. There are two issues in this new rights battle: the right of divorced parents who are gay to full legal rights to their children including visitation and custody rights; and the right of gay couples to adopt children. Though both areas have seen numerous test cases in the last few years, there is still tremendous bias against gay parents in the courts, and most decisions have gone against the gay parent involved.

The majority of cases have involved Lesbian mothers. Since mothers usually retain child custody in divorce cases, an estranged father will often sue for custody on the basis of his former wife's homosexuality. However, there is also some activity involving the rights of fathers who are gay.

from *Gay Source*, by Dennis Sanders, Coward McCann & Geoghegan. 1978. $6.95.

G Underlying the deep legal and social prejudices against gay parents is the unfounded assumption that a homosexual of either sex is *de facto* an unfit parent. There are, however, no scientific studies of gay parents and their children, and, therefore, no shred of evidence one way or another. The gay parent is presumed guilty before the fact.

Even the liberal judiciary and the social workers who advise them will agree that homosexuals can be (and usually are) healthy and well adjusted, but still refuse to give custody or full visitation rights to gay parents on the grounds that the social embarrassment children suffer from having gay parents is enough to warrant keeping them from their parents. Again, there have been no systematic studies of the validity of this assumption.

In fact, there have been a few cases of adoptions by gay couples, though the parents and adoption agencies have been understandably discreet and publicity-shy about the placements. In most of the cases, the adoption has been of a minority or problem child who could otherwise not have been placed in a comfortable home, and the adoptions have been by one of the pair in the marriage, with the placement agency tacitly understanding the domestic situation.

The following organizations are involved in various ways in the legal and social battle for the rights of gay parents. Contact them for information.

National Gay Task Force
80 Fifth Avenue
New York, NY 10011
(212) 741-5815

Gay Fathers
305 East 40th St.
New York, NY 10016
(212) 682-4167

Lesbian Mothers National Defense Fund
P.O. Box 21567
Seattle, WA 98111
(206) 325-2643

Lesbian Defense Fund
Box 4
Essex Junction, VT 05452
(802) 862-9046

A Gay Parent's Legal Guide to Child Custody
Anti-Sexism Committee of the San Francisco Bay Area
National Lawyers Guild
558 Capp St.
San Francisco, CA 94110
1978   44 pp. $1.00

Motherhood, Lesbianism & Child Custody
Francie Wyland
Wages Due Lesbians
P.O. Box 38
Station E
Toronto, Canada
1977   36 pp. $1.70

In the Best Interests of the Children
Resource Booklet
Iris Films
Box 26463
Los Angeles, CA 90026
1977   21 pp. $1.50

GIFTED CHILDREN

Every child is in his or her own way gifted. There are gifted children who are intellectually bright. They require special attention from their parents, as do children who are slow or who are having other difficulty. Gifted children have many needs, and the more understanding the parents have of their needs, the better. Some suggestions follow, as well as some recommended publications.

Gifted Children Newsletter
1255 Portland Place
P.O. Box 2581
Boulder, CO 80322
12 issues for $24.00

This newsletter is geared for the parents of gifted children with articles from how to raise your gifted child to how to get your child's school to listen, plus advice, tips and book, toy and game reviews, calendar of events and a pullout section for your child.

If You Think Your Child Is Gifted
Phyllis M. Pickard
Linnet Books (Shoe String Press)
1976   160 pp. $9.50

This book explains how to detect signs of exceptional ability and where to turn for advice and help in ensuring that your child receives education suited to her gifts.

. . . Parents are themselves beginning to recognize such indications of ability as early eye focus, control of movement well in advance of average, signs of early reasoning (with or without speech) and the short sleep period. There is no one sign of intellectual gift or artistic talent; but a cluster of signs has meaning to the experts. Colleges of education are just beginning to include reference to exceptionally able children, though usually as one of the special areas of study, such as physical disability, mental subnormality, etc.

The World of the Gifted Child
Priscilla L. Vail
Penguin Books
1979   202 pp. $3.95

In this lively, authoritative book, Priscilla Vail, a teacher and the mother of a gifted child, provides encouraging answers for the parents and teachers of these widely misunderstood children.

Through moving case histories, the author describes the unique emotional and educational needs of the exceptionally gifted child. She discusses how to recognize the gifted child and examines the types of schooling best suited to the individual child's needs.

The first things we have to remember about gifted children is *that they are children. Like other children, they grow, lose their baby teeth, cry, laugh, and suffer the glories and pains of growing up. People are sometimes intimidated by their intelligence and think that just because they have giant vocabularies or understand quadratic equations they have the world by the tail. Not so.*

Organizations
(See Appendix A)

G

Council for Exceptional Children

National Association for Gifted Children

National Foundation for Gifted and Creative Children

SOME SUGGESTIONS FOR PARENTS OF GIFTED CHILDREN

- They are still children. They need love but controls; attention and discipline; parental involvement plus training in self-reliance and independence.

- Emphasis on early verbal expression, reading, discussing ideas in the presence of children, poetry and music are all valuable. Parents should read to children.

- Parents can see to it that the gifted child age six or above has a playmate who is also gifted, even if he has to be "imported" from some distance.

- Parents should show initiative in taking able children to museums, art galleries, educational institutions and other historical places where various collections may stimulate and enhance background learning.

- Parents should be especially careful not to "shut up" the gifted who asks questions. Sometimes questions should not be answered completely; but the reply should itself be a question which sends the child into some larger direction. When the parent cannot answer the questions, he should direct the child to a resource which can.

- Though the gifted child usually has a wide and versatile range of interests, he may be somewhat less able to concentrate on one area for a long time. Parents should encourage children who have hobbies to follow through on them.

- Parents should avoid direct, indirect or unspoken attitudes that fantasy, originality, unusual questions, imaginary playmates, or out-of-ordinary mental processes on the part of the child are bad, "different" or to be discouraged. Instead of laughing at the child, laugh with him and seek to develop his sense of humor.

- Parents should avoid overstructuring children's lives so that they don't have any free time. Sometimes parents are concerned that gifted children spend some time in watching TV or reading comic books. While they should not spend all their time in doing so, they cannot be expected to perform at top capacity at all times.

- Respect the child and his knowledge, which sometimes may be better than your own. Do not presume on your authority as a parent except in crises. Allow much liberty on unimportant issues. Try to give him general instructions to carry out in his way rather than specific commands to carry out in yours.

- Whenever possible talk things out with him where there has been a disciplinary lapse. He is much more amenable to rational argument than are many children and usually has a well developed sense of duty.

- Take time to be with him, to listen to what he has to say, to discuss ideas with him.

- Be a good example yourself, and try to find worthwhile adult model figures of both sexes outside his family for him to know.

- Support the school efforts to plan for able children. Support study groups on gifted children. Form with other parents into cooperative activities.

Marda Woodbury
Author, Librarian

GRANDPARENTS

Grandparents usually enjoy playing with and spending time with their grandchildren. They have a great deal to teach them and children eagerly look forward to the time they have with their grandparents. The opportunities for older people and young children to be together are very important.

Although many grandparents like to take care of their grandchildren and babysit at specified times, it is important you not expect this as your right. Grandparents also need free time and have their own personal and social time needs, which should be respected.

See also the article "Old Folks and Little People Go Together" by Janet Gonzalez-Mena in the Growth and Development section.

The following are books to maximize the joy and minimize the problems of being a grandparent.

Book for Grandmothers
Ruth Goode
Macmillan
1976   199 pp. $7.95

With tips on how to grandmother in a lighthearted, lighthanded manner, this book answers questions on such problems as: What to give for birthdays, what to say when you haven't seen your children in a year, when to give advice, what rights you have as a grandparent in a divorce.

It is possible to keep the grandchildren even with a daughter-in-law who moves away and marries again. When the children's father still cares about them and maintains his visitation rights, we have not lost the children. And not all daughters-in-law turn away from a divorced husband's family. Some daughters-in-law feel closer to their mothers-in-law than to their own mothers, with whom they may never have learned to resolve old conflicts and become friends. Some divorced daughters-in-law continue to be regular visitors—with the children—to their ex-parents-in-law. But this can happen only when a direct friendship has grown between them, one that is more than simply in-law courtesy during the life of the marriage.

A Grandparent's Garden of Verses
Evelyn Barkins
Frederick Fell
1973   46 pp. $1.95

This collection of poems for grandparents to read to children contains rhymes and verses about the major incidents of life: "Play," "Learning to Read," "Afraid of the Dark," "On Being Sick," and the like.

*I watch you take to bed with you
A favored doll, a stuffed bear, too.
And in the battered, cherished toy
Know all of comfort and of joy.*

*Alas for me, that I am grown
And so must go to bed alone.*

GROWTH AND DEVELOPMENT

See also Emotional Development: Health and Hospitals.

Some Basic Principles

Changes do not occur at any one specific time but usually over a period of time. Each child's individual growth pattern is unique. The behavior of children goes from one extreme to the other before it is coordinated by the child himself. Growth is not straight but a forward-and-backward progression. Development in one area can affect the development in another area.

Growth is an important milestone-marking way of describing changes in children. We look at growth both in terms of physical changes and in emotional development in social areas, where children play first by themselves and gradually with other children. It is important to recognize that children grow at different rates, and for each of the different spectrums, the rate of change will vary. Be aware that your child will go through enormously difficult changes at times and should be supported in a calm, relaxed manner.

Growth and Development: Stages from Two to Twelve

Children grow at different rates although general characteristics express their specific ages. The information on growth trends given are to assist with an understanding of the average development of children. You should try not to make comparisons between children, but rather understand each child's individual rate of growth, physically, emotionally, socially, and intellectually. The information gives you a guide and helps in knowing more specifically where your child is on his or her own path.

For more information consult your pediatrician, child psychologist or child development specialist or review some of the suggested professional books given in Appendix F.

THE BUNNY WHO WANTED TO GROW UP

Once there was a little bunny who wanted to grow up to be a big rabbit. It tried as hard as it could, doing things like hopping, running, leaping, and playing. But no matter how hard it tried, it still remained a little bunny.

One day, feeling that it would never grow up, the little bunny had an idea. It would ask a big rabbit to tell it *how* to grow up!

The little bunny had to wait a long time before it got up the nerve to ask, but when it did, the big rabbit smiled.

"Little bunny," it said. "You might not know it, but you're growing bigger every day. Before long, you'll be a big rabbit too, without even trying."

The little bunny, happy to hear the words of the big rabbit, spent the rest of its days hopping, running, leaping, and playing, and sure enough, grew up without even trying!

Maytraya Stillwater
Windows of Nature
Troubadour Press
1978 80 pp. $3.95

---

2 Years

Sturdy on feet and bends at waist to pick up objects

Up and down stairs without alternating feet

Can kick a ball

Takes things apart and fits together again

Can rotate forearm, so turns doorknobs

Pinches, pushes, kicks, bites

Intrigued by water

Can copy a circle (imitate)

Can build a tower of 6 to 7 blocks

Usually dry at night

Negativistic—exercising powers

Fear of bedwetting, animals, being deserted—response is helplessness

Temper tantrums—exercising control

Fussy eater

Ritualistic and self-centered

Shows pity, sympathy, modesty, and shame and can evidence guilt

Can show great affection

Difficulty making choices

Possessions and physical ability more limited than ideas—main source of anger response

Vocabulary increases—300 words

Cannot share—"It's mine" (possessive)

Begins sentences—3-word phrases

Solitary to parallel play (when 2 children play alongside each other)

Shy with strangers

Vacillates between dependence and independence

Great imitation

Enjoys books, music, blocks

More responsive to humor or distraction than discipline

Puts two to three words together in sing-song sentences; knows his own name and can say it; questions "What's this?" "What's that?"; knows names of things, persons, actions and situations; uses some adverbs, adjectives and prepositions; asks for what he wants at the table using name of article; carries on "conversation"

with self and doll; tells needs but does not carry on real conversation with an adult.

Likes things to touch and look at in books and stories; can identify many pictures by name; enjoys repetition, talking animals, nonsense rhymes, but usually prefers the factual.

Likes humor games, such as peek-a-boo and chasing.

Sees and reaches out at same time; locates pictures in picture book; manipulates one hand, then alternates to the other hand; and fits nested blocks together; can take off shoes, stockings, pants; dawdles because he is not well coordinated. Can run, pull, push, drag, squat, clap in rhythm; can kick a ball and catch with arms.

Responds to suggestions better than commands; can accept imaginary pleasures in place of those denied him; likes independence but is not skillful enough to support it.

Spends a good bit of time absorbed in gazing; concentrates interest in small areas; interest is in present—

G

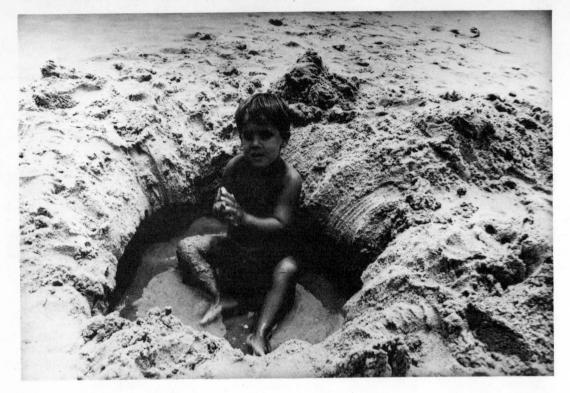

future is dim: attention span is two to three minutes, yet he may find it hard to shift to another activity.

Usually plays alone or watches; progresses to parallel play or playing with other children; needs to be near adult in play group situations, can't cooperate; engages in tug of war over materials; asks adult when he wants something from another child; is unable to share; collects and hangs on to toys.

Enjoys dramatic play because imagination can be vivid; is not easy for him to see difference between what he plays and reality.

Is warmly responsive, loving and affectionate and is dependent on mother or other adult; is lacking in self-confidence; responds to adults, holds hands while walking, helps around house; is shy with strangers; is possessive, aggressive, sensitive.

2¹/₂ Years

Jumps on both feet

Tiptoes

Tower of 8 blocks and simple bridges

Holds pencil more correctly and imitates vertical and horizontal strokes

Bowel and bladder control accomplished

Goes to extremes in all things

Capacity for voluntary choice weak, so tries both due to realization life has alternatives

Cannot be forced

Does not share willingly

Unpredictable

Dawdles when he can't make a choice

Vocabulary—1000 words

Dramatic and parallel play

3 Years

(Begins preschool years 3 to 5)

Nimble on feet—climbs, runs, turns well, swings arms more like adult

Can count to 5 and maybe 10 but can't understand

Knows night from day

Rides a tricycle

Dresses and undresses if helped with buttons and can brush teeth

Draws a man on request

Feeds self well

Full set of temporary teeth

Knows some nursery rhymes

Begins to show some self-control and can make simple choices

Tries to please and conform

Temper tantrums at peak

Imaginary worries—fears dark, dogs and death

Curiosity level rises rapidly

Frustrated with obstacles

Restless sleep

Enjoys praise

Responsive to verbal guidance

Playmates main source of anger response

Parallel play with small rudiments of cooperation

Begins to "wait his turn"

Likes to run errands

Speaks in sentences and uses pronouns

Sings

Distinguishes between girls and boys

Interest in own body

Loves to be with other children

Ritualism decreases

Highly imaginative

Begins to use words as tools and to comply with cultural demands

Loves to talk; uses plurals, past tense, personal pronouns, prepositions. Knows last name, sex, street on which he lives, simple rhymes. He is curious—asks "What?" "Where?" "When?" He understands simple explanations; asks frequent questions to which he already knows the answers; likes to learn new words; likes to compare two objects.

Is responsive to rhythm, has enough control to reproduce sound patterns; can recognize familiar melodies and sing simple songs, not always on pitch.

Is vague about time and space; is unlikely to stay with any activity more than a few minutes and has average attention span of ten minutes.

Has eye for form—knows circles, triangles and squares; can throw a ball without losing balance; can jump with both feet, use slide, climb, turn sharp corners, dig, ride trike easily; can gallop, jump and run to music.

Dresses partially—depending upon mood; puts on shoes and undresses almost entirely; holds cup by handle, tips head back to get last drop.

Has good eye muscles; can copy circle and cross; may "read" from pictures in book.

Can make choice and abide by it; asks help if he needs it; may not be able to do two things at once, as talk and eat; can suggest his liking for a meal; can run errands.

Likes paint, crayons and clay. Uses varied and rhythmical strokes in painting and drawing; likes to have his picture or art work saved.

May still play by himself quite happily, but is more likely to be playing beside other children (parallel play), and will later move into more cooperative play; is beginning to share; can adjust to taking turns; enjoys playmates; may help a shy child, if this is suggested; has no sex preference in play; begins to combine planes, trains and cars with his block play; shows order and balance in block building.

Your Child From Three to Four
Children's Bureau
446-1967
Reprinted 1968   24 pp.   25¢
Dept. of Health and Human Services

Brief and simplistic, this publication brings to light major points as to safety, medical care, and general upbringing.

Designed for quick and easy reading, it covers many important points parents need to consider for their child in his preschool years.

4 Years

Skips and does stunts

Climbs well

Can cut on a line, throw overhand, lace shoes, etc.

Holds brush in adult manner and paints in flourishes with running commentary

May know primary colors

Can usually count fingers

Uncontrolled aggression

Love of opposite sexed parent

Language added to tantrums—name calling

Acts out if he does not get his way

Defies parents, but often quotes them as authority

Boastful—dogmatic—bossy

Perceives analogies

Begins to conceptualize and generalize

Not as sensitive to praise of others

Moralistic judgments begin

Feels independence and often asserts

Some difficulty in separating fact from fancy

Concern for ghosts, goblins, etc.

Deductive thinking begins

Endless questions "why"—"how"

Great fabrication

Cooperative play with rapid change in friends

Swearing and silly words, i.e., "Batty-watty"

Concern for origin of babies and death

Loves an audience and talks to self if none available

Runs topics into the ground

Imagination vivid, rapid, varied

Rationalization

Total confidence in his own ability to do anything

Imaginary friend

Emotions at surface. Sometimes defies adults by hitting, throwing, running away, biting, etc., to test his own power.

Non-conforming, resists routines. Begins cooperative play but is more content in small group. Imaginative, enjoys dramatic play.

Uses sentences; has power of generalization and abstraction; exaggerates to practice words; tries out silly words and sounds; experiments with adjectives; speaks of imaginary conditions; can tell a lengthy story mixing fact and fancy; calls names and brags; asks many questions—not always interested in answers but in how answer fits into his thoughts; knows colors and can name them; has attention span of twelve to fifteen minutes.

G

G Can stand on one foot, skip on one foot, and then hop on the other; is very active—shovels, sweeps, rakes, climbs, slides every which way, races up and down stairs, throws ball overhand. Senses differences in gaps in skill and powers of adults and himself; wants reassurance that he is capable of being a strong skillful, capable person.

Can carry liquids without spilling; manages own clothes if they are simple; buttons and unbuttons; dresses and undresses dolls; works with precision in painting, but shifts ideas; begins to copy; tries to cut on line with scissors.

Watches to learn; reasons; shows dramatic ability; can talk and eat or talk and dress; is beginning to use talking instead of hitting in play.

Needs guidance and lots of materials; is physically aggressive—hits, kicks, throws and bites; is verbally aggressive, is rough and careless with toys; laughs wildly in play; indulges in name calling and bragging "I'll sock you"—with such silliness leading to tears and squabbling.

Shows little politeness at times; shows off and acts very badly before company; likes to play mother or teacher to smaller child; shows pride in mother though he may resist her authority; boasts about daddy.

Is able to accept turns and may share graciously; is able to accept rules and responds well to objective commands such as "It is time to . . ."

Has a great interest in music—in listening, dancing, or performing to it; has increased control of voice which allows him to sing on pitch; can recognize melodies.

Is beginning to be interested in other children and their activities; capable of group planning and play; can amuse himself alone; play reaches new heights of inventiveness and grows rich in detail; likes to act out his ideas; builds elaborate structures and names them; dolls are important, sharing experiences and having personalities; likes to arrange hazardous devices and does not like to be reminded of his limitations.

Can anticipate a tour or trip and help with preparations; talks about it afterward and reproduces his experiences; likes collecting—leaves, pictures, postcards.

Loves story time and enjoys turning pages; enjoys exaggeration, bubbling humor; interest in new experiences, in how and why; loves to talk about things of which the story reminds him.

Development of a 5-Year-Old

5-year-olds are at an exciting age. They are wondering about themselves and other people. They have played at home with toys, utensils, furniture and all kinds of other items and have had some contacts outside and away from home on trips. They have looked at books, listened to stories and watched a great deal of television. They are learning a lot of language and able to communicate and explain their feelings and ideas. They have self-confidence to develop relationships with others. They are sensitive to ideas—what is said and conversations. Each thinks about his own feelings and the way he is thinking. Likes to play house with fantasy. Is responsive to new ideas and has a lot of imagination. Has a relatively short attention span and enjoys building with blocks, playing with toys, doing drawing, music, numbers. Enjoys going from one experience to another.

5 Years

Agile

Draws a man

Poised and controlled motor ability

Self-help

Can tie shoe laces

Spontaneous drawing with definite ideas in mind—can copy a triangle

Knows full name and address

Knows primary colors

Knows morning from afternoon

Girls about one year ahead of boys in growth

Handedness well established (between 2 and 5)

Refines total gains

Much self-criticism

Where 4 rambles, 5 can stop—increase in self-control

He does not get lost; calm and self-confident

Likes to finish what he begins and brings projects home with pride

Temper tantrums end and courtesy high

Can separate truth from fancy

Thoughts are concrete

Strong sense of personal identity

Well adjusted and happy age

Individuality and lasting traits appear

Purposeful, constructive

Refines emotions

Vocabulary 2000 words well-utilized

Conforms—"angelic age"

Well organized

Self-contained and responsible

Obedient

Dramatizes life in play with detail

Likes group play

Likes experience outside the home

Wants to go to school

Socialized pride in appearance and accomplishments

Can share

Can now show anger to peer by exclusion rather than physical attack or name calling

Generosity increases

Emotions more stable. More able to verbalize than display physical emotion. Less fear. Self-critical.

Uses well defined sentences; likes to count and can count ten objects; answers questions; asks for information, not merely to talk; can carry a plot in a story and repeat a long sequence accurately: is interested in *why*; enjoys repetitive sounds; favorite questions—"How does it work?" "Why is it like that?" "What is it for?"

Fills dramatic play with dialogue and commentary having to do with everyday life; likes realistic props.

Draws crude but realistic reproduction of a scene; interprets meaning of a picture; can identify missing part of a picture; begins to paint with idea in mind.

Likes a limited time—has a sense of order; likes models for guides; likes definite task; is very good at problem solving; is not apt to attempt something unless he can finish it; likes something to show for his efforts.

Thinks before he speaks; thinks concretely; keynotes practicality and conformity; finds real world enough novelty for him because he has learned what is fantasy and what is not, and that now is a perfect time to absorb facts of everyday life; finds play is practice for life rather than invention; likes instruction to improve.

May be good or a pest with company; needs preparation for happenings as aid to good manners; sometimes asks permission—may ask ten times for the same thing.

Plays in social group without much conflict—most cooperatively with three children; feels protective toward younger ones; plans surprises and jokes; is better in outdoor play than indoor; shows flashes of resistance which are usually quickly overcome; uses verbal aggression; prefers playmates his own age; may cry if angry or tired.

Can march to music; ride on scooter; tries to jump rope and use stilts; wants to discard trike for bike.

Is observant, self-critical, self-dependent, proud of work, clothes, etc.; is factual, literal and has a remarkable memory.

Is impersonal—takes people for granted; mother is center of universe, although he has good relationships with daddy and enjoys grandparents' visits.

Can tie a bow, but not snugly, although he may not want to do it.

6 Years

Active and boisterous

Physical growth slows down

Large muscles better developed than small

Eyes not yet mature—tendency toward far-sightedness (not quite ready to read)

Permanent teeth begin to appear

Heart is in period of rapid growth

Copies a diamond

Names days of week

Knows right from left

Counts out any number up to 10 from a grouping of objects

Ambivalence

Has ideas of good and bad

Fears remote danger, ridicule, ghosts

Tense, upset, unpredictable

Shows off—less cooperative than 5

Keen for competition

Often less mature at home than with outsiders

Regresses when tired

Short interest span

Difficulty making decisions

Boys' and girls' interests begin to differ

Needs praise, warmth, patience Strongly embarrassed by lack of physical privacy

Has a great fear of supernatural and that parents will die

Indecisive

Group play (chaotic)

Independent

More interest in peer group than family

Learning competition and cooperation

Beginning social personality

Vocabulary 2,000 words in first grade

7 Years

Displays sudden spurts of active behavior in some task. Shoves desk, opens and closes desk top, gets up from chair or becomes rather talkative.

Likes to alternate outdoor play between extremely active and sedate.

Interested in developing various motor skills. Will concentrate on one activity at a time, then lose interest.

G

Some boys may favor activities involving bats and balls. Girls may prefer jump rope and hop-scotch games.

Enjoys climbing but has a new awareness of height that makes him cautious.

Finds pleasure in manipulating objects, creating with hands and building complicated structures.

Enjoys using pencils. Tends to grasp pencils so tightly he frequently drops them.

Is undergoing further visual development. Has difficulty in copying work from blackboard.

Is more serious and thoughtful about life. Shows increased awareness of relationships with people around him.

Is concerned that school may be too difficult.

Lacks confidence. Will approach new tasks or social situations with caution. Is concerned about how others perceive him. Is anxious for approval and acceptance by peers and adults.

Is easily confused about responsibilities but eager to accomplish them.

Can play fairly well with four or five friends.

Prefers realism to imaginative play.

Is not well organized in group activity.

May still prefer solitary play.

Begins to discriminate against opposite sex.

In Arithmetic:

- male prefers oral to written activities.
- female prefers concrete to written or oral activity.
- frequently reverses 2, 6, 7 and 9.
- delights in writing long numbers.

- is easily confused if addition and subtraction problems appear on same page.

In Writing:

- strives for perfection.
- uses the eraser a great deal.
- begins to recognize that he is reversing some letters.
- may still need widely spaced paper.
- worries if written work is not done.
- begins to control size and uniformity of letters.
- may find writing easier than printing.

In Reading:

- reads mechanically.
- omits or adds familiar or simple words.
- omits or adds a final *s* or *y*.
- can interpret story without knowing all of the words.
- substitutes vowels.
- hesitates or guesses at new words.
- needs to know how far to read.
- is interested in number of pages in a book.
- shows individual differences in reading speed.
- is beginning to be critical of reading materials.
- enjoys fairy tales.
- if male, appears especially interested in materials dealing with the army, navy, airplanes, electricity, earth and nature.
- if female, appears to enjoy books such as *Heidi*.

In Spelling:

- frequently lags behind reading skill.
- enjoys copying words.
- is interested in and beginning to grasp the sounds of letters.

8 Years

Has improved rhythm and grace in body movement.

Shows increase in speed and smoothness of eye-hand performance. May develop near-sightedness.

May display a gap between what he wants to do with his hands and what he can do.

Is improving in handwriting and printing. Likes to do neat work but frequently is in too great a hurry.

May react to disagreeable tasks or difficult school subjects with headaches, stomach aches or need to urinate.

Is accident prone (generally in connection with falls, automobiles and bicycles).

Has growing interest in games requiring small muscle coordination.

Enjoys group activities. Displays feelings of belonging.

Is generally more cooperative but still requires supervision in group play to prevent dissension.

Is interested in competitive games.

Is becoming selective in choice of friends. Is seeking a "best friend" of same sex.

Is quick to criticize.

Enjoys school. Is eager to attack new tasks.

Likes to talk.

Will interrupt work to socialize with peers. Generally returns to and completes assignment.

G

Is impatient for directions to be given but tends to forget them.

Is more exuberant in behavior. Is eager to tackle hard tasks. Will shift from one interest to another. Spends much energy anticipating events.

Tends to be argumentative and dramatic.

Can become emotional when fatigued, disappointed, when feelings are hurt, criticized and when he makes a mistake. Cries over dramatic stories or events.

In Reading:

- tackles new words by context or phonics.
- tends to omit unimportant words.
- reverses word in a phrase.
- can stop and talk about the story without losing thread.
- begins to prefer silent reading.
- likes stories with excitement and humor.

In Writing:

- shows individual differences in size and style of writing.
- begins to space words and sentences.
- has more ideas for a story than he can write.

In Arithmetic:

- prefers oral to written.
- is partial to new table he is learning.
- likes to shift from one process to another.

9 Years

Works and plays hard. Is apt to overdo.

Displays increased skill and interest in motor performance and competitive sports.

Eyes and hands are well differentiated. Gets tensional release through fine motor coordination.

Is eager to have a good relationship with those around him. Acts in the spirit of service.

Has special friends selected from his own sex. Enjoys verbalizing with peers.

Shows more organization in play than earlier. Organizes informal clubs which have a real purpose for short periods of time. Generally likes codes, secret language, bulletins. Wants to be part of organizations such as Brownies and Cub Scouts.

Displays fewer fears. Tends to be apprehensive about own activities. Worries about mistakes, failing, meeting standards. Will apply himself even if subject is too difficult.

Capable of planning daily activities. Will persist in completing what he has planned.

Is easily absorbed in what he is doing.

Is in initial stages of hero worship.

Is beginning to develop real feelings of empathy. Tends to be impressed with whatever he is told.

Enjoys school. Interested in achieving. Is easily discouraged by failure.

Displays independence, self-discipline, an ability to evaluate himself and his skills.

Individual differences are apparent in change from third to fourth grade. The child who earlier had difficulties in learning may now show a spurt in improvement. The pupil who had previously done well may now require special assistance in some areas.

Displays difficulties in immediate recall.

In Reading:

- prefers silent reading.
- likes to read for fact and information.

In Arithmetic:

- knows many combinations; still learning others.
- interested in discovering how he made his errors.
- displays a spontaneous interest in problem solving.

10–12 Years

A time for dramatic rate of growth. Is inclined to be clumsy if in a growth spurt; unaware of the space he now needs to operate in as reaching and stepping distance are different.

Very aware of body changes and the onset of puberty. Tends to undress in isolation as he is self-conscious about his changing body.

A time of great peer pressure for group conformity.

May display need to be independent and "growing up"; however, he may need more support than ever in his changing social world.

A time when he begins noticing girls. Puppy love and sexual exploration may take place; boys may experience wet dreams.

A time of extremes in behavior related to health habits; he will either want to bathe incessantly or never!

G This is a period in their lives in which sports may play a great role; street sports and organized sports seem to attract this age child.

Children of this age group like to live in Levis and sneakers, the shabbier the better!

Food likes as with other ages depend upon exposure to a variety of foods, experience with home and regular diet, and peer pressure.

The child is usually in preparation for graduation to Junior High School by the time he is passing through this age group. He is proud of his accumulated academic achievement yet is apprehensive about the upcoming new experience of Junior High and the potential peer pressures.

This is a time to be an active listener for the 10–12-year-old. They seek a non-judgmental listener. The parent able to meet this need will find a rich relationship awaiting him/her throughout their child's adolescence.

OLD FOLKS AND LITTLE PEOPLE GO TOGETHER

There is much talk of gaps between age groups. Infants and old people, who have so much to offer each other, seldom are together. Some mourn for the good old days when grandparents bounced babies on their knees and few people of any age spent their days (and/or nights) in institutions. More and more people at both ends of the age scale spend time in an institutional setting such as day-care centers. This fact tends to isolate both age groups from the society and from each other.

Old people and very young people can benefit from being together. An obvious benefit is the enjoyment they get from each other. Some early childhood educators have recognized this benefit and have brought senior citizens into their day-care centers and nursery schools to provide grandparent figures for the little people. It isn't too hard to find a center for young children with a rocking chair and a grandmotherly person seated rocking a youngster.

However, I see far beyond that picture. I see child development people and gerontology people getting together, working together. I see a pooling of knowledge about meeting the needs of helpless or semihelpless individuals of all ages in respectful and growth enhancing ways.

The rationale behind what I'm proposing here comes from the concept of the life cycle. We give lip service to this concept, write poems about it, sing songs about it, yet we tend to look at development as a straight line. We talk about a progression of stages, a series of transitions starting at the beginning (which can be either birth or conception depending on your point of view) and moving along to the end (death). A child's potential is as important as his or her present. Looking back from the other direction I've come to realize that the elderly person carries within him or her the child he or she was just as surely as he or she lives in the present condition. Past, present and future are together in every moment of every human life. We have a choice. We can acknowledge the cyclical nature of life and we can operate from that point of view. Or we can continue to see only the linear perspective and watch the end coming closer.

I feel there is a message in the work being done with split brain research and its implications for education. Science is throwing light on what people have been talking about for thousands of years—two ways of knowing. The logical, rational, verbal way of knowing is one. Infants and the very elderly may not show much evidence of using this mode of thinking. The other way of knowing involves intuitive, holistic, creative, nonlogical knowing thinking. I propose that the very old and the very young may engage in this second kind of thinking more than we realize. (But they may not be able to communicate it to us, or show signs of it in productivity.)

Janet Gonzalez-Mena
Director, Child Care Program

The First Five Years
Virginia E. Pomeranz
and Dodi Schultz
Doubleday
1973   312 pp. $6.95

This humorous, relaxed approach to child care deals with the practicalities of feeding, toilet training, hygiene, toys, medical care, sex education.

Flexibility, patience and resourcefulness are the overall parental qualities needed for getting necessary oral medication into a child. Each child, and each situation, is different. Some needed liquids are not pleasantly flavored and have a taste everyone agrees is disgusting. Others may be available in a choice of cherry, orange, and lime flavors—which takes care of most people's preferences, but your four-year-old may absolutely detest any and all fruit flavors.

The First Three Years of Life
Burton L. White
Avon
1978   275 pp. $4.95

White covers all areas of child development, dividing the first thirty-six months of a child's life into seven stages of growth, with a list of dos and don'ts for each stage. Topics include general behavior, motor skills, educational development and recommendations for toys and equipment for each stage of development.

Whenever you get a chance to do so, point out to the child what the world looks like to someone else. A good person to use in pointing out to a child what the world looks like from another viewpoint is yourself. It is relatively easy for most people to explain to children, even as young as two or two and one-half years of age, how they feel about something, particularly when there are concrete clues present to facilitate such an explanation. If you are talking about a pair of shoes that you are having trouble squeezing your feet into, you

can use that situation as an example by pointing out that although the shoes seem too small for you and hurt your feet, they would not hurt the child's feet because they are obviously not too small for him.

Growing With Children
Joseph and Laurie Braga
Prentice-Hall
1974   205 pp. $6.95

Drawing on works of noted authorities in child development, this book stresses parental influence on a child's behavior and development of positive self-concepts that will enable her to be successful in future interactions.

Children who have had generally positive experiences in their early years, who have been consistently made to feel that they are persons of value, will come to feel that way about themselves. They will assume that people like them and approve of them instead of worrying whether they do and trying to win their approval. Such a child will be able to be concerned about other people for who they are and for what they might need, not for what they can do to fulfill her needs or what they might possibly think of her.

Your Child From Three to Four
Children's Bureau
446-1967
U.S. Government Printing Office
1968   24 pp.   25¢

This pamphlet brings to light major points concerning safety, medical care and general upbringing.

Designed for quick and easy reading, it covers many important points parents need to consider in the preschool years.

After your child's third birthday, he begins to do many more things for himself. He has more imagination. He plays well by himself. More often, though, he likes to be with boys and girls of his own age. He doesn't say "no" so

often. He says "yes" a great many times. He has learned a new word —"why?" Answer him simply and honestly. He learns then. If you don't answer him, then you won't help him learn.

Your Child From One To Six
Children's Bureau
30-1962
U.S. Government Printing Office
1973   97 pp. $.75

This pamphlet helps parents understand child development and gain confidence in their own ability to cope with problems. Provides an essential section on medical care, including directions on how to care for a sick child, childhood diseases and what to do for emergencies such as broken bones, bites, burns, poisons and the like.

The infant who snuggles willingly into bed may become a toddler who puts up a fuss. Going to bed interrupts everything he values —play and the nearness of people. He lives in the present moment and feels that he is being deprived forever. Tomorrow seems not to exist. Tired after a busy day, even groggy with fatigue, he battles to stay awake to keep his parents near and "the show on the road." Some toddlers fight against bed because they aren't sleepy. A toddler may have somewhat lower sleep requirements than the baby and is ready to omit one of his daytime naps. Just which one will vary from child to child, and may be unsettled from day to day.

G

G

Your Child from Six to Twelve
Children's Bureau
324-1966
U.S. Government Printing Office
1966   98 pp.   25¢

This pamphlet offers guidelines for dealing with and aiding a child going through the various and confusing changes of physical, sexual and emotional development. It covers such topics as social development, childhood diseases and community services.

Even though you do your best to promote good feeling in your family, one or more of your children might accuse you of playing favorites.

It might be worth your while to think this over. Maybe, without realizing it, you do show more favor to one child than to another. You might have especially high standards for one because he is so much like you. Perhaps you understand him best, but perhaps you get particularly cross with him when he shows traits that you have —and wish you didn't—like a hot temper, for instance, or a tendency toward shyness or carelessness. It may well be that you are more severe with this child than you really ought to be.

See Appendix C for Films and Audio-Visual Aids

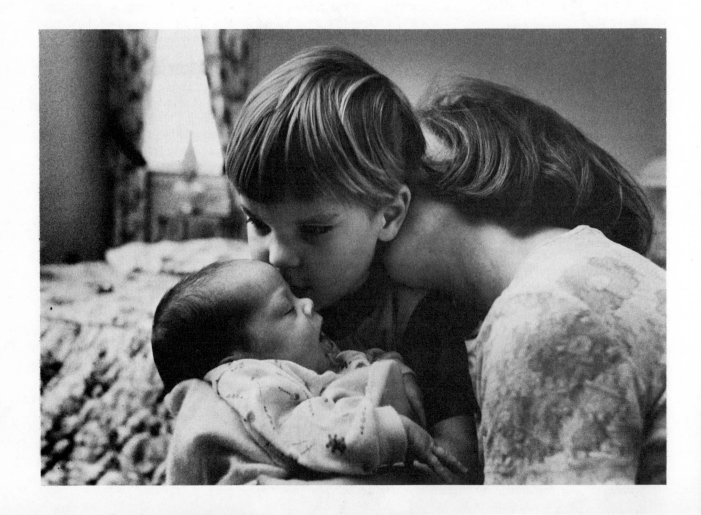

HANDICAPS. SEE DISABILITIES.

HEALTH AND HOSPITALS

See also Death; Dental Care; Disabilities; Eyesight; Mental Health.

A child's health is determined by environment, exposure, health habits and basic attitudes. A healthy, positive attitude is a great boon to good health. But when your child becomes ill, she requires understanding and support. These resources will aid you as you help your child grow to be a strong and healthy adult.

Visits to the Pediatrician

Call a doctor immediately when there is breathing difficulty, bleeding, severe pain or the child seems to be unconscious or in convulsions. Also watch for bumps or bruises that do not heal rapidly, frequent urination, dramatic changes in energy or moods and aches or complaints that remain or recur. Discuss these with the pediatrician over the phone before making an appointment. Remember to keep accurate records of the treatments, vaccinations and medications your child receives in case you should be away from home when she becomes ill or if your child's school should request medical information.

When your child enters preschool, be prepared for a period of what seems like endless colds and minor illnesses. Have faith, as this too will pass, usually during the first year of school. Some parents claim that breast-feeding may arm the child with antibodies which make this period pass more easily. If you find yourself minding a sick child for a long period of time, invest in a baby-sitter for an afternoon or arrange a mutual exchange of time with another parent. Your mental health is very important to your well-being as well as your child's.

Preparation for a Hospital Stay

If your child has to go into the hospital, prepare him in advance. Explain what is going to happen, tell him you will be there and reassure him that he will be coming home again. If he is going to have a surgical procedure, make sure he understands that he will be anesthetized, that he will be unaware of actual surgery and will be unable to feel any pain and that when he comes out from under the anesthetic, the operation will be over. Plan to be with your child as much as possible. Now that many hospitals allow parents to room with children, you may be able to spend the night. Bring books, toys and other items that will be fun and familiar for your child.

Find ways to alleviate your child's anxiety. A trip to the hospital to meet the nurses and doctors and see the equipment can make the real visit much less terrifying. Give him a toy doctor's kit. On the other hand, it is important not to overprepare most kids. Too much solicitousness may make the child more anxious because of the intensity of your concern. Above all, don't lie about procedures or pain. If you lie once, the child will not trust you the next time you attempt to reassure him.

WHAT PARENTS NEED TO KNOW ABOUT GOOD HEALTH PRACTICES

In these days of high medical costs and a shortage of doctors, more responsibility for judging the need for expert care and for carrying out medical instructions may well be required of parents. The mystique that traditionally surrounded medical knowledge is gradually disappearing. Parents are asking to be told what symptoms mean, what the treatment or medicines are expected to accomplish, and what side effects or complications they may expect. Sometimes parents have felt left out of the decisions that were being made about their child's care and treatment because of their own lack of knowledge about medical techniques. At other times, parents become so dependent upon the doctor's opinion and advice that they are unable to exercise any initiative of their own. Times are changing; parents are becoming much more sophisticated about diseases and medical techniques. Many parents want and should be able to use their own common sense in handling minor illnesses, and can do so with a few guides.

Richard Feinbloom
Child Health Encyclopedia
Dell Publishing
1975   568 pp. $7.95

Use this guide to keep track of your children's immunizations. Be sure to note any adverse reactions your child may have to these. Note—Your physician's schedule may be slightly different.

Immunization Record

FIRST YEAR	Recommended age	Date given to your child
DPT*	1½ to 2 months	
	3 months	
	5 months	
Polio vaccine	5–8 months	
Smallpox vaccine	Before 12 months	
Measles vaccine	12 months	

SECOND YEAR

Give any injections not started or completed in first year.

Additional injection of DPT.	12–18 months	

Polio vaccine may be recommended by your doctor.

BEFORE GOING TO SCHOOL

DPT and polio vaccine	4 years	
Smallpox vaccine	5–6 years	

THEREAFTER

Booster doses of DT (whooping cough no longer needed) and polio vaccine.	At intervals recommended by your doctor.	

Smallpox vaccine every 5 years, before the child leaves the United States or if there is an epidemic.

*DPT stands for diphtheria, pertussis (whooping cough), and tetanus.

Communicable Diseases

Disease	First signs	Incubation	Prevention	How long contagious	What you can do
Chickenpox	Mild fever followed in 36 hours by small raised pimples which become filled with clear fluid. Scabs form later. Successive crops of pox appear.	2–3 weeks. Usually 14–16 days.	None. Immune after 1 attack.	6 days after appearance of rash.	Usually not serious. Trim fingernails to prevent scratching. Dilute alcohol or a solution of baking soda and water may ease itching.
German Measles (3-day measles)	Mild fever, sore throat or cold symptoms may precede fine rose-colored rash. Enlarged glands at back of neck and behind ears.	2–3½ weeks. Usually 18 days.	None. Immune after 1 attack.	Until rash fades. About 5 days.	Not a serious disease, complications rare; give general good care and keep baby quiet. Avoid exposing any woman who is, or might be, in the early months of pregnancy unless she is sure she has had the disease.
Measles	Mounting fever; dry cough; running nose and red eyes for 3 or 4 days before rash which starts at hair line and spreads down in blotches. Small red spots with white centers in mouth (Koplik's spots) may occasionally be seen before the rash.	1–2 weeks. Usually 10 or 11 days.	Vaccine can be given to provide immunity. A baby not vaccinated if exposed can be given gamma globulin to lighten or prevent measles.	Until 5 days after the rash has appeared.	May be mild or severe with complications of a serious nature; follow doctor's advice in caring for a baby with measles, as it is a most treacherous disease. If other children who have not had the disease are exposed, ask the doctor about protective inoculations for them.

H

Disease	First signs	Incubation	Prevention	How long contagious	What you can do
Mumps	Fever; headache; vomiting; glands near ear and toward chin at jawline ache and these develop painful swelling. Other parts of body may be affected also.	14–28 days. Usually around 18 days.	None. (It is apt to be milder in childhood than later.)	Until all swelling disappears.	Keep child quiet until fever subsides; indoors unless weather is warm.
Roseola	High fever for 2 or 3 days which then falls to normal before appearance of a fine rash or large pink blotches on back and stomach or sometimes the whole body. Child may not seem very ill despite high fever (103–105), but he may convulse.	Not fully known.	None. Usually affects children from 6 months to 2 years of age.	Until the child seems well.	No special measures. Give plenty of liquids during high fever.
Whooping cough	At first seems like a cold with low fever and cough which changes at end of 2d week to spells of cough, accompanied by a noisy gasp for air which creates the "whoop."	5–21 days. Usually within 10 days.	See that your baby has DPT shots. If an unvaccinated baby is exposed the doctor may want to give a protective serum promptly.	At least 4 weeks.	A baby needs careful supervision of doctor throughout this taxing illness. It is especially dangerous under 6 months of age.

Child's Body
The Diagram Group
Paddington Press
1977   150 pp. $6.95

The information in this book covers almost every aspect of child development and care, presented free of medical jargon, in carefully planned chapters, with a full index and cross-references. It covers diaper changing, problems with sick children, first aid, play, party-giving and selecting clothing for the child, and includes an important chapter on caring for children who need special attention because they have physical, mental, social or family problems.

For certain types of handicaps, feeding equipment such as suction-based plates, dishes with lips, and specially-shaped cutlery encourage valuable independence. Devices that can be operated with minimal movement—perhaps only a toe—have been perfected and are now applied to a wide range of equipment such as page-turners, type-writers, and tape recorders.

Doctor and Child
T. Berry Brazelton
Delacorte Press
1976   231 pp. $8.95

A pediatrician relates his experiences with children and offers suggestions for dealing with problems such as colic, discipline, sibling rivalry, how much television a child should watch and the like.

Discipline can be built into a relationship with a child. Consideration, respect for family rules, acceptance of family duties—all can be natural results based on expectations of how people in a family behave. Discipline is part of learning to live with others. In our society, however, it is often easier for parents to give in to their chil-

dren's whims than it is to see the opportunity that's offered for teaching them social behavior. But if parents don't pass on their firm expectations about behavior, the children must spin their wheels more, waste precious energy searching for a "bedtime," find out the limits of danger for themselves. This is why I look upon the permissive era as anxiety-producing.

Holistic Health Handbook
Berkeley Holistic Health Center
And/Or Press
1978   480 pp. $9.95

This comprehensive, multidimensional view of the revolution in ideas about health and disease presents healing systems, techniques, practices, legal and social issues and a bibliography.

Growing Up Healthy
Diego Redondo and Edith Freund
Condor Publishing
1976   170 pp. $1.75

You are a first-time parent—when do you call the doctor? Where do you go for help? What do you do about the generation gap? This paperback deals with such questions concerning the infant to the twenty-year-old in a query-and-reply format.

Parents sometimes make the mistake of overscheduling their child's day, giving the child no time to sit and think or daydream. One mother, when told this, added one hour for daydreaming on the family blackboard. This is not the way. Let your son wander a bit after school. He may find his own special place to sit and think.

H

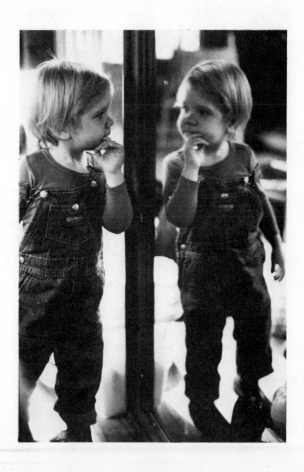

H The application of holistic practices to families naturally involves, for most of us, a major change in lifestyle and a conscious planning for wellness. Health becomes a deliberately created basis for life, rather than a passively experienced effect of life. Family members should be educated in the practices of self-responsibility for wellness. This practice can begin at any age; younger members should be taught their responsibilities as early as possible. These include: nutrition, stress awareness and management, physical fitness, environmental health, and spiritual sensitivity.

How to Live with Diabetes
Henry Dolger and Bernard Seeman
Schocken Books
1978   211 pp. $4.95

Designed to help the reader understand diabetes on a medical as well as a personal level, this volume is a realistic approach to an illness suffered by thousands of children and adults. The authors stress how a child or adult with diabetes can relate to growing up, work, marriage and sex, aging and the emotional demands of the disease.

. . . The parents should become intelligently informed about diabetes; disregard the mysticism, mumbo-jumbo and old wives' tales and seek out the latest scientific information. They should avoid being either overrestrictive or overindulgent. They should avoid bribery, cajolery, or intimidation to make the child accept injections and other necessities of treatment. They should accept the fact that the injections, while painful, are necessary.

Mother's and Father's Medical Encyclopedia
Virginia Pomeranz and Dodi Schultz
New American Library
1977   687 pp. $2.50

Over two thousand topics are arranged in alphabetical order and cross-referenced. Information ranges from infancy through college and includes helpful appendices for choosing doctors, locating poison control centers and obtaining information from other books and magazines.

The color and condition of the skin can also be a helpful diagnostic barometer in a number of ailments not specifically affecting the skin itself. Yellowing of the skin, for example, may reflect problems in the liver or circulation; unusual dryness can signal certain endocrine difficulties affecting the body's chemical balance; certain eruptions are characteristic of specific infectious diseases.

Parents' Encyclopedia of Infancy, Childhood, and Adolescence
Milton I. Levine and Jean H. Seligmann
Thomas Y. Crowell
1973   619 pp. $10.00

This large, single-volume, comprehensive encyclopedia provides information and instruction on all aspects of child care from colds and thumb sucking to homosexuality. Included are appendices on poison control centers, mental health clinics, genetic counseling centers, government and charitable agencies, calorie charts and immunization centers.

Hiccups are caused by a spasm of the diaphragm, the large muscle of breathing between the chest and abdomen . . . they last only a short time and can generally be quickly relieved by giving the baby warm water. Hiccups occasionally

occur in older children and if troublesome, can usually be treated by having the child hold his breath as long as possible or breathe in and out of a paper bag while the nostrils are held together.

Parents' Medical Manual
Glenn Austin, with Julia Stone Oliver and John C. Richards
Prentice-Hall
1978   401 pp. $8.95

This down-to-earth manual covers all aspects of health care needed to raise healthy, happy children. Early chapters emphasize things parents should know so they can act responsibly at home to prevent or treat many conditions.

An important factor in understanding illness and sorting out disease is the age of the individual. At times, the differences in response between newborns, toddlers, children, adults, and old people are so great that the same infection can cause markedly different diseases. Only recently, for example, has it been discovered that many small children seem to get infectious mononucleosis—and get over it without problems. It is entirely a different disease than teenagers have; in fact, we rarely recognize it in children even when they have it.

Taking Care of Your Child
Robert H. Pantell, James E. Fries, Donald M. Vickery
Addison-Wesley
1977   378 pp. $10.95

A commonsense guide to medical problems from birth through adolescence, this book includes information on earaches, measles, how to stock the home pharmacy, alternative schools, sexuality and so on. Easy-to-read charts help the parent decide when to take the child to the doctor and when to treat her at home.

Long-standing weakness and tiredness in children may result from depression. It is a common mistake to assume that only adults are subject to emotional stresses and therefore capable of becoming depressed. Children may react severely to a move, the loss of a pet or friend, an inability to keep up in school, an inability to be successful with friends, or an inability to compete in sports, by withdrawing. Depressed children often have little energy, feel tired all the time, refuse to eat or eat too much, have trouble falling asleep at night or sleep too much, and may complain of a number of physical ailments. These symptoms should be treated seriously. The longer a child spends away from school or from normal activity, the harder it is to begin functioning normally again.

Child Health Encyclopedia
Richard Feinbloom and The Boston Children's Medical Center
Dell Publishing
1975 568 pp. $7.95

Authoritative, nontechnical information and sound advice for parents who want to educate themselves about their responsibilities for the health of their children are presented in this book. Information includes caring for the sick child at home, what to do if your child must go to the hospital, as well as information on childhood diseases and safety.

Medical specialization has received overemphasis in response to the explosion of medical knowledge. Experts in all parts of the body have been developed. Too often the person with the complaint has been forgotten. Patients themselves must choose from a smorgasbord of specialists, each of whom disclaims responsibility for anything but his own increasingly narrow area of concern.

For Children

A Hospital Story—An Open Family Book for Parents and Children Together
Sara Bonnett Stein
Walker
1974 47 pp. $6.95

The Open Family Books help adults prepare children for common hurts of childhood.

This one is also helpful in preparing for visits to the hospital. From the child's text:

Jill doesn't want her tonsils out. She doesn't want anyone to do anything to her.

From the parents' text:

When a child's very own body must be intruded into, we might as well agree it is unpleasant and hard for a child to go through. We might even say that it is quite all right to be mad at the nurse who jabs a hole in his finger. It is quite all right to be mad at the doctor who is too interested in what's up his nose or in his belly. It is quite all right to be angry, if that is how he feels.

My Friend the Doctor
Jane W. Watson, Robert E. Switzer and J. Cotter Hirschberg
Western Publishing
1971 28 pp. $1.95

This read-together book encourages parent/child discussions about illness, pain and visits to the doctor.

My friend the doctor knows I sometimes get a little scared. He doesn't mind if I cry or can't sit still. He has felt the same way himself, he says. Sometimes my friend the nurse gives me a shot. She is very gentle. It almost doesn't hurt at all. Or she takes a little bit of my blood to look at closely.

Visit To The Hospital
Francine Chase
Grosset & Dunlap
1958 20 pp. $.49

H

This story about a boy's first hospital experience is for school-age children who will be entering the hospital.

Then they all went to Stevie's hospital room. His daddy showed him that the hospital bed had handles attached to it. By turning the handles, the ends of the bed could be raised or lowered.

"This is fun," he giggled, as his daddy made the bed go up and down with Stevie in it.

Later, a nurse gave Mommy a little white jacket, and said, "This is for Stevie to put on. It looks like the one his doctor will wear in the operating room." Daddy helped him put on the jacket. "Well, hello, Dr. Stevie." he said.

"Will I be in the operating room long?" Stevie asked.

"No, it takes only a little while," Mommy answered, "about as long as it takes us to walk to the playground and back to the house again."

"Will it hurt?"

"No," Mommy said. "Remember, I told you that you won't feel anything—because you'll be fast asleep."

H Organizations (See Appendix A)

American Academy of Pediatrics

American Alliance for Health, Physical Education and Recreation

American Dietetic Association

American Foundation for Maternal and Child Health

American Medical Association

American National Red Cross

American Podiatry Association

Appalachian Regional Commission

Association for Sickle Cell Anemia Research

Asthma and Allergy Foundation of America

Children in Hospitals

Epilepsy Foundation of America

March of Dimes Birth Defects Foundation

National Institute of Child Health and Human Development

U.S. Department of Health and Human Services

See Appendix C for Films and Audio-Visual Aids

Drug Abuse: A Threat to Your Child's Health

See also Part I—Diet, Drugs, X-Ray and Illness.

In my ten years of teaching, I have become aware of the growing problem of drug abuse now facing the elementary school teacher, parent and child.

Two areas in drug prevention where problems exist are: 1. children coming from chemically dependent homes, 2. children faced with peer pressure to experiment with drugs at an early age.

Children coming from homes where chemical abuse is taking place have a much greater chance of developing behavior patterns which may lead to their own chemical abuse.

Most school systems don't know how to deal with this problem even though four out of five families are affected by it. There is little guidance in the schools and there are very few drug prevention programs at the elementary level, where it should begin.

Self esteem is important in promoting the social and emotional growth of children before they enter the drug-experimenting years of adolescence.

Positive support and feedback along with accepting the child in a loving and caring way are some of the best early preventive measures that can be taken.

When children at an early age feel good about themselves and are clear about what's going on around them, they may try a drug(s) out of curiosity but run a much lower risk of becoming abusers. Most drug abuse is associated with low self-esteem.

In the past year or so more prevention programs have been introduced to the elementary school systems. There drug prevention programs focus on raising self-esteem and promoting mutual respect and acceptance among students and adults. They are hoping that this will promote the social and emotional growth of children, thereby developing healthy, contributing members of society.

Shelly Itman
Elementary School Teacher

Resource Material

"What's 'Drunk,' Mama?"
A book approved by the World Service Conference Al-Anon Family Group, P.O. Box 182, Madison Square Station, N.Y., N.Y. 10010.

Prevention Programs

Project Charlie
5701 Normandale Rd., Edina, Minnesota 55424. A drug abuse prevention program for grades one through six.

Me Me Program
Cooperative Educational Service Agency Number 8, 107 North Douglas Street, Appleton, Wisconsin 54911. A drug abuse prevention program for grades one through six.

HUMOR

Although having children is usually joyful and fun, it is not always that way. We hope that if parents do understand and have information, they can make their experience with their child as joyful as possible. There are many ways to encourage humor and joy in your children. By talking, singing, having fun, playing activities, having a good time and being as positive (yes!) as possible!

HUMOR

Laughter and merriment are the most conspicuous signs of a happy childhood. Most young children enjoy playing, and this playfulness leads them to see more humor in their world than do adults. As adults, we learn that we must face up to the many grim realities of life, and this takes many of us out of the playful frame of mind that seems to be so important for the development of a healthy sense of humor. Since most adults take pride in having a good sense of humor, is there anything that parents can do to help assure that their children reach maturity with a well developed ability to "look on the light side" of things?

Perhaps the most important thing a parent can do to help develop a child's sense of humor is to support the child's natural interest in fantasy or imagination. Many parents worry about the amount of time their children spend in pretend play and games, and try to lead them into "more constructive" activities. These activities may be of real value to the child, but research by social scientists has shown that early imaginative play activities also play an important role in the child's development. This early fantasy play helps the child explore the boundaries of reality, producing a firmer grasp of the nature of things, including what is and is not possible. It also appears to foster the development of creative thinking. The child who has a lot of early experience constructing strange or incongruous worlds in fantasy remains more open to unusual ideas and is likely to be generally more flexible in thinking. Children with well-developed fantasy skills are also better at channeling aggressive feelings into more constructive forms of expression; they are less likely to be physically aggressive toward other children. In addition to these benefits of fantasy activity, playful forms of fantasy are likely to evolve into a heightened sense of humor.

Parents might also strengthen their child's sense of humor by showing some form of positive reaction to the child's early attempts at making people laugh. One reason for clowning or joking is that it gains attention and affection from others. So the parent who shows some appreciation of the child's efforts at humor is actually reinforcing the tendency to initiate humor. Adults must remember, of course, that children's humor tends to be simpler than that of adults because of their more limited level of intellectual development. This difference leads some parents to the conclusion that their child's humor is just silliness and a waste of time. It is parents who happily join in and share the child's humor, in spite of its lack of sophistication, that are most likely to nurture the development of a strong sense of humor in their sons and daughters. Similarly, parents who provide models of humor and laughter in their own interactions with each other and other adults are probably indirectly strengthening this pattern of behavior in their children.

Psychoanalytically-oriented writers noted decades ago that a well developed sense of humor helps children cope with the normal conflicts and stresses associated with growing up. The child who is able to see the humorous side of problems is less likely to be overwhelmed by them, and may actually be in a better position to deal with them. In this sense, a good sense of humor should promote good mental health.

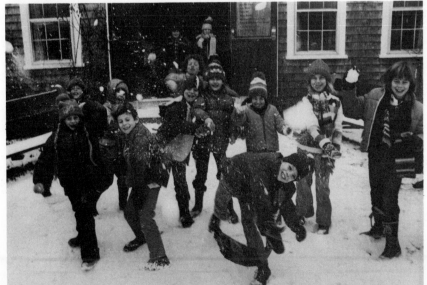

Paul E. McGhee
Humor: Its Origins and Development
W. H. Freeman
1979   251 pp. $8.95/$15.95

I

INTELLIGENCE

See also Developmental Disabilities; Education; Gifted Children; Growth and Development; Learning

Intelligence is a measure of learning accomplishments that your child has achieved and may look forward to achieving. Intelligence may be measured by a child's ability and mental development. These measures are dependent upon the child, the life-style and culture as well as its relevance to the language of the test, not to mention how the child feels the morning of the test or what he or she had for breakfast.

Children who are accustomed to the inner city, its street language and experiences may fail a standard intelligence test prepared for suburban middle-class children.

Questions may deal with subjects the child has not been exposed to, thus invalidating the test results as a measure of his or her intelligence, rather than the accumulation of experience. Another child who lives on Nantucket Island off Cape Cod, Massachusetts, may fail a test designed for the Harlem child for the very same reason. A national study has proven this to be true. Intelligence tests should be regarded as a partial picture of your child's development and potential.

Your Child's Intellect
T. H. Bell
Olympus Publishing
1972   191 pp. $4.95

Bell advocates that preschool learning should take place in the home rather than in institutions; the book offers a year-by-year program of home-based teaching for the growing child from birth to five years, utilizing ordinary household items and readily available materials.

Only after we know that a child can count at least to ten and only after we are certain that he understands that the sound symbol made with the vocal cords represents a number, will we be ready to teach written number symbols. Parents should think about the sound symbols made with the voice and the written symbols of the numbers. The child has often learned that the sound made with the vocal cords for the number three represents that number. He knows that this sound means something, and he knows what it means. It is then a simple matter to teach that the written number "3" is merely another means of communicating the basic idea for three.

JEALOUSY

Children experience feelings of jealousy, sometimes due to the birth of a new baby. The older child can be helped to overcome these feelings by the loving support of his or her parents. The child will express jealousy by getting angry, reverting to being baby-like in behavior, or seeking other attention.

It's better if the child expresses his feelings and parents reassure him that he is still loved even if he does feel jealousy. Parents can express other forms of attention to the older child and support his needs without being anxious or overly protective.

Helene Arnstein in her book *What to Tell Your Child** says:

No matter what you do or how hard you try, you cannot completely spare your child from experiencing feelings of jealousy— expressed by him overtly or covertly. Jealousy, like love, is a universal emotion encountered by each and every one of us at some point. We run into jealousy in our love, work, and social experiences. Yet there are some of us who seem to be able to handle these pangs fairly well, while others are thrown by them. Whatever we can do now to help our very young child face and learn to deal with such feelings (without making him feel guilty about them) will help prevent these feelings from becoming unmanageable or destructive now and later in life.

---

*(page 138, Condor Publishing, 1978, 302 pp., $2.25)

JOY

Having a child is a joyful experience most of the time with lots of responsibility. The child usually expresses joy and laughter, but as with any person feelings change and shift and range from joy to sadness, laughter to tears. Enjoy your child as he or she is and understand that feelings do change.

K

KISSES

Children need lots of them. So do parents. Express your love and affection for your child through your words and actions.

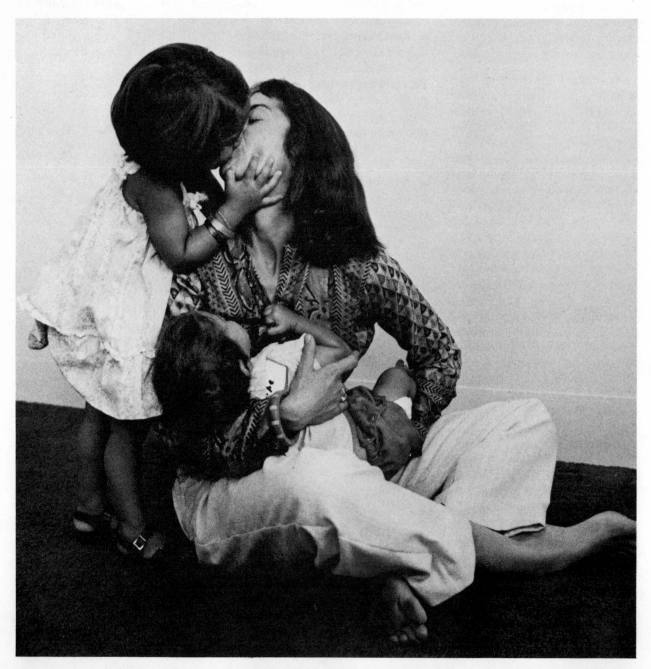

LANGUAGE AND SPEECH

See also Disabilities; Gifted Children; Growth and Development.

Children learn language by listening to parents and others speak. They respond to recognition and rewards for their behavior. Children can learn more than one language and can communicate by their behavior as well.

Some children develop difficulties expressing themselves, but with the suggestions included in the books listed below, parents can provide the assistance needed to help correct the problem.

Is Your Child's Speech Normal?
Jon Eisenson
Addison-Wesley
1976   158 pp. $3.95

This book traces the development of speech from babbling to the first sentences. It covers such topics as hearing loss, delayed speech, minimal brain damage, stuttering, why some children do not talk, why others do not speak distinctly.

Suppose, however, that either the adolescent boy or girl is trying to sound like a pre-adolescent child. The voice tends to be a falsetto, high in pitch, but without the quality of the child's voice. This may suggest that the physically adolescent boy or girl may still want or need to be a pre-adolescent child. We strongly recommend, however, that this possible conclusion not be made by the parents or any other relative. It should be made only by a physician who understands young adolescents and their growing-up problems.

Language and Thought of the Child
Jean Piaget
New American Library
1974   251 pp. $3.95

This classic study by the eminent Swiss child psychologist incorporates his previous theories about the nature of children's cognitive processes, with a new assessment of the realm of child's thought as symbolic and essentially different from the adult world.

The explicatory functions arise out of the need felt by the child, as soon as he becomes conscious of intentions, to project these into the world around him. On the one hand, he finds himself surrounded by people whose actions can be foreseen and whose motives can be detected; on the other hand, he is faced by a world of phenomena and events which up till now have never resisted his thought and therefore required no explanation, but which have now become as great obstacles to his fantasy as are people themselves. This duality has to be abolished; since there is a "why" to human actions, the same treatment must be applied to everything which presents itself. Hence this universal desire for precausal explanations which comes from confusing psychological intentionalism with physical causality. Thus the explicatory function has two poles—psychological explanation and material explanation. These two poles are close together at first and not easily distinguishable, but as time goes on they grow more and more distinct, though always held together by the fact that both are rooted in one and the same desire for explanation.

Teach Your Child To Talk
David R. Pushaw
Dantree Press
1976   248 pp. $9.95/$5.95

Covers typical speech and language development from birth to five years. Suggests activities for parents to provide good speech models and encourage the development of language and a healthy self-image. A section on the child with special needs is included.

When your child is nearby, talk out loud about what you are hearing, seeing, doing or feeling. Let him know there are words to describe all sorts of activities and feelings. For example, as you are hanging up clothes, dusting the furniture, making the beds, washing the car, or setting the table, talk about the things you are doing. Be sure to talk slowly and clearly, and use simple words and short phrases. "Romper Room" and "Captain Kangaroo" are television programs that use this kind of self-talk. Watch them to see how it is done.

Stuttering And What You Can Do About It
Wendell Johnson
Doubleday (Dolphin)
1961   279 pp. $.95

Johnson describes some of the known causes of stuttering and gives concrete advice on how parents can help children and adult stutterers help themselves.

What does a child learn that makes him do the things and have the feelings that lead him and others to take for granted that he "is a stutterer"? He learns to doubt and to fear, and to do certain things because he feels doubtful and afraid. He learns to doubt that

L he can talk smoothly enough to please the people he talks to, mainly his parents. He learns to fear what will happen if he doesn't. What this amounts to is that he learns to be afraid that "he will stutter" and that if he does, he along with "the stuttering," will be disapproved. Naturally, therefore, he learns to do anything and everything he can think of "to keep from stuttering."

Stuttering Solved
Martin F. Schwartz
McGraw-Hill
1976 178 pp. $4.95

This documented book of case studies explains Dr. Schwartz's new "airflow technique" for stutterers. This volume describes the physical mechanism that triggers stuttering—conditioned laryngospasm or locking of the vocal cords in response to stressful situations. Chapters focus on such things as: the types of stress that usually provoke stuttering and how to deal with them, treatment and therapy and success rate.

The second self-imposed speech stress, called the stress of uncertainty, arises as the child attempts to use new vocabulary and grammatical forms. He becomes uncertain about which form or word is appropriate for what he wants to say, resulting in a tensing of his vocal cords that causes a laryngospasm.

When speed stress is combined with the stress of uncertainty the problem is substantially compounded. On the other hand, if the child slows his speech markedly, he usually allows himself enough time to program his speech properly and thereby eliminates almost all the stress of uncertainty. Given enough time, the child can usually deal successfully with most of the self-imposed demands for adultlike speech.

Organizations (See Appendix A)

American Speech and Hearing Association

See Appendix C for Films and Audio-Visual Aids

LEARNING

See also Creative Expression; Disabilities; Education; Games and Activities; Growth and Development; Intelligence; Language and Speech; Literature for Children; Playing; Toys and Play.

Children learn from the moment they are born; language, social behavior, similarities, differences, likes and dislikes.

They must learn how to learn in a world that will not stand still. You play an important role in this continued learning cycle—a most important role, because you the parent will be there long after schoolteacher Jones or whoever has come and gone.

Learning does not stop when the school bell rings to go home from school, nor did it start when the bell rang that morning. Most parents hope to help their children by challenging them and preparing them for more complex tasks. The school's task is to provide the drive to reach this goal with parents, making it a common endeavor. If you feel that this drive is being slowed or hampered by your child's teachers, you have every right to demand change.

Learning and Play

Children work as hard in school as we do at home or in the office. They are eager to explore the world. They learn through direct experience. They like to travel, to use their imagination, to ask a lot of questions. Play is one of the ways children develop the abilities to listen, speak, write and read.

Play

Young children learn best through play. They gain in their intellectual and social development through games, talk, sharing and being with other children. Games are often as simple as tossing a ball back and forth or jumping on chalk numbers; they may involve game boards, drama and puppets.

Organized Play

Children learn a great deal through dramatic play. They play house or dress-up as characters that they would like to be. Parents should not interfere with children's play. They should encourage and allow children to develop spontaneity. It is a good idea to let kids know some time ahead when you want them to stop, so they have an opportunity to complete their games. It is very difficult for them to make the transition suddenly if they are totally engrossed in their play, as it would be for you to break off one of your activities abruptly. Respecting a child's need for play is important.

It is important to differentiate play, which is active and creative, from television, which is passive and receptive. Play stimulates children's healthy development.

Toys

Children learn in different ways. These include:

- physical activities and exercise
- fantasy and dramatic play (with dolls, toys, animals)
- creative play (manipulation, learning extractions, reading, counting, educational toys)
- Cognitive play (manipulation, learning extractions, reading, counting, educational toys)

Toys can be educational as well as fun. Choose toys that will not fall apart and are well constructed. Be selective. Have a place for the child's toys to go; toy shelves or boxes are useful. Children should be expected to pick up their toys after they finish using them and to put them back in the toy area.

Teaching Your Child Basic Skills

You can help your child by developing games and activities that you can share. Teach your child numbers by counting objects, fruits and vegetables. Use a clock; show a child the big hand and the little hand. Explain the concept of "first," "before" and "after." Play games following recipes; look at telephone numbers and explain how to dial; figure out how much food is needed for different numbers of people; set the table; use measuring units—cups, spoons, tapes. Add, subtract, measure. Count the number of candles or utensils in your kitchen. Use a thermometer, a calendar and dates. In the car, talk about mileage and how long you have driven and how far you are going.

Go over basic concepts like "more than," "less than," "equal to." Can your child separate out shapes like squares and circles? Can she count and give examples of numbers? Count numbers of cookies or napkins at home. Help your child learn to listen, to follow directions, to listen to an adult who is talking, to a story, or to music. Play listening games with records in which your child isolates distinctive sounds made by instruments.

Be sure you have given her opportunities to be creative and to discover finger paints, poster paints, chalk, clay and other materials. Talk about new experiences with your child and let her share her feelings, ideas and creativity. When preparing for school, explain that learning is fun. Talk together during a drive or walk, while doing housework or during a meal. Listen to and respect your child's opinions and support her feelings. Try to answer questions that she asks.

Read to your child each day, even if it is only for a few minutes. Give your child opportunities to pick out books and go to the library with you. Be sure that your child feels she can ask questions of the teacher in class and listen for the answer.

When you send your child out each morning, send along a lot of love.

Basic Skills Techniques

1. Before starting the activity, give the child time to familiarize himself with the task materials.

2. Before starting the activity, explain what you are going to do.

3. Allow the child to ask questions.

4. Ask questions that have more than one correct answer.

5. Ask questions that require more than one word as an answer.

6. Encourage the child to enlarge upon the answer.

7. Praise the child when he does well or takes small steps in the right direction.

8. Let the child know when the answer or work is wrong, but do so in a positive or neutral way.

9. Encourage the child to make judgments on the basis of evidence rather than by guessing.

10. During the activity, give the child time to think about the problem; don't be too quick to help.

L

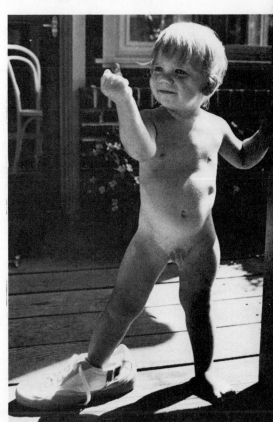

L

Feely Bag Game *

Equipment: Small drawstring bag and two sets of cut-out shapes. Each set has these four shapes: a circle, a square, a triangle and a rectangle.

Purpose: To help the child identify a shape by touch and by sight.

- Take one each of the four shapes and put them in the bag; then place the other four shapes on the table so the child is able to see them.

- Pick up the circle from the table and say to the child, *"Find a shape in the bag that is the same shape as this circle."*

- If the child chooses a different shape, hold up your circle and the shape the child took from the bag and say, *"These two are not the same."* Put the shape the child selected aside. *"Try again."*

- If the child chooses a circle, say, *"These two shapes are the same. They are both circles."*

- After the child has found the circle, place the four shapes in the bag again. Pick up the triangle from the other shapes, and say, *"Find a shape in the bag that is the same as this triangle."* Continue until the child has identified all four shapes.

NOTE: If the child looks in the bag while playing the game, say, *"Now find the shape WITHOUT looking in the bag."*

---

*Feely Bag and similar games for learning were developed by Dr. Glen P. Nimnicht as part of the Parent/Toy Lending Library (General Learning Corporation)

Finger Plays

Witch's Cat
I am the witch's cat (Make a fist with two fingers extended for cat.)
Meow! Meow! (Stroke fist with other hand.)
My fur is black as darkest night.
My eyes are glaring green and bright. (Circle eyes with thumbs and forefingers.)
I am the witch's cat. (Make a fist again with two fingers extended and stroke fist with other hand.)

The Bunny
This is the bunny with ears so funny. (First two fingers of right hand held up, slightly bent.)
And this is the hole in the ground. (Hole made with thumb and first finger of left hand.)
If a slight noise he hears
He pricks up his ears (Straighten fingers.)
and hops in the hole in the ground. (Put ears through hole.)

Soldiers
Ten little soldiers standing in a row. (Hold up 10 fingers, spread.)
Along came the Captain and they all bowed so. (Close hands.)
They marched to the left. (Hands open, move to left.)
They marched to the right. (Hands open, move to right.)
Bang! went the gun and they ran out of sight. (Wiggle fingers like running behind back.)

The Beehive
Here is the beehive. (Closed fist.)
Where are the bees?
Hidden away where nobody sees,
Soon they'll come creeping out of the hive.
One, two, three, four, five. (Put up a finger as you count each number.)

Math

- Count objects in the home, seen on trips, or belonging to a particular person, as "We have six straight chairs in our home." Make comparisons between and among things—of the six chairs, four have plastic seats and two have cloth. Are there more chairs with cloth or with plastic seats?

- Meal preparation is a good time to help your child with measurement and fractions. A measuring cup is fun to play around with and also educational. Ask questions about the quantities —is there more water in $1/2$ cup of water than in one cup? How many halves does it take to make a whole? Timing the cooking or baking of foods involves the ability to tell time and gives parents a chance to help their child develop a sense of time lengths.

- One-to-one matching is an important math concept. Help your child realize that we put one milk glass for each person, one knife, one spoon, one plate, etc. The same is true for eggs if everybody eats only one egg. You can extend this to addition—if you can eat two eggs, Daddy eats three eggs, brother eats two eggs and I eat one egg, how many eggs will we have to fix? Begin by adding the number of eggs for just two family members and gradually work up to where your child can help you find a total for all family members.

L

- Collections of various numbers can be fun to make. Have your child find one of something, say a large thread spool. Then ask for two of something, perhaps bottle caps. These can be assembled into a counting group. If the objects are no longer needed, they could be glued to paper and the numeral and word for each number written on the paper. After your child has finished, he will have an example of the number of objects each number stands for. Use the numbers from one through ten to begin with.

- The concentration game idea is a good one to use in math and word recognition. Take twenty cards about 2" × 2" (for numerals) and write the numerals 0, 1, 2, 3, 4, 5, 6, 7, 8, and 9 on them. You should have two cards with 0, two with 1, two with 2 . . . and two with 9. Twenty cards may be too difficult at first so start with ten cards. Make sure you are using five matching pairs of cards. Turn all ten cards face down so the numeral doesn't show. Arrange the cards in neat rows. Each child asks for two cards to be shown. If they make a match and he can identify the numeral, he takes the pair. If no match is made, the cards are turned back over. The winner is the child with the most pairs. After this version becomes too easy, use all twenty cards. Another variation has a set of numeral cards and a set of matching number words on cards. The child then must match the numeral with the word for that numeral.

Reading and Language Arts

Recognizing common signs

- While riding the bus, in a car or walking, read signs to your child (One Way, No Parking Any Time, Stop, Women, etc.). Talk with your child about what a One Way sign means. Ask about letters and the words as well as comparing these signs with others he knows or sees.

- Use old cardboard, sheets of paper or whatever you have and write down the words from signs your child has seen. A pencil or crayon will do. Talk about the cards. "Read" them to one another.

Other Words in Our World

- Talk with your child about words he sees on billboards, box labels, books, magazines, on the T.V., etc. Take time not only to read and define the words but to compare them for size, beginning or ending letters, rhymes, or maybe number of letters.

- Games using the bingo idea could be made with cards listing common household words. Several children can play. For instance

milk	eggs	grits
soap	salt	bleach
bread	butter	corn

This game takes at least two to play—one to call the words and one to cover them with dried beans or bits of paper as the words are called. More children can play if you make more cards. Mix up the order of the words on the different cards.

Oral Communication

Talk with your child about the time of day. You can do this while preparing meals, setting the table, getting ready for bed or whenever.

PARENT: We eat breakfast in the _____.
CHILD: morning.

PARENT: We set the table for dinner in the _____.
CHILD: evening.

PARENT: You went to school before you ate _____.
CHILD: lunch (dinner)

PARENT: The first thing you did this morning was to _____.
CHILD: (any appropriate answer).

PARENT: What did you do next?
CHILD: (Whatever happened next.)

Other topics to discuss:

- The order of the favorite T.V. shows

- The order in which family members come home in the evening; leave in the morning; get up; have birthdays; etc.

- The difference in certain things as, soup is hot, ice cream is _____. Jim is a boy, Ann is a _____. The table is hard, the pillow is _____. I sit on a chair, I sleep on a _____.

- When you bring groceries home let your child help you sort the food—by color, by kind (fruits, vegetables, meats), by shapes, by place of storage (on the shelf or in the refrigerator), things to eat and things not to be eaten, etc.

L

Noises you hear—what makes them, how do they sound (as loud or soft, high or low), how do they make you feel?

Play an observation game, "Can I trick you?"

PARENT: Let's see if I can trick you. I'm going to name some things here in the bedroom. Stop me if I name something that's not in the bedroom. Ready . . . bed, lamp, chair, window, tree . . .

CHILD: Stop. There isn't a tree in here.

• Play a rhyming game. Use sentences you already say to the child anyway as:

PARENT: I'm going to fix dinner.

CHILD: dinner—spinner (or any word rhyming with dinner)

PARENT: It certainly is hot.

CHILD: hot—pot

• Cooking time is a good time to talk about the order for doing things, especially if you are making something from a recipe. A child can help read the recipe in order to know what happens when and how much of things to use to make that dish.

Help Your Child Learn to Write Letters and Numbers

Teach Me, I'm Yours!
Joan Bramsch
Liberty Publishers
1979 194 pp. $12.95

For parents who are concerned about the quality of individual education their children are

receiving, this book offers over a hundred tested lesson plans, songs and games with which you can teach your children. This book includes skill practice in body control, reasoning, memory, creative imagination, movement, problem-solving, and positive thinking.

Play Pegs*

Use for audio, visual and tactual perception, small muscle manipulation skills, eye-hand coordination, directionality, left-right recognition, reasoning, problem-solving.

Materials Needed:

• One pegboard, 5 holes across and 5 holes down—25.

• 31 pegs—8 red, 8 blue, 5 green, 5 yellow, 5 white.

• A frozen juice can with plastic lid for storing pegs.

• A flat box or pie pan or cake pan to use while working. This type container will allow for easy eye contact when choosing the correct peg color.

You can buy a pegboard made from plastic with plastic colored pegs at a creative children's store. Or you can make a board yourself by using a piece of pegboard which has 25 holes in it—5 across and 5 down. Make a simple frame in the back to hold the board up off the table. Make pegs from doweling bought at a hobby shop and cut into 2 inch pieces. One end of each can be shaped a bit smaller than the other end for easier manipulation into the peg holes (gently turning them in a pencil sharpener can do the trick, but do not make them pointed for safety's sake).

Instructions:

• Give your child the peg board. Encourage him to examine it and place it before him on the table. Give the child the can of pegs. Tell him to open the lid and pour the pegs into the flat container.

"This is a game to help your eyes and fingers be the best they can be. This game will be fun for your good listening ears, too. It's like an 'echo game' because I say something and then, you do it. Let's begin."

• Make ONE ROW of YELLOW pegs across the TOP of your board. Begin at your LEFT and go toward your RIGHT.

• Make ONE ROW of BLUE pegs at the BOTTOM of your board. Begin on the LEFT and go toward the RIGHT.

• Make ONE ROW of RED pegs across the board right UNDER the YELLOW row. Begin at the LEFT.

• Make ONE ROW of GREEN pegs across the board right ABOVE the BLUE row. Begin at your LEFT.

• Make ONE ROW of WHITE pegs across the board right IN THE MIDDLE BETWEEN the YELLOW row and the BLUE row. Begin LEFT.

• You have made FIVE rows of colored pegs. Count them. 1–2 –3–4–5. Clear the board and put the pegs in the work box.

These and other learning activities appear in *Pointers for Parents*, Florida Department of Education, Tallahassee, Florida.

*from *Teach Me, I'm Yours!*

More Learning Resources

Challenge of Achievement
Shirley Gould
Hawthorn Books
1978   135 pp. $7.95

Based on the principles of social psychologists Alfred Adler and Rudolf Dreikurs, this book examines the use of television, books, music and games to help children explore their capabilities. Topics covered include how values affect achievement and interpersonal relationships.

In many families, elaborate plans are made, expensive outfits and equipment are bought, and the budget stretched because a parent wants a child to excel. Thus the way is paved for endless family arguments about the investment of time and money. It is similar with hobbies and clubs. They can be healthy and satisfying, especially if the child finds and wants them, but they can quickly lose their appeal to the youngster if parents overemphasize them.

Decisions, Decisions, Decisions
Barbara Kay Polland
Celestial Arts
1976   109 pp. $4.95

The author examines ways in which children learn decision-making skills. An introductory text in each section is followed by photographs and questions for children, providing a catalyst for open communication.

It may be difficult for us to understand a child's motivation but even toddlers frequently state a strong preference for certain clothes. Rather than forcing our will on a small child's choice of clothing, it would be much better to acquiesce until there is opportunity to discover and evaluate the

child's reasoning. Instead of causing tears over a favorite shirt that needs to be washed, it might be worthwhile to purchase a similar or identical shirt, or arrange to launder it at night. These phases of needing the same clothes, day after day, fade in and out during childhood and should be respected whenever possible.

Don't Push Me, I'm No Computer
Helen L. Beck
McGraw-Hill
1973   171 pp. $2.95

Beck looks at alienation, lack of concentration, hyperactivity and other physical and psychological effects of mechanical devices and techniques used in education and emphasizes that human relationships are essential to learning, particularly for preschoolers.

For many a child whose early learning and experiences centered around the television with little parental involvement, school becomes an enlarged TV set. It is to provide entertainment and to be turned on and off at will. The teacher and the other children can be screened out of consciousness like the shadows on the TV screen. In many a home, the set is on all day. Parents defend this by stating that the child pays only sporadic attention to it. He thus is trained for inattentiveness.

Help Me Learn: A Handbook for Teaching Children From Birth to Third Grade
Mary F. Rice and Charles H. Flatter
Prentice-Hall
1979   398 pp. $13.95/$6.95

The authors cover every facet of early childhood learning and

show how to create a stimulating environment for children, one that will fill their childhood with a wealth of learning experiences.

There is no doubt that memory is enhanced by repetition and positive reinforcement. There are both repetition and positive reinforcement in recognizing the familiar in new situations. When one hears a familiar theme in the middle of a symphony one has never heard in its entirety, the symphony will be remembered. The pleasure of recognition is positive reinforcement. On the other hand, fear hampers memory. School tests can be frightening for conscientious children. When he is doing his homework, help your child learn to test himself so that when he has to take tests in school, fear will be less likely to interfere with his ability to recall. Treat school tests casually and avoid making too much of an issue of grades. Rather, use school tests as indications to you and your child of what facts and skills need further reinforcement.

Made in Summerhill
Humphrey A. Truswell
Hawthorn Books
1975   104 pp. $3.95

Over a hundred projects mostly for older children are illustrated in this book of ideas derived from the Summerhill School workshop. The whole concept of the workshop program is to let children work out an idea creatively, and not to give them a set of instructions to follow. Among the ideas for children in this innovative book are: construction games, pegboard games, paddle boats and wind machines.

L *Freedom, as opposed to license, is a large part of the Summerhill philosophy, and this is especially so in the workshop. Visitors often ask me about the safety aspect of the workshop, possibly imagining that children given a free hand with sharp tools will inflict damage on themselves and those about them. This isn't so. Children are sensible, and, so long as they don't interfere with anyone else, they are free to work as they see fit—although this doesn't mean that if I see a kid sawing laboriously I won't show him an easier way. I am very firm about safety with machinery and power tools. When someone needs to use a power tool he checks with me first, and it is understood that he is solely responsible for operating the machine until he is finished. I find that the simple act of asking me first makes the child more consciously careful.*

Magical Child: Rediscovering Nature's Children
Joseph Chilton Pearce
E. P. Dutton
1977   257 pp. $10.00

The rising toll of brain-damaged children, the increase in autism, childhood suicides and the rebelliousness of children are seen as indications of the "biological plan" thwarted by a "monstrous misunderstanding" in our culture —where stress is unrelieved, where bonding is conditional, and where anxiety aborts intellectual growth.

Intelligence is the ability to interact, and this ability can grow only by interacting with new phenomena, that is, by moving from that which is known into that which is not known. Although this seems obvious, this movement from the known to the unknown proves to be both the key and the stumbling block to development.

Most intellectual crippling comes from the failure to observe the balance of this movement. In our anxieties, we fail to allow the child a continual interaction with the phenomena of this earth on a full-dimensional level (which means with all five of his/her body senses); and at the same time, we rush the child into contact with phenomena not appropriate to his/ her stage of development. That is, either we block the child's movement into the known and so block intellectual growth, or we propel the child into inappropriate experience.

Revolution in Learning
Maya Pines
Harper & Row
1966   237 pp. $5.95

In a nontechnical description of numerous experimental programs designed to stretch human minds through early learning, the material in this book deals with experiments in early learning, such as the Head Start program. Studies are examined and programs evaluated, showing that children as young as three can learn to read and even compose poetry. The author assures the reader that even the severest educational problems in our society could be solved if we started teaching children in the early years—before first grade.

What we need is a better intellectual diet for each child. . . . We can hook babies on learning, developing a life-long need for it. We can feed the toddler's drive to explore, allowing a variety of talents and interests to flourish. . . . In well-baby clinics and pediatricians' offices, we can provide regular check-ups on intellectual development for every young child. By means of Children's Houses on every block, where mothers can leave the young for half an hour or

a full day, and a network of home tutors, we can prevent the intellectual crippling of millions of youngsters.

Successful Children
Raymond T. Coppola
Walker
1978   196 pp. $11.95

The author assures us that parents can reinforce a child's learning experience and make education fun, then provides over nine hundred activities as further proof and incentive. Specific tips cover how to get the most from family conversations, how to use and enjoy the public library and how to use games and songs in everyday routines.

Some parents make the mistake of having children only do the chore aspects of cooking—setting the table, cleaning up, drying the dishes. While these chores must be done and are good responsibilities for children to have, a great deal of enjoyment and learning are related to the food preparation in the kitchen. Hook your child on cooking —he'll use his skills all his life. And what a palatable way to practice reading, math, and science. Have him read the recipe to you so that you can make sure that it is being correctly interpreted. He can learn the measurements of ounces and pounds as well as the differences between beating and whipping, blending and stirring. He will learn about the various states of matter —solid, liquid. . . . Boiling eggs and spaghetti and freezing desserts and stored foods can teach your child something of the Fahrenheit and Celsius scales. Changing substances such as flour into dough and dough into bread will show your child how outside forces (heat and water) will cause a chemical change to occur in certain substances.

L

Your Child Learns Naturally
Silas L. Warner and Edward R. Rosenberg
Cornerstone Library
1977   214 pp. $2.95

This book discusses the learning process in the child's early years, how and what she learns and how a parent can prepare her for school. The authors provide insights into learning theories and suggest practical methods of adapting theories to bring children to learning readiness.

A child enjoys repetition. In time he will choose a favorite toy, puzzle, or book. The act of making his own choice, even a repeated one, assures him of the strength of his wishes. Besides, an adult cannot know what element of newness a child can find in the same object or the same situation. What appears to be simple repetition to a mother or father can be a new aspect of familiarity to the child.

Montessori and Piaget

The Montessori teaching system, which Maria Montessori created by working with young children, develops children's particular language skills and abilities from birth to three years of age. She stressed the child's love of order and ritual around two years of age, and learning writing and reading between four and five and one-half. Montessori's approach allows children to develop sensory and motor skills, understand counting and develop self-image. She saw that children would focus on learning if they were provided with specially designed materials that support the child's own innate abilities. Schools that practice the Montessori approach have teachers specially trained in this method.

Another early learning approach introduced by Jean Piaget indicates that the stage of development of the child's mind is important in determining what the child learns. Children, says Piaget, go through different phases: from birth to two, they focus on touch and smell; from two to seven, they are able to learn language and to gain understanding of the world; after seven, they are ready for abstract concepts. He saw how children adapt between the social and physical environments. You can read a description of Piaget's book, *Language and Thought of the Child*, in the Language and Speech section of this book.

Child's Work
Paul S. Shakesby
Running Press
1974   112 pp. $4.95

Shakesby utilizes the Montessori method for constructing toys and games to encourage the child's natural development.

Playing can be hard work for a child. But the difference between a child's work and an adult's is largely one of attitude. Children do not approach their hard-working games with the kind of negativism that our society has conditioned many of us to associate with the idea of work. For the very small people in our world, experience is not so narrowly defined. Let us try to get inside our children's heads, where work can be fun while fun may be work— where playing, working and learning are all one and the same.

Montessori And Your Child
Terry Malloy
Schocken Books
1976   96 pp. $3.95

This illustrated manual to help parents of young children understand the theories of Montessori education contains practical suggestions for Montessori materials that are useful in the home, along with observations concerning child development.

In a Montessori school, your child teaches himself through his use of the specially designed Montessori materials. These are attractive, generally simple, child-sized materials that are self-correcting; that is, if a child makes an error, he can see it by looking at the material itself. In this way, no adult is needed to point out his mistake and perhaps injure his self-esteem.

Your child learns to work alone and with others in a Montessori school—he can usually make this choice himself. He learns to follow the class ground rules and may often remind other children to follow them. Because he can choose his own work and do it at his own pace, your child has many opportunities for success; the Montessori classroom is an attractive place in which your child can be free from adult domination and can discover his world and build his mind and body.

Teaching Montessori in the Home: The School Years
Elizabeth G. Hainstock
New American Library
1971   176 pp. $3.95

This is a guide for older children's learning which stresses Montessori methods to supplement and complement the child's education regardless of the type of school he attends. It includes instructions for making teaching materials.

L*Encourage your preschool child's curiosity by answering his seemingly unending questions, and give him every opportunity to develop and strengthen language skills by talking to him. Always speak distinctly and use clear and accurate pronunciation. Remember that this is a stage when much is learned by imitation and both good and bad language habits will be readily copied. Teach the correct names of people, places, and objects. Try to avoid baby talk. Don't be afraid of introducing large or unfamiliar words, for this is how children learn them. The young child loves to talk about parallelograms, rhododendrons, cumulus clouds and so on. In fact, I remember one three-year-old I taught in school who knew all of the dinosaur names and pronounced them with no difficulty at all. Give names and meanings to everything in the child's environment, and talk to him about numbers, colors, etc.*

General Techniques and Skills for Parents

Helping Children Learn
Barbara Cabell Wilcox
Vantage Press
1975   201 pp. $6.95

In this do-it-yourself book to help children acquire knowledge, acquisition of knowledge is related to the child's total environment. The author emphasizes that preparedness for learning should begin before conception, with the parents' optimal health providing the foundation for the child's well-being. Stressing that the home should be a learning center, the author provides exercises and information to aid a parent in guiding the child in neurological development, in reading and writing development and in building a good self-image.

There is no more creative role than that of parenthood in the physical and psychological nurturing of other human beings. Few parents consider that they function as designer, fashioner, architect, artist, builder, yet all kinds of creation go into evolving of personality. To bring into being an individual one must be positive of one's differences. . . . this parent seeks to animate the child's personality.

How to Double Your Child's Grades
Eugene M. Schwartz
Frederick Fell
1975   269 pp. $7.95

The difference between being the class failure and at the top of the class is not intelligence but techniques—rapid study and flash-reading, for example. The author offers a plan to aid parents in improving their child's school grades, stressing skills such as organization, note-taking, listening and speed-reading. Chapters deal with such subjects as test-passing skills, problem-solving skills to make math easy and skills to help a child increase vocabulary.

As you remember, your child is reading to find specific answers to specific questions. . . . Does it answer his questions, or does it not?

If it does not, he flash-reads it, and searches on for his answer.

If it does, however, he slows down, concentrates his full attention on that sentence, and picks up his pencil to underline the answer.

This aggressive underlining of answers in the textbook as they are read . . . makes your child's concentration automatic.

It converts routine reading into active, physical thought. It prevents his mind from wandering. It makes the dead, lifeless material in the book come to life with the thrill of personal discovery. It forces him to evaluate, weed out, judge, emphasize. It is the first great step in turning that material into his own personal acquisition. . . .

How to Help Your Child Get the Most out of School
Stella Chess, with Jane Whitbread
Doubleday
1974   292 pp. $7.95

This guidebook for parents shows how children learn, the differences in normal learning rates and styles and common problems in the early years of a child. Using case histories the authors offer answers to such questions as: when is a child ready for school? What does psychological testing tell? Does competition make children work harder?

Children have a right to learn about reality from their parents. If you protect them from everything negative, you give them a false picture of the world.

If you insist on complimenting him indiscriminately for every paper, artwork, athletic performance, he will get a phony idea of his abilities, and no experience in judging his work or himself. Worse, if he's perceptive, he'll recognize your comments are valueless and decide that 1. you don't take him seriously enough to pay attention to what he is doing, or 2. you think so little of his effort that you are afraid to tell him the truth.

L

Learning Can Be Child's Play
June Mather
Abingdon
1976 62 pp. $3.95

Mather tells how parents can help the slower-than-average preschooler develop through play experiences. The book includes large black-and-white drawings.

There is a very thin line between having a child do as well as he possibly can and pushing him beyond his capacity. One of the best ways to be sure that you are not putting too much pressure on your child is to be on the watch for signs such as Amy's stutter or Therese's wetting. These signs may be outward indications of inward frustrations.

Once children begin saying words, the important thing to do is to talk to them. Conversation is the way children learn how to use words. It is one thing to learn the names of people, objects, numbers, colors, sizes, and actions; but only in conversation do these words begin to have real meaning.

Thinking Is Child's Play
Evelyn Sharp
Avon
1969 143 pp. $1.45

A guide to learning and teaching games for preschoolers that emphasizes learning as a thinking process rather than memorization, this is based on the work of psychologists Piaget and Bruner.

After looking around the house and supermarket, I used materials I found there to devise some games for the home. None of them is meant to be mastered in the way a lesson is. They are play, but play with a purpose. In most, the purpose is to give your child explicit firsthand experiences of a kind that will provoke thinking. Some are intended to give you an indication of the level of mental development your child has reached, in order to

help you understand his way of reasoning as contrasted to an adult's.

The Three Rs Plus: Teaming Families and Schools for Student Achievement
Dorothy Rich and Cynthia Jones
Home and School Institute
1978 128 pp. $9.00

Stressing that everywhere can be a classroom for a child, this manual offers suggestions for building basic skills at home with exercises aimed at improving math, writing and reading skills.

IMPORTANT: Do let the children trade places with you and give these idea-generating tests. After taking these yourself, you'll be duly respectful of a child's inventive imagination.

Encourage children to conjecture: what would happen if the automobile had not been invented, etc. A whole new world opens up. Ask children to name five inventions the world could use that have not been invented yet.

Supertot
Jean Marzollo
Harper & Row
1977 155 pp. $11.95

Featuring specific learning activities for supertots—children who feel loved, who like the world and who continue to want to learn about it, this book also gives suggestions to parents for taking care of their own needs.

Keep a few favorite toys put away for times when friends come by and you want to give them your undivided attention. Don't make a big deal about it; but after they've said hello, played with your child a bit, and settled down for a cup of coffee, bring out a favorite toy and set it on the floor nearby. With luck, your child will play contentedly alone for a while. But don't expect miracles. If you can get this

technique to work half the time, you're batting 500, and that's good.

Up from Underachievement
Barbara E. Biggs and Gary S. Felton
Charles C. Thomas
1977 183 pp. $6.95

In this nontechnical book for people who are underachievers or work with underachievers, the authors offer clearcut steps for changing underachieving patterns into success-oriented behaviors.

Since the underachiever fears failure, success or both, she relies on a behavioral pattern that prevents risk taking and consequent change. Experiencing failure demands change if a person does not wish to fail. Experiencing and acknowledging success at least suggests that further investment in responsible behavior might lead to continued success. And that's the rub. When an underachiever succeeds, and admits that her success is not accidental, she and others around her begin to have expectations about her success in future tasks. This places a difficult demand on her. Helping the student to deal with her feelings about such demands is an important task for any program designed for underachievers.

Dear Mom and Dad—Parents and the Preschooler
Barbara J. Taylor
Brigham Young University Press
1974 175 pp. $5.95

This collection of simple ideas for group or home use helps the child develop socially, physically, emotionally and cognitively. Activities included teach children about music, colors, their bodies and making friends.

Because a young child is unskilled and inexperienced in the use of his hands, he needs easy tasks

L

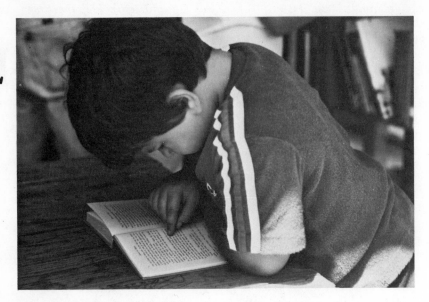

first and then increasingly more difficult ones to help him grow. He will develop his small muscle coordination as he has the opportunity. He can sort buttons (by size, color, or number of holes), toothpicks, thread, nails, hair rollers, or paint brushes; he can put macaroni, rice, or cereal into small containers; he can screw lids on various kinds of jars; or under supervision, he can cut fabrics and different kinds of paper. If possible, the child should see where his father, mother, an adult friend or relative works and observe how different people use their hands as they perform different tasks. The adult can talk to him about how different occupations require hand involvement (for example, dentist, artist, mechanic, baker, assembler, sales clerk, architect, carpenter, typist).

Fun with American Literature
E. Richard and Linda R. Churchill
and Edward H. and Kay Reynolds
Blair
Abingdon
1968   249 pp. $4.95

The authors have assembled scores of games and puzzles in an effort to provide entertainment for children in their discovery of American literature. Games and quizzes range from those dealing with poetry (name the poet who wrote these lines) to filling-in-the-blank questions about twentieth century novelists.

To aid you in your task, we have divided the authors and their works into four groups of seven books and writers. Remembering something of the place each writer holds in American history as well as the period in which he lived should enable you to make a perfect set of seven associations every time. After all, seven is a lucky number!

Home Guide To Early Reading
Toni S. Gould
Walker
1976   162 pp. $9.95

Gould emphasizes Structural Reading, a system of relating

sounds to words, to teach preschoolers. Learning games are included.

A child should learn through thinking as early as possible, for it is the thinking, and not the amount learned, that will contribute to his intellectual growth. We should evaluate his knowledge by how well he can apply it in new situations or in tasks he has been taught. Only in this way do we allow for creativity in the intellectual areas as we do in the arts. The child who is helped to figure out words on his own, to think out a sentence, practices thinking and will get better and better at it. And, in this process of learning to use his mind and discovering that he can depend on his ability to think, he develops an ever increasing motivation for learning more.

How to Teach Your Baby to Read
Glen Doman
Random House
1964   166 pp. $8.95

Fascinating case histories illustrate that tiny children desire to, and actually can, learn to read. By relying on the author's method, which he clearly presents, a child at one year will learn to read individual words; a two-year-old, sentences; and a child of three, whole books—with joy, curiosity and keen perception.

The cardinal rule is that both parent and child must joyously approach learning to read, as the superb game it is. The parent must never forget that learning is life's most exciting game—it is not work. Learning is a reward, it is not a punishment. Learning is a pleasure, it is not a chore. Learning is a privilege, it is not a denial.

Parent's Guide to Children's Reading
Nancy Larrick
Doubleday
1975   409 pp. $8.95

This book stresses the use of words in conversation by encouraging children to ask questions and listen to answers. It includes activities to help parents develop children's love of reading and provides information for the selection of magazines, film strips and records as well as the creation of a home library.

Parents interested in their children's reading development should be sure he is physically fit. Good food and plenty of sleep are all-important. Watch out for bad tonsils, poor vision, impaired hearing following a heavy cold, and undue fatigue. Help him to know other children. This may be especially important if the teacher reports he is shy in school. A hot-dog picnic in the backyard may help to build confidences that the child needs in reading aloud. Get him accustomed to speaking distinctly by showing a decided interest in conversation with him. If the two of you join in reciting poems, he may gain facility in talking quickly and easily. Answer his questions about the meaning of words, but don't push him into reading words from a ready-made list. At this stage one of the most important things you can do is to show that reading is fun. When the child is convinced that stories and books mean pleasure, you have made a real contribution.

Preparing Your Child For Reading
Miles A. Tinker
Holt, Rinehart, Winston
1971   157 pp. $1.88

Tinker presents a program for parents to develop a child's early reading skills by turning everyday chores into learning experiences, playing vocabulary-increasing games, helping the child distinguish sounds or pick out subtle visual differences.

If the parent and child have developed a sound, comfortable relationship, full of love and mutual respect, the child will be ready to set forth confidently on his first day of school. He will expect to like his teacher and the other children, and he will be ready and able to apply himself to the major undertaking of the first grade—learning to read.

Programming Your Preschooler for Reading: A Book of Games
Brandon Sparkman and Jane Saul
Schocken Books
1977   113 pp. $7.95

Designed to guide parents in teaching their preschoolers to read, this book contains eighty-four visual games and fifty-six listening games. The authors have included a list of recommended reading and listening materials to further aid the parents in developing visual and auditory skills in their child.

Learning to read requires the ability to see likenesses and differences in detail. We see largely what we are trained to see. You can help your child grow in ability to discriminate visually by pointing out how various things are alike and how they are different. For example, you can find a great deal of pleasure and satisfaction in taking walks with your child and in spending time discovering things and talking about the things which you discover together. Grass, leaves, bugs, and dogs are just a few examples. But, more important are the details of each item which you discover. Note the likenesses and differences in the leaves.

See the veins, the size, and the color, the way they feel on each side, and on and on. The more minute details one is able to see, the nearer one is to being able to read.

L

Teaching Young Children to Read at Home
Wood Smethurst
McGraw-Hill
1975   224 pp. $7.95

Beginning with a summary of the history of home-reading education, the author proceeds to offer his step-by-step program for teaching children to read. A useful guide at the end of the book offers information on teaching materials that are available to parents (with prices and ordering information) for use in the home-teaching environment.

A striking fact about early readers is that they are often children who have been read aloud to a great deal. Not only are they read to often (daily or better) by parents, sitters, siblings, or someone else; presumably they also sit so that they can see the pictures and the words as the reading goes on. Other factors in the homes of most early readers are the presence of lots of books, especially children's books, and people in the house who value reading and books. One more point about the early reader's environment: Since early readers are often also early scribblers, there usually are writing materials in abundance that the child can get at—paper, crayons, pencils, markers, chalkboard and chalk, maybe even a typewriter. Some early readers are also TV fans; it is interesting to speculate about the number of readers who have been inspired by "Sesame Street" and "The Electric Company."

Science

L

*Whole Cosmos Catalog of Science
Activities*
Joe Abriscato and Jack Hassard
Goodyear
1977   134 pp. $9.95

For children, teachers, parents, this is a sourcebook of creative scientific learning including both articles and activities in such areas as cell biology, ecology, geology and chemistry.

Observing the moon on a clear night can be a wonderful experience. Several types of studies are suggested, including locating the moon each hour and making a calendar based on the moon.

Make a drawing on an index card of the landscape around your home. Draw it from southeast to the southwest. At twilight go out and find the location of the moon. Draw it on your card. Go out every hour for at least two more hours and do the same thing. In what direction is the moon moving? Did it change shape? Compare your cards to those of other people who do this activity.

*Bees and Honey
The Butterfly Cycle
The Spider's Web
The Stickleback Cycle
Common Frog
The Chicken and the Egg
Dragonflies
The Wild Rabbit*
Oxford Scientific Films
G. P. Putnam's Sons
1977–80   each book 32 pp. $7.95

Oxford Scientific Films, a team of British filmmakers and zoologists, has written this series of magnificently photographed, full-color nature books which can be used by children of all ages.

Organizations
(See Appendix A)

American Association of Elementary-Kindergarten-Nursery Educators

American Library Association

American Montessori Society

Appalachian Regional Commission

Association for Childhood Education International

Education Development Center

National Alternative Schools Program

National Association for Gifted Children

National Association for Retarded Citizens

National Association for the Education of Young Children

National Education Association

National Foundation for Gifted and Creative Children

Magazines
(See Appendix B)

*Day Care and Early Education
Early Years*

See Appendix C for Films and Audio-Visual Aids

LITERATURE FOR CHILDREN*

A child's book is something special. A book is uniquely rewarding and pleasurable to a child. Choosing that book can be great fun for you.

Here are a few things to keep in mind to help you in your selection:

---

*from *Choosing A Child's Book*, Children's Book Council, Inc., 67 Irving Place, New York, N.Y., 10003

Babies and pre-nursery schoolers are attracted by brightly colored pictures of simple objects. It is never too soon to introduce children to the joy of sturdy, boldly illustrated books. Try to choose simple texts with a good rhythm for reading to the very youngest children. Many of these picture books are wordless thereby stimulating children's visual perceptions to a greater extent.

Nursery school and kindergarten children like Mother Goose, nursery stories and other simple picture books, with little text, depicting familiar objects and experiences. If you will be reading to the child, slightly more complex texts with good rhythm and effective word repetition are good choices.

Early school years (ages 5–8) Some children begin to read independently as early as nursery school, but generally they are not reading until the end of their first year of grade school or later. It's fun for adults and children to read together, so select picture books with strong story lines and character development. If children read by themselves, choose a book with a good story employing words that will be reasonably familiar from everyday use. Third graders can frequently handle stories with a good deal of content but the vocabulary should still be relatively easy. A substantial amount of non-fiction books have been published for this age enabling children to explore the natural and realistic elements of their environs.

Older children (ages 9–12 and older) A child's personality and preferences are the most important factors in selecting books for older children. Give some thought to the child's special interest, then choose a non-fiction book or novel in this subject area.

L

Frequently, publishers indicate in a book or on its jacket the age levels for which they think that book is most suitable. Don't hesitate to choose a book suggested for a slightly older child. If a book is actually beyond a child's reading ability, it can be read to him or her now, and independently later. A beautiful, well-illustrated picture book with an interesting story offers the child an esthetic experience to enjoy over and over again.

Some children's books have become classics. They have great appeal, in part because they have stood the test of time and should be a part of everyone's reading history. For many children, however, a book that is contemporary in every way may be a far more pleasing reading experience than a classic would be. So that children will enjoy reading, it may be wise to select books that are sure to appeal to *them*.

Don't overlook paperbacks. Thousands of children's books— older titles, many new books in reprint and originals, as well, are now available in paperback editions and are especially good values.

Always look for quality. This is not automatically the biggest or most expensive book on the shelf. It *is* a book that is written, designed and illustrated well. There is a difference between garish pictures and simple, bold illustrations. You will be able to tell by taking a few moments to look at the books. A book is an unlimited investment in the human mind and spirit. Its selection deserves at least as much time as we devote to choosing clothes for our children.

If you have not been in touch recently with the children for whom you want to buy books and so do not know what books they already have or what their current interests may be, ask your local bookstore about Give-A-Book certificates. This nation-wide program allows you to buy certificates in varying denominations and send them to your young friend or relative to redeem in a bookstore in his or her community. While it may not be as satisfying as choosing the book yourself, it does assure that you have given that child the opportunity to experience the unalloyed pleasure of choosing, owning and reading books.

Some Children's Book Selection Resources

There are many sources of information for guidance in choosing children's books. Some communities are fortunate to have regular reviews of new books in local newspapers. Certain newspapers with regional as well as local distribution review children's books regularly. Many of these newspapers can be examined at public libraries. Even newspapers without regular coverage frequently have special features about children's books in pre-Christmas or late spring issues, or in November for Book Week.

Most general interest magazines do not review children's books regularly, even though many have articles about them from time to time. The articles customarily include the titles of current books of interest to young readers.

Booksellers are usually very knowledgeable in respect to giving assistance in choosing children's books; and so, of course, are children's librarians. They are always pleased to give guidance to readers —both to the youngest and to those adults selecting books for children. In addition to giving personal counsel, most children's librarians will be able to share bibliographies of children's books, professional magazines and reviews.

Some other sources of information about new children's books are:

American Library Association (50 E. Huron St., Chicago, IL 60611)

- A professional association deeply involved in the evaluation of children's books through its publication *Booklist* and the activities of its Association for Library Service to Children (ALSC)

- *Booklist* published on the 1st and 15th of each month includes reviews of recommended books for children and young adults.

- "Notable Children's Books of the Year" selected annually by members of ALSC. Single copy of annotated list available in late spring for a stamped, self-addressed envelope.

- *Let's Read Together: Books for Family Enjoyment* substantial, annotated bibliography revised irregularly.

- ALSC administers the prestigious, annual Newbery and Caldecott Awards for, respectively, the author of the most distinguished contribution to literature for children and the illustrator of the most distinguished picture book for children.

L

Bulletin of the Center for Children's Books (University of Chicago, 1100 E. 57th St., Chicago, IL 60637)

- Evaluates a substantial number of new children's books; published eleven times a year.

Children's Book Council (67 Irving Pl., New York, NY 10003)

- A publishers' association encouraging the reading and enjoyment of children's books. Sponsors National Children's Book Week each November. Prepares materials for various programs for encouraging reading year-round.
- *The Calendar*, a miscellany of news and information about books, publishing and children's literature, mailed at eight-month intervals to persons paying a one-time-only charge to be added to mailing list.
- Distributes three annual bibliographies: "Outstanding Science Trade Books for Children" and "Notable Children's Trade Books in the Field of Social Studies," available in the spring; "Children's Choices" available in the fall. Free for a stamped (2-oz. postage), self-addressed envelope for each.

Children's Books (Supt. of Documents, U.S. Government Printing Office, Washington, DC 20402)

- Annual annotated list of books for preschool through junior high school age children compiled by a committee under the direction of the Children's Literature Center, Library of Congress.

The Horn Book Magazine (31 St. James Ave., Boston, MA 02116)

- About books for children and young adults. Includes informative and critical articles, reviews of new children's books. Published six times a year.
- "Fanfare" a short listing of the previous year's books considered most outstanding by the magazine's reviewers is published in the June issue annually. "Fanfare" reprints, and other bibliographies and books, are available.

A Catalog of Horn Book Publications is available free from the same organization, describing such books as:

- BOOKS, CHILDREN AND MEN by Paul Hazard. Translated by Marguerite Mitchell. An eminent French scholar discusses the children's books of different countries.
  Hardcover $5.00, postage 15¢
  Paperback $3.00, postage 10¢
- THE HEWINS LECTURES, 1947–1962 Edited by Siri Andrews. Valuable source material on children's literature and on some outstanding authors.
  $10.00, postage 20¢
- NEWBERY MEDAL BOOKS, 1922–1955 Edited by Bertha Mahony Miller and Elinor Whitney Field. Acceptance speeches by winners of Newbery medal, awarded each year to the author of the most distinguished contribution to American literature for children. Biographical sketches of authors and descriptions of award-winning books.
  $10.00, postage 20¢
- CALDECOTT MEDAL BOOKS, 1938–1957 Edited by Bertha Mahony Miller and

Elinor Whitney Field. Acceptance speeches by winners of Caldecott medal, awarded annually to the artist of the most distinguished American picture book for children. Biographical sketches of artists and descriptions of award-winning books.
  $10.00, postage 20¢

International Reading Association (800 Barksdale Rd., Newark, De 19711)

- Eight small, accessible publications directed to parents are available: *Why Read Aloud to Children?, What Books and Records Should I Get for My Preschooler?, What is Reading Readiness?, How Can I Help My Child Get Ready to Read?, How Can I Help My Child to Read English as a Second Language?* (also in Spanish), *How Can I Encourage My Primary Grade Child to Read?* and *How Can I Get My Teenager to Read?*

School Library Journal (1180 Avenue of the Americas, New York, NY 10036)

- Reviews nearly all new children's books. Includes articles about librarianship and literature. Published monthly September–May. May issue contains the editors' selection of "Best Books for Spring"; December issue, "Best Books of the Year."

Unless otherwise noted, there is a charge, often nominal, for the materials mentioned. Information is available directly from each source.

A Guide To Non-Sexist Children's Books
Judith Adell and Hilary Dole Klein
Academy Chicago Ltd.
1976   149 pp. $3.95

"Stories for children are like dreams that we share with our kids. And since dreams can be rehearsals for reality, it's important what roles they find in those stories," says Alan Alda in the introduction to this guide which offers a wide range of children's and young-adult books dealing with boys and girls in nontraditional roles. Contained in this annotated guide are the names of publishers, dates of publication and price of each book, along with the grade and/or age category.

To be sure, there's some pleasure to be had in winning, but not when half of us are considered to be incapable of winning and the other half of ever losing. The stories listed in this book are the kind that treat boys and girls as people who have the same kinds of frailties and strengths. I think one of the great advantages of children's literature like this is that some day soon men and women will think of each other less as strangers or aliens from another planet and more like the brothers and sisters we really are.

Human and Anti-Human Values in Children's Books
Prepared by CIBC Racism and Sexism Center for Education
Council on Interracial Books for Children
1976   268 pp. $7.95

This book urges new children's literature to respond to a changing world and to be a tool for the conscious promotion of human values free of sexism, racism,

classism and materialism. Hundreds of books are rated for artistic quality, language and presentation of values.

We must be concerned above all with the effects of a book on the children who read it. What happens to children from the racial group depicted when they look in that mirror and see sameness, ugliness, dependency on whites, lack of resistance, acceptance only on the basis of an endless willingness to suffer? What happens when they

see something they can never have —whiteness—embodied with superiority and desirability? What happens when they see a pretty world free of racism, which they know to be unreal? What happens when they see their own kind always "in trouble with the law"? What happens when they see none of their own kind showing strength? What happens when they see their culture and language reduced to quaintness, at best, and more often to inferiority?

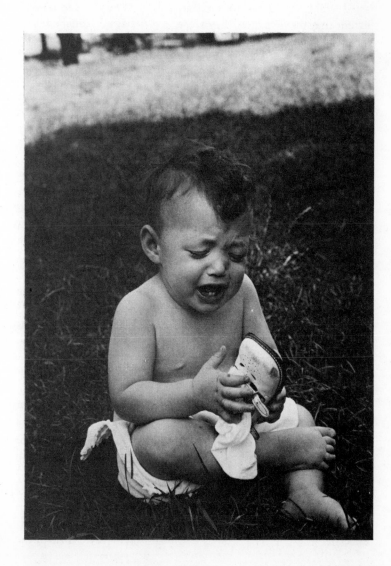

Thirty Twentieth-Century Children's Books Every Adult Should Know*

L This list—for adults who may be familiar only with the children's books they met in their own childhood—is intended to give a sampling of the freshness of approach and the variety in setting, mood, style, treatment, and plot to be found in good children's books. This is not a basic list; it is merely a selection from many fine books of a few about which this reviewer is especially enthusiastic. However, all these books have proved themselves with children, have interested college students to such an extent that they "forgot" they were "reading children's books," and have given much pleasure to many other grownups.

Poetry, legends and traditional fairy tales, translations, and creatively written informational books should have their own lists and are not included here.

These are all fiction and all books in which the writing is of primary importance, illustrations, if there are any, being subordinate or unnecessary to the actual telling of the story. Because of the trend to overemphasize illustration, most adults are familiar with picture books, so none are listed here. This is an attempt to show that the good writing of a good story is still enough to charm and excite.

Literary Fairy Tales and Fantasy

- THE CHILDREN OF GREEN KNOLLS by Lucy M. Boston. Illustrated by Peter Boston (Harcourt)

    A small boy comes to live with his great-grandmother in

an old English mansion filled with the past.

- THE CAT WHO WENT TO HEAVEN by Elizabeth Coatsworth. Illustrated by Lynd Ward (Macmillan)

    Although cats, alone of all animals, did not accept the teachings of Buddha, one patient little cat and a compassionate Japanese artist bring about a miracle.

- A PENNY A DAY by Walter de la Mare. Illustrated by Paul E. Kennedy (Knopf)

    A varied selection of this poet's fairy tales, including "The Old Lion," which has also been published as a separate book, *Mr. Bumps and His Monkey* (Holt).

- THE TWENTY-ONE BALLOONS by William Pène du Bois, Author-Illustrator (Viking)

    The amazing adventures of Professor William Waterman Sherman, who takes off from the Pacific Coast in a balloon and three weeks later is picked up in the Atlantic Ocean among the wreckage of twenty balloons.

- THE LITTLE BOOKROOM by Eleanor Farjeon. Illustrated by Edward Ardizzone (Walck)

    This poet's own selection of her stories mixed of "fiction and fact, fantasy and truth," written over many years.

- THE DOLLS' HOUSE by Rumer Godden. Illustrated by Tasha Tudor (Viking)

    A "novel in miniature" and the first of this writer's stories about dolls.

- RABBIT HILL by Robert Lawson, Author-Illustrator (Viking)

    Excitement and humor attend the efforts of the small ani-

mals to learn about the new family in the Big House.

- A WRINKLE IN TIME by Madeleine L'Engle (Farrar)

    An adventure in time and space in which three children accomplish a heroic rescue.

- THE LION, THE WITCH, AND THE WARDROBE by C. S. Lewis. ILlustrated by Pauline Baynes (Macmillan)

    The first of the seven stories about the mythical world of Narnia.

- THE BORROWERS by Mary Norton. Illustrated by Beth and Joe Krush (Harcourt)

    The first of four books about the race of tiny people who live by borrowing from human beings.

- THE HOBBIT by J. R. R. Tolkien, Author-Illustrator (Houghton)

    The story of a quest in which the home-loving little hobbit finds himself involved in adventures which are uncomfortable, exciting, and sometimes of epic proportions.

- CHARLOTTE'S WEB by E. B. White. Illustrated by Garth Williams (Harper)

    A story of Fern, the little girl, Wilbur the pig, and Charlotte the spider, written with humor and wisdom and overtones of mysticism.

"Realistic" Stories with Varied Settings

- THE WHEEL ON THE SCHOOL by Meindert De Jong. Illustrated by Maurice Sendak (Harper)

    The children of a little North Sea village in Holland search for a wheel on which the storks might nest.

*Horn Book, Inc., 31 St. James Avenue, Boston, MA 02116

- GONE-AWAY LAKE by Elizabeth Enright. Illustrated by Beth and Joe Krush (Harcourt)

    Two children discover an abandoned summer resort on the shores of a marsh which was once a lake.

- THE MOFFATS by Eleanor Estes, Author-Illustrator (Harcourt)

    The first of three books about an engaging family in a little Connecticut town in the Twenties.

- BLUE WILLOW by Doris Gates. Illustrated by Paul Lantz (Viking)

    Janey, a child of migratory workers in California, longs above everything else for a permanent home.

- MY SIDE OF THE MOUNTAIN by Jean George, Author-Illustrator (Dutton)

    A boy spends one complete year alone in the Catskills and proves to himself that he can live entirely off the land.

- HOMER PRICE by Robert McCloskey, Author-Illustrator (Viking)

    A typical American boy in a typical American small town has adventures which are far from typical in their humor and exaggeration.

- DAUGHTER OF THE MOUNTAINS by Louise Rankin. Illustrated by Kurt Wiese (Viking)

    A Tibetan girl leaves her home high in the Himalayas to search for her stolen dog.

- CRYSTAL MOUNTAIN by Belle Dorman Rugh. Illustrated by Ernest H. Shepard (Houghton)

    The setting is Lebanon, where English, American, and Lebanese children together solve a mystery.

- ROLLER SKATES by Ruth Sawyer. Illustrated by Valenti Angelo (Viking)

    Ten-year-old Lucinda on roller skates explores New York of the Nineties and makes many friends.

- BANNER IN THE SKY by James Ramsey Ullman (Lippincott)

    A Swiss boy has to struggle for what he believes is his inherent right—to be a mountaineer.

- LITTLE HOUSE IN THE BIG WOODS by Laura Ingalls Wilder. Illustrated by Garth Williams (Harper)

    The first of eight family stories drawn from the author's memories of her pioneer childhood.

Historical Fiction

- THE COURAGE OF SARAH NOBLE by Alice Dalgliesh. Illustrated by Leonard Weisgard (Scribner)

    After their log house in the wilderness is built, Sarah is left with the Indians while her father returns to the old home to get the rest of the family.

- CALICO BUSH by Rachel Field. Illustrated by Allen Lewis (Macmillan)

    A gently reared French girl arriving in the American colonies as an orphan becomes a "bound-out girl" on a Maine farm.

- JOHNNY TREMAIN by Esther Forbes. Illustrated by Lynd Ward (Houghton)

    The story of Revolutionary Boston is an integral part of the story of an orphan apprentice boy's growing up.

- ISLAND OF THE BLUE DOLPHINS by Scott O'Dell (Houghton)

    An Indian girl alone on a California island for eighteen years makes a life that has beauty and dignity.

- RANSOM FOR A KNIGHT by Barbara Leonie Picard. Illustrated by C. Walter Hodges (Walck)

    Two children have adventures and hardships as they journey across medieval England to ransom Alys' father from the Scots.

- THE BRONZE BOW by Elizabeth George Speare (Houghton)

    A story of Jesus' time and of a boy obsessed by hatred of the Romans.

- CALL IT COURAGE by Armstrong Sperry, Author-Illustrator (Macmillan)

    A South Sea Island boy sets off alone in a canoe to cure himself of his fear of the sea.

Organizations (See Appendix A)

American Library Association

Magazines (See Appendix B)

Career World

Children's Digest

Humpty Dumpty's Magazine for Little Children

LOVE

L

See also Emotional Development; Mental Health.

Roots of Love
Helene S. Arnstein
Bantam Books
1975   220 pp. $1.95

Arnstein concentrates on the feelings of infants, young children and parents, showing how the capacity to love and form human attachments develops. Love should be stressed in all activities, including control of anger, spanking, sex development, overcoming fears and guilts if parents divorce.

With all of this stimulating and playing, the baby also needs to have periods when he can play quietly in his crib or playpen with an object or two, or lie on his back and maybe kick or pull at some dangling toy. He does not need someone in the room all the time.

Being able to remain alone at times and not feel lonely is a great achievement, an asset for living itself. This capacity has its origins in early infancy, and starts out through the experience of "being alone." Although mother and child may not be exchanging words, the baby physically knows his mother is there emotionally as well as physically—even if she isn't constantly in the room.

SPOIL WITH LOVE

We used to think that a baby did not see or smile until he was three months old. Now we know that babies can see at birth. They can make eye contact within the first minutes after birth and react and interact with people from the very beginning of life. These early emotional and social interactions are the foundation for all other growth. All development is interdependent—intellectual capacity, emotional strength and physical development are interconnected.

First there has to be the trust and love that makes a child feel he is somebody special and that others care about him. Intellectual development follows this emotional security. Parents often worry about spoiling their baby, but we now know that the children who are most secure and confident are those who were responded to when they cried. They are the ones who are free and secure enough to reach out and explore the world independently. Those whose cries were unanswered often feel insecure and low in self-esteem. They are the ones who always check to see if mother is there before embarking on any activity.

There is no such thing as a spoiled baby. He has needs. Crying is the way he gets those needs met.

Therese Lansburgh
Maryland Committee for Children

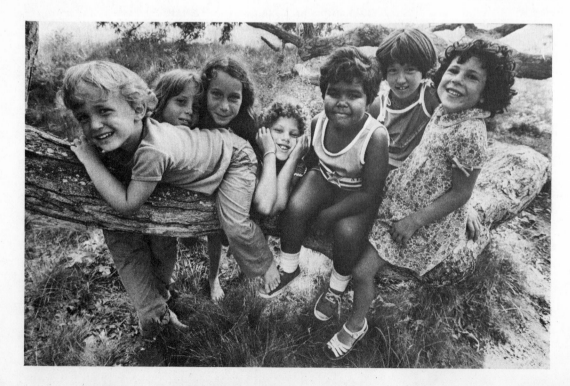

MARRIAGE AND SHARED ROLES

See also Fathering; Mothering; Parenting; Working and Family Life; and Part I—Sharing Roles/Working and Parenting.

Parents need to define and agree upon their respective responsibilities for their children. Responsibilities include attending to basic needs, such as care and feeding, as well as social trips and visits.

If you and your husband are divorced or separated, you should be able to arrange shared custody. Some people are able to do this by working out an amicable relationship after the separation. It is a good idea to share the responsibility, allowing the child some free time each week as well. Visitation rights also need to be worked out. Trying to develop a plan that works best for the children is essential.

Employed wives and husbands who want to work toward egalitarian role-sharing, may need, each, to define themselves and each other as competent both in paid work and in householder tasks.

What do we know of children who grow up in shared-role families? They do not see their two parents as neuter, or identical in their characteristic behaviors. Children of employed mothers are more likely to value both traditionally male and traditionally female characteristics, although on most measures they do not differ from the children of mothers who are not employed. We have little data, but there will soon be more answers because the topic is of considerable current interest.

Mary C. Howell
Helping Ourselves: Families and the Human Network
Beacon Press
1975   231 pp. $4.95

BALANCING ROLES

In the last few years there has been some pressure for men to change their family responsibilities. Much of the housework may be shared, paternity leaves have become more acceptable, and fathers probably do participate more in child care including diaper changing. Certain jobs still seem to remain mostly the province of the mother, unless the man is pressured into them. For instance, the managerial functions and the organization of the household are characteristically the woman's sphere. Men may be willing to do any specific household task and care for the children, but rarely of their own volition do they take over the coordination of children's social life, transportation, clothes shopping, or many of the decisions which determine the children's life-styles, and in a sense their standard of living. The school conferences with teachers may sometimes be attended by fathers, but it is the mother who is in touch with the details. If she is working, it is she who is expected to—and generally does—take the time off from work. Many women do not feel comfortable unless this is so, and exhaust themselves attempting to maintain full participation in both roles.

Malkah Notman
Psychiatrist

189

No-Fault Marriage
Marcia Lasswel and Norman M. Lobsenz
Ballantine
1976   278 pp. $1.95

This no-fault approach to marital problems provides guidelines to help eliminate defensiveness, to argue constructively and to recognize early warning signs. The book includes a six-stage program to reinstate lost intimacy, plus quizzes to help define trouble areas.

The essential element in marriage talk is the feeling behind the words.

Effective communication between spouses depends not so much on what is said as why and how it is said.

To hear beyond the words, to hear the emotion behind them, is basic to understanding what they actually mean. There are so many possible ways to react to another's remarks that we often respond inappropriately. The key to appropriate response is a single question that should always be asked—silently, if not openly: "Why are you telling me this?"

Magazines

MOMMA
Marriage and Family Living
Women Who Work
Working Mother
Working Woman

MENTAL HEALTH

See also Disabilities; Emotional Development.

What Every Child Needs for Better Mental Health

To grow healthy and strong, children should have good food, plenty of sleep, exercise and fresh air. Children have emotional needs, too. To have good health—to be both healthy and happy—all children require . . .

Love

Every child needs to feel

- loved and wanted
- that he matters very much to someone
- that there are people near him who care what happens to him

Security

Every child needs to know

- that her home is a good safe place she can feel sure about
- that her parents or other protective adults will always be on hand, especially in times of crisis when she needs them most
- that she belongs to a group; that there is a place where she fits in

Control

Every child needs to know

- that there are limits to what he is permitted to do and that he will be held to these limits
- that though it is all right to feel jealous or angry, he will not be allowed to hurt himself or others when he has these feelings

Acceptance

Every child needs to believe

- that she is liked for herself, just the way she is
- that she is liked all the time, and not only when she acts according to others' ideas of the way a child should act
- that she is *always* accepted, even though others may not approve of the things she does
- that she will be able to grow and develop in her own way

Guidance

Every child needs to have

- friendly help in learning how to behave toward persons and things
- adults around him who show him by example how to get along with others

Independence

Every child needs to know

- that she will be encouraged to try new things and to grow

Protection

Every child needs to feel

- that she will be kept safe from harm

Faith

Every child needs to have

- a set of moral standards to live by
- a belief in the human values—kindness, courage, honesty, generosity and justice

Publications Available

from your local Mental Health Association or from the National Headquarters of the Mental Health Association:*

- *Some Things You Should Know About Mental and Emotional Illness* (English and Spanish)
- *How to Deal with Mental Problems*
- *How to Deal with Your Tensions*
- *Mental Illness Can Be Prevented*
- *The High Cost of Mental Illness*
- *Mental Health Is 1, 2, 3* (English and Spanish)
- *Growing Up Ain't All That Easy*
- *Depression: What You Should Know About It*
- *A Child Alone in Need of Help*

(There is a slight charge for these publications. Contact the organization for prices.)

How to Find Help

There are a number of organizations in your community that can help you determine if you need assistance with a mental problem, and then help you find mental health services. They will vary from community to community, but at least one of them is sure to be in your area.

1. *Mental Health Association.* By its own description, "The Mental Health Association is a nationwide, voluntary, nongovernmental organization dedicated to the promotion of mental health, the prevention of mental illness and the improved care and treatment of the mentally ill. Its 850 chapters and divisions, and more than one million citizen volunteers, work toward these goals through a wide range of activities in social action, education, advocacy and information. If you need help, or can help others, get in touch with us."

   This group can give you information about mental health and mental illness, help you find services in your community that are best suited to you or the member of your family who needs help, or help you if you feel that you are not getting the kind of treatment you need. Mental Health Associations do not offer direct therapy services, but can refer you to the people in your community who do offer services. They know about the facilities that are available, and the fee schedule for each of them. There are about 1,000 Mental Health Associations across the country, in large cities and rural counties. Look in your phone book under Mental Health for your local Mental Health Association. If you are unable to locate a Mental Health Association in your community, you might contact the state Mental Health Association (they are usually located in the state capital) or The Mental Health Association at 1800 North Kent Street, Arlington, Virginia 22209.

2. *The Family Service Association of America* includes over three hundred agencies in large and medium-sized cities. Family Service agencies offer direct services for family problems such as marital difficulties, school drop-outs, emotionally disturbed parent or child, or other problems which seem to affect the entire family. The agencies operate on a sliding fee scale, based on a family's ability to pay. Look in your phone book under Family Service Association or contact their national office: Family Service Association of America at 44 East 23rd Street, New York, New York 10010.

3. The local branches of your American Psychiatric Association and American Psychological Association can help you find *psychiatrists* and *psychologists*. Your family doctor or the county medical society can put you in touch with the local branches of these organizations to help you find a psychiatrist or psychologist who would suit your needs. If you are unable to locate a local branch of these organizations, you might contact your Mental Health Association or the national offices of the two organizations. They are the American Psychiatric Association at 1700 18th Street, N.W., Washington, D.C. 20009 and the American Psychological Association at 1200 17th Street, N.W., Washington, D.C. 20036.

4. *Child Welfare Agencies* can refer you to appropriate resources and facilities in your community to help with child problems. Some child welfare agencies run day care or residential centers for emotionally disturbed children, but usually do not offer out-patient care.

5. Almost every community does have a mental health service that offers treatment on an out-patient basis. These in-

*The Mental Health Association, 1800 North Kent Street, Arlington, Virginia 22209

M clude psychiatric departments of general hospitals, community mental health centers, veterans' hospitals and clinics (for those eligible), and a wide variety of public and private out-patient clinics. There are about 2,250 of the latter across the country, along with about 600 community mental health centers. While the fees for these services vary, a great many of them, especially those which are operated by public funds, have a sliding fee scale, so that they may offer services to anyone in the community. Most of these services will offer emergency diagnostic out-patient treatment and referral services. Again, you can usually find these facilities through your telephone book under mental health, or the city or county health or mental health department. Another way to locate local services is to contact the state department of health or mental health in the state government.

Children At Risk
Gary A. Crow
Schocken Books
1978 280 pp. $13.95

A handbook for alerting teachers and parents to symptoms that point to difficulty in the lives of children aged five to eight, this book focuses on behavior problems that can almost always be pinpointed by specific signs or symptoms, such as temper tantrums, cruelty to animals, inability to follow simple instructions.

The principle is that some problems are only problems relative to the age of the child, while others are problems regardless of age. Generally, physical problems are not age related, while emotional, social and academic classroom problems or symptoms are. . . . A five-year-old may experience difficulty negotiating new relationships in the world of peers and playmates. Second and third graders, though, should be showing fairly good social skills and involvements. A five-year-old may become noticeably emotionally upset when mother leaves him or her at school. A seven-year-old, though, will usually involve himself or herself in school with some enthusiasm while mother remains at home, goes to work, or is involved in other activities.

Dibs—In Search of Self
Virginia M. Axline
Ballantine
1964 220 pp. $1.25

This is a moving story of a deeply disturbed child's emergence from darkness and confusion, describing the process of psychotherapy and Dibs' search for the beauty within.

As for Dibs' mother, it seemed to me that it was highly unlikely that she could have been unaware of her child's intellectual endowment—at least to some degree. Out of her total experience, intellectual achievement alone had not been a very satisfactory answer. Her failure to relate to her child with love, respect, and understanding was probably due to her own emotional deprivation. Who can love, respect, understand another person, if they have not had such basic experiences themselves? It seemed to me that it would be more helpful for her to have learned in this interview that she was respected and understood, even though that understanding was, of necessity, a more generalized concept which accepted the fact that she had reasons for what she did, that she had capacity to change, that changes must come from within herself, that all changes—hers, her husband's, Dibs'—were motivated by many accumulative experiences. How had she phrased it? "Two frightened, lonely, unhappy people with their defenses crumbled and deserted . . . a relief to know that we could be human, and could fail and admit that we had failed."

Help For Your Child
Sharon S. Brehm
Prentice-Hall
1978 165 pp. $4.95

In this useful book guiding parents to the mental-health services available for children from birth through adolescence, the author not only covers conditions such as autism and hyperactivity, but also explains how parents can determine if their child needs professional help and which type of facility (crisis center, private hospital, emergency room, etc.) best fits the child's needs.

Parents ask themselves, "At what point should I take my child to a mental health facility?" Children ask themselves, "Why are they taking me here?" And these concerns are just the beginning. Once the decision is made to go to a mental health facility, parents must try to find one. Once a facility is located and contact is made, parents and children may meet a variety of mental health professionals, and the variety itself can be quite bewildering. Many people do not know the difference between, for example, psychiatrists and psychologists; moreover, they aren't sure whether they need to know the difference.

Psychotherapy With Children
Clark E. Moustakas
Ballantine
1959   365 pp. $1.65

Moustakas records dialogues with normal, gifted, handicapped and disturbed children, describing the hidden world of children in crucial moments of psychic development.

Perhaps the most important aspect of the play therapy experience for the normal child is the concentrated relationship with the therapist. In the busy life of children the opportunity rarely exists to be alone for one hour with an adult once or twice a week. Furthermore it is rare for a child to have a relationship in which he is the center of the experience, where he can express his feelings and be understood as a person, where the adult is fully attending the child, watching, listening, making statements of recognition, and being present in a deeply human sense.

Signals—What Your Child is Really Telling You
Paul Ackerman and Murray Kappelman
Dial Press
1978   281 pp. $8.95

Temper tantrums, school phobia and frequent physical complaints are signals—that is, messages to parents from their children that special attention is needed. The authors provide a guide to help parents identify the message and act on it in a loving and constructive way.

Lies can produce results! Children know this: you must be prepared to ask yourself a very sensitive question after your child has lied to you: "Is my child looking for something from me? Attention? Praise? Recognition? Have I given this 'something' in the past, when my child has lied to me?"

Children, You Are Very Little
Betsy Drake Grant
Atheneum
1971   245 pp. $6.95

This is a novel about the discovery of life's wonders and cruelties from the point of view of a nine-year-old girl. Set in New York, New England and Virginia, the heroine attempts to survive the trauma of an emotionally disturbed family.

Now Lucia knew how to approach Henrietta, because Henrietta would love being part of a happy family so pleased to be back together. Henrietta could bring her baby, when it was born, and they could all live happily, rolling around. They could take baths together or play hide and seek, or take turns washing the baby squeaking in the bathtub, or Daddy could hide surprises, and they could follow a secret thread that went around and behind things, over and under up down finally leading to Mother, who would say, "Good night, I'm in a good mood tonight, and love you very much." She'd turn out the light. "Sweet dreams, sweet child, my dearest child." And there would be peace.

Organizations (See Appendix A)

National

American Association of Marriage and Family Counselors

Black Child Development Institute

Council for Exceptional Children

Jewish Board of Family and Children's Services

National Institute of Mental Health

National Society for Autistic Children

U.S. Department of Health and Human Services

Local:

Bananas Child Care Information Service

Children's Council of San Francisco

Devereux Foundation

Erikson Institute for Early Education

Parents Preschool Resource Centre of the National Capitol Region

MONEY

Children learn the value of money at an early age. They learn to save and spend, depending on their early experiences. Earning money is a good way for children to learn how to obtain and save money for their own uses. Allowances are also a good way to help children budget for their needs.

The Consumer Union of the United States has recently begun publishing a magazine called *Penny Power*, which was created to assist children in their understanding of money. Articles appear on many topics of interest. (Write to *Penny Power*, 256 Washington St., Mount Vernon, NY 10550 for more information.)

Children and Money
Grace W. Weinstein
Schocken Books
1976   224 pp. $2.50

From infancy through adolescence, America's children spend enormous amounts of money.

Weinstein explains how parents can teach the principles of budgeting and setting priorities, and help children view money as a tool and not as a symbol of love or security. Chapters deal with such topics as the impact of advertising on children, children's use of credit, the temptation to shoplift and the difference between males and females in handling money.

A school psychologist in Connecticut tells of an unhappy fourteen-year-old who . . . has saved seven hundred dollars of her babysitting money toward college, but knows nothing at all about spending. When she wants to buy her mother a birthday present she flounders with not the least idea what things cost or how to shop. "She squeezes the dollar," says the psychologist, "it's a mystical thing to her. But it would be better if she understood money as a practical tool, something to be used in daily life, not something which exists for itself alone.

Good Cents
Amazing Life Games
Houghton Mifflin
1979   128 pp. $7.95/$3.95

An excellent source of information for children on the subject of money and handling it.

MORAL DEVELOPMENT AND VALUES

Children easily make mistakes. The way in which you respond to the mistakes is important in helping a child develop to the next level of understanding. When a child lies, you need to realize he may be afraid of being punished. It is necessary to show him what has happened and suggest what he

might do. Your support will make a big difference in expanding his ability to be honest and fair. It is important that you explain values to your child and show him the difference between right and wrong.

Allow your child to assist you with different jobs. Make sure he gets his job completed. Give him lots of praise. Give him activities that he can do and feel good about. Do not over criticize your child. Make sure that you provide opportunities geared to his own individual ability. Give the child a variety of things to do. Give him the opportunity to earn and save money and point out the value of giving you honest answers. Use punishment sparingly. Allow your child to express his feelings. Reward the behavior that you want the child to continue and try to ignore that which you would like to change. Establish limits and make sure you enforce them. Show respect for your child. Be sure you talk nurturingly to your child.

Anticipate problems beforehand and try to divert your child's attention. Set a limit when necessary and stick to what you say you are going to do. Help your child expand his vocabulary and show him how things work. The most important thing is to have energy, patience, the ability to enjoy your children and to encourage your children to get along with each other.

Obviously, not all children get along with each other all of the time. Brothers and sisters learn to cope with the rest of the world by fighting often with each other. Sometimes they are in competition with each other and you can reduce the amount of conflict and stress. Sometimes they are merely out of sorts; they are tired or hungry or have shared too much

time together. It is important before a second child is born to have the older child know he is not going to lose your attention. Each child is different and unique. The age of your child and his position in the family is going to make a difference, so you should not compare your children with each other. Spend time with each child individually. Give each child equal opportunity for responsibility and special attention. Develop respect for your children by letting them have their own place and time. Allow your children to solve their own disagreements unless one is getting bullied by an older one.

Helping Your Child Learn Right from Wrong
Sidney B. Simon and Sally W. Olds
Simon & Schuster
1976   220 pp. $7.95

This book is a collection of aids to help parents find the values they want to impart to their children. Through gamelike experiments, the authors strive to show parents how to teach children to determine their own values concerning such things as money, love, friendship, work, honesty and responsibility. Chapters stress teaching children to examine life rationally, weigh alternatives and foresee consequences.

A child learns more by making the wrong decision by himself than by making the right one because we told him to. . . . If Denise ignores her social studies report and fails the course; if Eli loses a valued friendship because he went to the ball game—then these children will be learning far more than they could ever learn from all our advice and admonitions.

The classroom or the home with several children provides opportunity to have the child participate in positive acts toward others. This can be done independent of development of moral thought, but moral reasoning will advance more smoothly and quickly when children have concrete experiences to discuss and can relate these experiences to the concepts proposed in later lessons. Such acts would include sharing, working with others, completing work already started, and helping to attend to others' injuries, either psychological or emotional.

My Mother/My Self
Nancy Friday
Delacorte Press
1977   475 pp. $9.95
Dell Publishing
1978   475 pp. $2.50

Today, when mothers are involved in more than one job, children need more than one mother. Not just someone who sits with them as coldly as a television set, but a person to whom they feel free to turn, who will be there for them, and from whom they can openly take in warmth without feeling they are making mother jealous. Young women, particularly, are going through great changes in manners, mores and expectancies; they need all the love

they can find from as many different people as possible; they need access to a variety of role models other than mother.

M

That's Not Fair—Helping Children Make Moral Decisions
Larry C. Jensen
Brigham Young University Press
1977   177 pp. $6.95

For parents and teachers of kindergarten and first-grade children, this book provides specific instructional goals and techniques to help direct moral development while focusing on how children's concepts and goals emerge. It offers aids to cope with aggression, discipline, sharing and respecting others' property.

MOTHERING

See also Marriage and Shared Roles; Parenting; Single Parents; Working and Family Life; Part I—Sharing Roles/Working and Parenting.

Mothers and fathers play a crucial role in the development of their children, but because mothers so often spend more time with their children, it is they who determine their baby's emotional and social response. Usually, if a mother is happy and supportive of her baby, the child will tend to be more open and responsive to others. Because mothers usually form this first emotional bond for their children, they need all the support they can get from the extended family to enable them to express their nurturing feelings. These feelings and attachments to the child are not necessarily innate in all mothers and often must be developed over time.

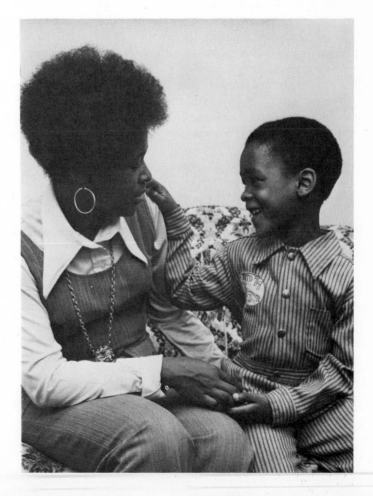

THE GENTLE REVOLUTION

Mothering is the world's oldest profession.

A group of mothers at our center recently were deeply concerned about the apparent collapse of the school system so evident on every hand. These mothers, quietly, individually, but in ever-increasing numbers decided simply to take matters into their own hands. Their husbands quietly agreed. Neither the school systems, the Parent-Teacher Associations nor the school boards of the Action Committees seemed able to do more than to stem the tide of ever more expensive and ever less productive schooling.

They decided that they would be, not just mothers, but Professional Mothers.

And it was about this time that their gentle revolution discovered the other gentle revolution. The results have been truly incredible.

When this new kind of mother discovered that they could not only teach their babies to read, but to teach them better and easier at two years of age than the school system was doing at seven, they got the bit firmly in their teeth—and a new and almost indescribably delightful world opened up. A world of mothers, fathers and kids. It has within it the potential to change the world, in a very short time and almost infinitely for the better.

This handful of young, bright and eager mothers, who happened to live near Philadelphia, discovered The Evan Thomas Institute, which is one of The Institutes for the Achievement of Human Potential, and The Evan Thomas Institute discovered them. Together they taught their babies to read, superbly in English and adequately in two or three other languages. They taught the kids to do math at a rate that left them agog and in shocked but delighted disbelief. They taught their one-, two- and three-year-olds to absorb encyclopedic knowledge of birds, flowers, insects, trees, presidents, flags, nations, geography and a host of other things. They taught them to do Olympic routines on balance beams, to swim and to play the violin.

In short they found that they could teach their tiny children absolutely anything which they could present to them in an honest and factual way.

Most important of all, they found that by doing so, they had multiplied their babies' intelligence.

Most interesting of all, they found that doing so was, for them and for their babies, the most delightful experience they had ever enjoyed together. Their love for each other and perhaps even more important, their respect for each other, multiplied.

Not only was it true that mothering was the oldest profession, but it was also true that mothers have been the first teachers and they remain the best. It was mothers, after all who had brought us from the Australopithecine caves to the Age of Reason. One wonders if we professionals, who brought us from the Age of Reason to the Atomic Age (in itself a questionable bit of progress) are going to take the world as far in the next hundred thousand years as the mothers have brought us in the last. How then were our new Professional Mothers different from the mothers who had always been?

They were different in two ways. My own mother and father seem to me to be typical. They had raised their own children, of whom I am the oldest, with profound love and with an intuitive balance of just the right mixture of parental spoiling and parental discipline. They had, however, done so at great personal sacrifice and had found *their* reward solely in vicarious appreciation of *our* personal progress.

To those ancient virtues and intuitions our Professional Mothers had added two new dimensions. Those dimensions were professional knowledge of what they were doing, added to ancient intuition, and taking their pleasure now, in the doing, added to the vicarious pleasures to come later.

I looked around me at the mothers, now seated with me in the advanced math room. No drudgery here among these young and glowing mothers. They had still to deal with dirty diapers and household chores as had my own mother. But no longer did they face a lifetime which had only such chores to offer. Not by a long shot. At a time of life which had been my mother's peak, their life was, in a very real sense, just beginning.

Glenn Doman
Educator

Every Child's Birthright: In Defense of Mothering
Selma Fraiberg
Basic Books
1977   156 pp. $8.95
Bantam Books
1979   154 pp. $2.50

Intelligence, a sense of identity and the ability to make genuine connection with other human beings all depend upon a bond of love between the infant and a person committed to giving it nurture.

As more and more mothers of young babies go to work, the author fears the infants' need for love is not being met. In this slim but important volume, the author argues for restoring infants' birthright of maternal care. Human attachments in infancy, as well as the effects of such conditions as poverty on human bonds, are discussed.

During the first six months, the baby has the rudiments of a love language available to him. There is the language of the embrace, the language of the eyes, the language of the smile, vocal communications of pleasure and distress. It is the essential vocabulary of love before we can speak of love. Eighteen years later, when this baby is full grown and "falls in love" for the first time, he will woo his partner through the language of the eyes, the language of the smile, through the utterance of endearments, and the joy of the embrace. In his declarations of love he will use such phrases as "When I first looked into your eyes," "When you smiled at me," "When I held you in my arms." And naturally, in his exalted state, he will believe that he invented this love song.

MOMMA
The Sourcebook for Single Mothers
Karol Hope and Nancy Young
New American Library
1976   388 pp. $3.95

This sourcebook is a natural outgrowth of the MOMMA organization, sharing all the helpful, practical information so crucial to the survival of the single mother—the day-by-day things that a woman can do to put her life, and her children's lives, back together. This book contains interviews with and statements from single mothers all over the country.

When the house is full of people, children, adults, into things, talking, moving around, I sometimes get lost in all the activity. I get absorbed in what we're all doing—ninety million demands from ninety million directions. But when I get off alone, close the door, I have a chance to be with myself. I lie on my bed and think, or read, without distraction, get a real sense of myself. And then I can spend time with one or a couple of kids privately, really concentrate on them.

Mothercraft
Margaretta Lundell
Simon & Schuster
1975   151 pp. $4.95

The classic mothercraft tools assembled in this volume date back to the pre–World War I era and include recipes and household suggestions designed to help a mother save her energy and yet have a sense of accomplishment at the end of the day. The author recaptures the older, slower sense of mothering calm while retaining the benefits of twentieth-century education, technology and change.

Aside from the nutritional aspect, constantly depending on pre-packaged and frozen foods robs a child of a learning experience. Stirring canned beans is not very interesting. But if a mother is snapping real beans, she can show the child the stalk end, how to break off the tips and snap in the middle. The helper may decide to become a bean thief, popping uncooked pieces into his mouth when she isn't looking. He offers one to the cat, or builds a log house of beans. He laughs and learns. Even though he is slowing down the process, his mother laughs with him.

Mothering
Rudolph Schaffer
Harvard University Press
1977   120 pp. $2.95

The infant is an active participant in continuous behavioral interchanges between itself and mother. The essence of good mothering lies not in rigid schedules but in the sensitivity the mother brings to her part in the mother-child dialogue.

Do babies need mothers? Yes—if it means that they need to be involved in a love relationship, that satisfaction of their physical wants alone is not enough. No—if it means that mother must be the one who gave birth, that no other person can take her place. No again—if we take mother to involve an exclusive care relationship that must encapsulate the child's total social and emotional life; on the contrary, there are many arguments for allowing a child to widen his interpersonal horizon from the beginning and for not discouraging other attachments. And finally yes—if we mean that a limited range of familiar people should provide consistent care throughout the years of childhood.

M

Mothering: The Emotional Experience of Motherhood After Freud and Feminism
Elaine Heffner
Doubleday
1978   177 pp. $7.95

A strong case is made here for the role of mothering as a professional choice. To make the difference in a human life is a significant accomplishment, one deserving of self-esteem and the esteem of others. Motherhood today has been shaped by psychoanalytic theory, which gave mothers the responsibility of raising healthy children without teaching them how to achieve that, and by the women's movement, which sought to rescue women from this plight by liberating them without helping them to be successful at both roles.

While staying in charge of her child's development, a mother learns to stay in charge of herself. She learns to see herself as an adult and to accept adult responsibilities. She develops independence of thought and the capacity to function as an effective force in the world beyond the nursery. She strengthens her understanding of human behavior and of the nature of human interactions. Strengthened in this way, she is well equipped to meet whichever of life's challenges await her. She is no longer a helpless child-mother. She is her person—and a mother.

Survival Handbook for Preschool Mothers
Helen Wheeler Smith
Follett Publishing
1978   161 pp. $2.95

Surviving the preschool years is the main topic of this book for mothers, which stresses a positive approach to parenting in dealing with problems such as sibling rivalry and temper tantrums. The emphasis throughout is on the im-portance of the mother-child interaction in the molding of self-sufficient and creative children.

A child's attitude toward life and learning is formed by the reactions of his parents. When he pulls all the pans out of the cupboard and his mother smiles and says, "What have you found?" he will feel very different than if she scolds, "You're making a mess." This is the period when he learns that curiosity is good or bad. If it's bad, learning is thwarted.

Woman At Home
Arlene Rossen Cardozo
Doubleday
1976   156 pp. $6.95

This book shows women how to integrate personal interests and activities into a total life scheme without working outside the home. Topics include liberating oneself from being the family servant, trading services with neighbors and establishing personal relationships with each child.

Who is most qualified to raise a woman's child? She is. What qualified her? Those parts of her which are unique to her. Every woman is a specialist in the area of raising her child—whether she knows it or not—because of her special background, interests, and heritage, which are hers to transmit to her children. The best schools, the most expensive lessons, do no good if later on a woman says, "I can't talk with my children, yet I've done everything for them."

Magazines
(See Appendix B)

Handbook for Working Women
MOMMA
Mothering
Mother's Manual
Women Who Work
Working Mother
Working Woman
Young Mother

MOVING

Moving from one residence to another can be traumatic for a child, as it involves separation. This separation from roots and ties to others needs to be planned, discussed and implemented with the child involved, if possible. Try to have special items belonging to your child to be transported by him. For example, a special stuffed animal can travel on your child's lap. The toys in your four-year-old's room can be boxed by him. He might even draw a picture on the box so he will recognize which is his when he arrives at the new house. There are many such techniques you can use to help your child through this period.

If your move is local, visit the new neighborhood and nearby houses. You might find a neighbor with children the same age as yours. If you're like many of us, that's one of the criteria for a new home—to find a neighborhood with children for yours to play with. Your child might find a new friend to look forward to being with. That will make the move much easier for all of you.

It is important to recognize that your child will need to have his feelings about the move recognized and supported. He will probably have some of the same feelings you have. Working this through together can be an opportunity to grow closer.

For Children

I'm Moving
Martha Whitmore Hickman
Abingdon
1974   27 pp. $5.25

Written for the school-age child whose family is soon to move, this book gives parents ideas on how to make moving a positive adventure.

The moving man left us some boxes folded flat. After he was gone, my mother and I sat on the pile of boxes and talked some more about the moving. I asked her if we would take everything with us, and she said, "Almost everything." We'd take my dresser, but not my closet. We'd take my rug, but not my floor. We'd take my bike, but not my sidewalk. We'd take my baby brother, but not my friend Jimmy. We'd take my turtle, but not the squirrel that eats at the windowsill. We'd take my sandbox, but not my apple tree.

City, Sing for Me; A Country Child Moves to the City
Jane Jacobson
Human Sciences Press
1978   32 pp. $6.95

When Jenny's family moves from a rural environment to the city, Jenny, like many school-age youngsters, feels anxious displacement in her new neighborhood. The contrast between the peace of the country and the chaos of the city is awesome, and her first experience outside is frightening. On the way home, while frantically seeking the right apartment building, Jenny meets Rosa, a young native urbanite. A series of charming episodes follows as Rosa endeavors to give Jenny the necessary street-smarts.

They were greeted by another fabulous smell. It was from a store that had cheeses and smoked fish and sausage and pickles. Rosa called the store a Deli, short for Delicatessen.

"Let's go in," Jenny sighed.

"I take you to see the sights and you just smell the smells," Rosa laughed.

Inside the Deli, they discovered the pickles floating in a big wooden barrel with a heavy lid. They lifted the lid a crack and whiffed the most fabulous whiffs. And Rosa whiffed with her.

"I'll get one of those pickles, girls, if you want," a woman said. Jenny and Rosa could hardly see her. She was hidden behind a row of sausages that hung from the ceiling, and a case of cheeses that stacked under the counter.

"We're just smelling them," Rosa said.

MUSIC. SEE CREATIVE EXPRESSION.

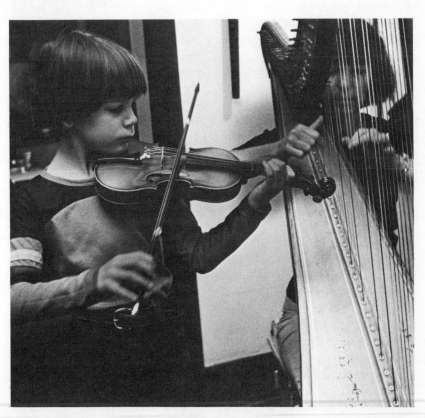

N

NURSERY AND PRE-SCHOOL CARE

See also Child Care; Education; Playing.

Nursery school or preschool provides an important opportunity for children to socialize with other children and to have a first comfortable school experience away from home, in an environment designed for use by young children with trained, experienced teachers and administrators. Preschool is a wonderful place for children to have fun, learn and grow, explore and begin to develop their potential in a supportive environment. It is very advantageous for children to have exposure to the kind of learning that takes place in a preschool, preparing children for later education in elementary school. Children are usually between three and five years of age in these programs. Programs are usually three hours in length. Most preschools confine hours to mornings as young children often nap in the early afternoon.

Preschools may be offered as part of a comprehensive program to serve families and children by a community center, a city recreation program or a child-care center. These programs must meet government regulations, which vary depending upon who is sponsoring the school and who is paying for the program. Quality of

staff, space, quality of program, safety and health are among the important issues, which vary with federal, state, county and local regulations. For example, in California, a school does not have to adhere to state regulations unless it is accepting state funds. This exemption may affect the quality of city-sponsored preschool offered through the recreation or leisure offices.

It is most important to visit many programs before making your selection. Don't be intimidated by who sponsors it. Look for quality that meets your child's needs. There may be a variety of programs to choose from, if you are lucky. Some federally sponsored programs may include Head Start, Title Twenty funded programs, as well as others with demonstration programs for special groups.

Some states provide funding for programs. For information, contact your state welfare department or state department of education. Counties and cities may also provide programs. Check with your local information and referral office or your elected official's office. They will usually be happy to provide you with such information.

Private agencies and religious groups also sponsor preschools. Check your local telephone directory for information.

All programs, regardless of who is funding or sponsoring them, have some requirements. While some charge full fees, others charge on a sliding scale and still others do not charge much but require your participation in the program. Requirements change from time to time. For example, you may not have been eligible for a program in the past due to income, and may be eligible now due to change in the sliding scale.

For Children

Betsy's First Day At Nursery School
Gunilla Walde
Random House
1976   24 pp. $1.95

This book is intended to be read aloud to young children encountering day-care for the first time. It has an entertaining text and funny, colorful illustrations.

When they get to nursery school, Robert says hello to them. Mommy and baby brother say hello. But Betsy doesn't want to . . . because all of the other children are staring at her. Betsy keeps her snowsuit on while Robert shows them around the school. One of the rooms has lots of pillows to jump on. Betsy would like to jump on them, but she doesn't know any of the children who are playing there.

For Parents

Living with Preschoolers
Willard Abraham
O'Sullivan, Woodside
1976   145 pp. $3.95

In this commonsense book to help parents better understand their children and their children's needs, the author discusses discipline and punishment as well as creativity in children. In various chapters the author tackles such problems parents face as watching television, coping with death and how to change the behavior of young children.

If your child is mildly hyperactive preschool encouragement and supervised play may be helpful. If severely hyperactive, you shouldn't expect teachers to provide one-to-one help. You'll need the necessary combination of medical, psychological and psychiatric support. Your doctor may be the one with whom to start.

However, the first approach to the problem should begin even earlier, at home. Among the specific things you can provide are these:

—A structured routine of dressing, meals, and cleanliness.

—His room kept in order, with your help.

—Tasks at which he can succeed, and rewards when he is successful.

—Consistent discipline that makes sense to him.

—Time your schedule alone with him.

—A substitute for mother or father if either one is missing.

—A record of your child's behavior; when, where and under what circumstances does the hyperactivity occur?

Parent Guidance in the Nursery School
Margarete Ruben
International Universities Press
1973   72 pp. $1.95

This handbook applies psychoanalytic educational principles to specific problems of preschoolers, utilizing nontechnical language to solve such common problems as thumbsucking, aggression, jealousy, masturbation, etc.

Children, growing up, cannot assimilate their total environment all at once. They take in bits and pieces of the world in digestible amounts. Often the mind distorts the facts into forms acceptable to the child in terms of his own past experiences, feelings, or wishes. These distortions are perfectly logical to the childish mind.

Parents As Playmates
Joan Millman and Polly Behrmann
Human Sciences Press
1979   139 pp. $8.95

This delightful book provides parents with a wide variety of creative and educational activities which can be shared and enjoyed with pre-school children. These entertaining games not only turn trying times into enriching ones but they stimulate children to exercise their imagination and learning potential at the same time they are having fun.

Ask your child to try to describe his own feelings: How do you feel when you walk past a beautiful garden? How does it feel to watch the sun go down? What do you think about when you see so many people hurrying home? What does it make you feel like to stretch your neck to look up to the top of the highest building? What are you thinking when you look down at that tiny ant burdened with food for her family?

Pre-School Play
Kenneth Jameson and Pat Kidd
Van Nostrand Reinhold
1974   111 pp. $7.95

The authors give suggestions for offering children the magic of real play. They cover activities ranging from arts and crafts to cooking, music and storytelling. Designed for children in a group, the book can also be applied by parents in a home environment.

As for constructors, the mechanics, the imaginative children, they will need no prompting to join things together to make things. They will, however, benefit if they are shown how adhesive works. A technical tip of this kind helps and is valid, but let the adult's intervention stop there. If the play-leader is tempted to go further and show the child how to make a lighthouse out of a toilet roll middle the effect will be self-defeating. We do not want to see how well a child can copy the adult. We want to release the individual inventiveness of each child. If we cause him to imitate we put him in a straitjacket and prevent the free flow of his own imagination, and he may become dependent upon the adult for a lead every time.

Your Pre-School Child—Making the Most of the Years Two to Seven
Dorothy Kirk Burnett
MacFadden-Bartell Corp.
1971   256 pp. $.60

Written by a mother who has been meeting the challenges of her own preschoolers with energy, ingenuity and good cheer, this book provides ideas for toys, games, crafts and rainy-day activities. This book also includes a list of recommended reading.

Although we acknowledge cabin fever, or too much closeness, in almost every kind of living, we still expect children to live, eat, sleep, play and be with each other (and us!) twenty-four hours, seven days, fifty-two weeks per year without contracting this malady.

O

ONLY CHILD

More and more couples are making the decision to raise a single offspring, but few have any knowledge of how difficult it can be to grow up as an only child. Only children do not have to be the self-absorbed, overprivileged child of popular myth if parents are prepared for the pressures and pitfalls and learn to avoid them.

Unique problems do exist and can have severe behavioral consequences if they are improperly handled. They are the overconcentration of parental focus and expectation, the child's sense of hav-

ing constantly to choose one parent over the other, the missing companionship and loyalty of another nonadult, the need to invent peers to love and punish and otherwise practice living with, to name a few.

Play groups are an excellent resource for the single-child family. When your child is ready for preschool, a cooperative nursery school is excellent. It provides your child with companionship and opportunities to practice socialization skills. It also gives you the opportunity to work with other children and develop a better sense of who your child is and who you are as a parent. It can be a

wonderful support system for parents.

Raising the Only Child
Murray Kappelman
New American Library
1975   164 pp. $1.75

A comprehensive guide to raising an only child, including benefits and drawbacks for parents or potential parents to consider. Some areas covered are the advantages, disadvantages and problems faced such as sex education, exaggerated independence, extreme dependence, divorce or death of a parent, social interaction and other areas of concern.

How often have I been asked by only children whose parents literally paralyzed their own growth in order to be totally accessible, "Doctor, when will they ever wise up?" They're still living twenty years ago. Sadly, the only child is right; the parents have stunted their own lives through their misguided dependency on their children for stimulation and nourishment.

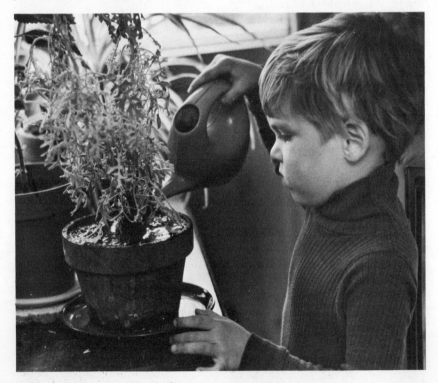

PARENTING

See also Family; Fathering; Marriage and Shared Roles; Mothering; Working and Family Life; and Part I—Sharing Roles/Working and Parenting.

A child is a person full of many wonders and ideas.

A child can express and reason in family discussions and decisions.

A child is a person worthy of the warmth of love and affection.

A child should be taken seriously, respecting his desires and dislikes.

A child is a person who shouldn't be pushed in a direction that he doesn't think he would enjoy or be happy in.

A child is a person who learns from the surroundings he lives in,

And those surroundings should be of love, trust and understanding.

Parenting is the art of creating an environment for children that allows them to grow into wholesome and healthy adults. Parents have an enormous reponsibility to provide for all the basic needs of children who are totally dependent upon them, at least for the first ten years of their lives. Parenting re-

quires patience, understanding and knowledge. Parenting is the recognition by each individual of his or her responsibility to protect, care for and nurture the young. One does not need to have conceived a baby in order to be a good parent. One does not even have to have children to be a good parent. One can provide parenting support or parenting feelings by caring for the children of a relative or friend. Parenting is a specialty which carries with it many responsibilities, and it is important to provide information to parents.

Parenting Guidelines

Here are some guidelines to follow with your child: Children need a balance of experiences and educational opportunities. They need freedom, structure and support. Let your child know how you feel and give her the opportunity to have her own experiences. She needs reassurance and control. A child's dependency is greater when she is under four years of age. After four, it is important that you do not reject your child, become too aggressive, express things too strongly, or overprotect your child. You want your child to build trust, explore her own ideas, develop her curiosity and ability to try new things. Do not reject or

punish in a way which might affect how she feels about herself. Threats, physical punishment or deprivation of privileges are all tools to get what you want, but be cautious about using them. Try to be consistent, reasonable and loving to your child.

Try to explain things before they become a problem. Explain why you think something is important and let your child understand the consequences. Be realistic. Set clear standards. Allow your child to have freedom, and show respect for your child. Give your child the opportunity to explore his own or her ideas and activities.

Parent Relationships

Parents need to continue their close adult relationship after a child is born. They need to work continually on enriching their own relationship without either losing identity to the other, and in mutual appreciation and support.

Children are usually able to delay their need for gratification, though many parents never test this. Demands may be made for "Juice now!" or "I want that toy and I want it now." Other familiar ones are "I want to sleep with you tonight" and "why can't I come too?" What often happens is that parents' needs take a back seat to

P the instant needs expressed by their children. This martyrdom can be habit-forming and grow to include others outside the immediate family. It is important for parents and prospective parents to be aware of this process. Those who sacrifice their own relationships and communication for what they consider the good of the child may ultimately be sacrificing their lifetime relationship with their partner.

The needs of children are not to be dismissed; they are to be recognized for what they really are and then put into your priorities. If you do this, you will be enriching your child by modeling healthy, thoughtful decision making, not decision making from guilt or desperation.

Parents should have, as needed, opportunities for time away from their children, time alone and individual time with their children. Time spent alone with a child can be an enriching experience. It gives you an opportunity, depending upon the activity you two choose to engage in, to listen to your child's expansion of her concepts of how her world works.

Some Tips for Parents

- Recognize and respect that each child is different in abilities.
- Allow each child to feel good about his or her uniqueness.
- Set reasonable limits.
- Mean what you say and don't threaten your child.
- Assist child to understand himself and others.

- Provide support through praise, encouragement and understanding.
- Provide many varied opportunities to learn. Recognize that your child will have many teachers including those in school, other relatives and friends and others in your community.
- Assist child to learn self-help skills—putting away toys, clean-up, preparation of parts of meals, setting table, and cleaning room.
- Make child safety-conscious and as he or she grows, to understand what to do in emergencies.
- Encourage child to read and enjoy learning of all kinds. Listen to child read aloud.
- Provide reassurance and praise.
- Provide learning experiences which reinforce and extend concepts pertaining to self, growth and development, disease, dental and physical health.
- Provide opportunities for the child to reflect upon what he is seeing, hearing and reading. Expose him to a variety of sights, sounds, books and people. Be available when he desires to share his concerns and questions.
- Give child encouragement as he faces new situations. Offer quiet guidance and praise. Avoid embarrassing him unnecessarily. Be sincere, reasonable and honest in relationship with him.
- Be tolerant of feelings of the child. Act as a listener and clarifier of emotions.

- Be specific in establishing responsibilities with the child. Guide him in the right directions. Encourage and support him as he endeavors to meet objectives.
- Expose child to a variety of peers from which to select friends. Provide opportunities for child to socialize.
- Recognize need for some children to be alone. Be alert to child who needs help in becoming a member of a group. Encourage participation in group activities but do not demand it.
- Provide opportunities for child to "let off steam" but pace activities so he does not get overstimulated.
- Plan for learning experiences in crafts and shop work.
- Be accepting, encouraging and appreciative of child and his efforts.
- Enrich conversations through stimulating experiences.
- Help child discriminate between justifiable and unfair criticism. Teach child how to express constructive criticism.
- Discuss with the child the things he hears to help him interpret and clarify his impressions.

CONSCIOUS PARENTING

Conscious parents are responsible adults. They have completed the transition from childhood and adolescence—from looking to another adult for nurturance, approval, and caring—to real adulthood in which they have assumed these functions for themselves, hopefully improving on their original models in the process. They live in nourishing, harmonious, and non-judgmental relationships with themselves and are able to extend this way of relating to others.

People mature by developing an awareness of, and responsiveness to, their own feelings and needs. Conscious adults treat themselves with love and deep respect and speak to themselves with kind, caring inner voices. They use their "inner critics" to review and to evaluate what they do, in order to learn, not to judge themselves. Conscious adults who are parents treat their children with the same respect and awareness. They are alert and alive, willing to be responsible and response-able with their children.

Responsible parents have established credibility, trustworthiness, accountability, involvement, and commitment. They do what they say they will do within defined time and situational boundaries, are aware of their power and carry out their obligations. They are honest and direct, emotionally engaging and understanding. They see their children as separate people and are willing to fight for the right of these small human beings to experience directly life's vagaries and riches. They allow their children to speak for themselves, to voice their feelings and needs in the absence of critical judgments or insensitive ears.

Conscious parents also are "response-able": able to respond to people and to life as it ebbs and flows about them. They are present. People who keep emotional and other "business" up to date are less likely to be distracted from fully attending to present experience than are people who are struggling with yesterday's conflicts or tomorrow's expectations. When commitments have been fulfilled, people are more aware of their current feelings and their responses are likely to be appropriate and satisfying. Children can observe in their parents and experience in themselves the freedom, exuberance, and assurance which come from "being" in the present, trusting their feelings and the responses which stem from them.

On the other hand, when people are encumbered by unfinished "business"—emotional and otherwise—they are less free to respond to a here-and-now exchange. Flooded with demands, they may shift off center and blame others for their felt pressures. When children witness such behavior, they learn that the center of responsibility is exterior to the person, and therefore do not become responsible themselves.

The freedom to be and to explore is essential to conscious parenting. This freedom is for both parents *and* children. Parents need to develop a sense of what is important in their own lives, to maintain a balance between fulfilling their own needs and meeting the needs of their children. This is not easy! Ultimately, conscious parenting means not giving in totally to your children all the time and also not going with your own needs all the time at the children's expense.

> Barbara Biggs and Gary Felton,
> Parent Educators

VALUE OF PARENTS

Between parents and children there evolves a reciprocal humanizing relationship. A parent helps a child sustain himself or herself in an unfamiliar world, helps a child learn to moderate impulses and move away from egocentrism, helps a child achieve a sense of personal identity and integrity, and helps a child find loving bonds with others. And that is precisely what a child also does for a parent, even though each differs in behavior, roles, responsibilities and levels of consciousness.

Certainly, there are burdens in living with a child. There is a period of prolonged dependency which makes it difficult for parents to always do what they want. Sacrifices in time, money and space, including some psychic space, may have to be made. There is the keen, continual anxiety as to whether even our best efforts are good enough for this new person we are to guide through childhood. But the exchange is wondrous and weighted on the side of parents. Their child thinks of them as the most important people in the universe. No one else will ask them how many grains of sand there are in a play pail, or ask if they stay up all night, will they be able to see the stars move in the skies? No one else will turn to them for answers about what is a rainbow or where does a sound go when you don't hear it any more? No one else will ever believe what they say in the same way that a child does.

> Olympia D. Tresmontan
> Teacher/Therapist

P

Conferences for Parents

Many communities plan parent days, or special meetings. These days there are often opportunities to hear speakers, to look at exhibits of materials and to talk with one another. Having a parent conference in your community can be an exciting way to come together and learn more about parenting and resources.

Perhaps an author of one of the books that is presented in this Sourcebook lives in or near your community, and might be available to speak to a parent group. If you are looking for speakers, contact local colleges and universities, the departments of early-childhood education, psychology or other areas of interest, or write to us c/o The Institute. Leave ample time for discussion among the participants and for parents to ask questions and to discuss concerns among themselves.

PARENTING AS AN OPPORTUNITY

Guiding is different from bossing. It might be very helpful for parents to remember that from the very moment of birth, each child has his or her own eyes, ears, brain, feelings, body, and skin. The problem is that infants do not have the words to communicate directly what is going on. Each person is always seeing, hearing, feeling, and thinking from birth to death and must be discovered by himself and help others do the same. It is probably easier for parents to accept this for their child when they have accepted it for themselves.

Child rearing is an adventure which has pain, struggle, joy, and lots of Solomon-like situations. There are no recipes for solving situations, but there are resources present in the individuals that parents and children can use if they know how to communicate with each other, human to human.

Parenting is an adventure with responsibility, an almost daily risk-taking where there are no experts, really, but only your own wisdom, awareness, knowledge, and love. Keeping this in mind will take you a long way toward making that three-person experiment among mother, father, and child a rewarding experience.

Virginia M. Satir
Peoplemaking
Science & Behavior Books
1972   305 pp. $7.95

PARENTING AS AN ART

Every human being's experience on this earth is unique, and where parents err is in trying so hard to make their child's experience the same as their own . . . or even just the opposite.

Parents are so unbelievably omnipotent anyway, with their tremendous unspoken power, that the major contribution a parent can make to a child's life is to permit him to have his own experience—whatever it is—whether joy, sadness, anger. Never, never keep a child from being free enough to tell you what he is really feeling, and never set a value judgment on what they tell you.

How many parents have screamed in fury "You are bad," because a child says, "I wish you were dead, Mommy or Daddy," when all the child is doing is expressing some angry feelings with the only vocabulary he/she has.

If parents see a child as a circle of love, within which there are many kinds of feelings, and many ways of expressing them, then they can better handle the problems that arise.

My other rule of parenting is to bring up children with what I call "intelligent neglect." Focusing on every minute detail of a child's life robs him of dignity and the sense that life is a total adventure.

P

My two children (now grown-up) were my experiment: we fought and frolicked and screamed and admired one another, and the result—in their adulthood—is honesty in communication. Some communication of course is positive, though not all. But most importantly, there is no estrangement, just a sense of on-going openness and honesty for all of us.

This, in my heart, is the essence of what a parent has to offer a child: truth and love and the freedom for the child to share his truth, as well.

> Adelaide Bry
> *Est, 60 Hours That Transform Your Life*
> Harper & Row
> 1976   96 pp. $1.95

PARENTING

Parenting means loving and caring for children, helping them to grow. The process is not confined to relationships between adult and biological offspring, but occurs whenever an individual takes an active role in helping a child develop.

Parenting is an intense, exciting experience that exercises us in all areas of functioning. We develop physical stamina as we care for infants with few hours of sleep. Our physical agility and speed increase as we chase toddlers. Our athletic abilities grow as we don roller skates, ride toboggans, play baseball, and become active members of the sports world. Our minds are stretched in many directions. We master science and math to answer questions about where the stars go in the daytime, what makes rain, why do people grow old. And then the questions only a child can ask—after all, why can't a girl grow up and marry a dog she loves? Where are children before they are born? Emotional responsiveness gets a real work-out. Our range of emotions is extended—there are fine gradations of joy and frustration never known before. Our depth of feeling is intensified, and we gain incredible speed in emotional reactions. We can go quickly from joy to tears, rage to delight, happiness to despair in a matter of a few minutes.

Strange to say, in helping a new life grow, we gain for ourselves an inner vitality and a richness in all our relationships that is truly amazing. Parenting is indeed the best all-round exercise for being human.

> Jane B. Brooks
> *The Process of Parenting*
> Mayfield Publishing
> 1981   326 pp. $10.95

WHAT KIND OF PARENT AM I?

"How effective am I as a parent?"

Do you ever ask yourself that question? Perhaps you do, and your answer may be "So-so," 'Pretty bad" or perhaps "Great!"

Here is a self-rating scale that may help you look at yourself a little more objectively. It will just take a few minutes to complete.

Rate yourself on each item: Good—2 points; Fair—1 point; Poor—0; I don't know—✔. (Circle your answer.)

1. *Communication.* Young children try to use a lot of words, but not always accurately. Nor are they always easy to understand. But correcting them isn't as important as listening, exchanging ideas, and actually carrying on a conversation. Do I let them tell me what they did at their day care center or preschool? Do we have some "Talking Time" every day? Do I answer their questions, in words they can understand? 2 1 0 ✔

P

2. *Time.* Merely spending time together is less important than enjoying or laughing at things together. Do we really like each other's company? Do I regularly take time for playing a game, taking a walk, going to the park or seeing a movie with my preschool child? 2 1 0 ✓

3. *Example.* Children learn by copying their parents. Do I set a good example by following through on *my* job, being honest in *my* relationships, and showing moderation in *my* T.V. watching, drinking, eating, sleeping and other habits? Nibbling grapes from the supermarket fruit bin may seem like such a small thing, but it's too important to be seen by a young child. What kind of example do I set in controlling my temper and moodiness? 2 1 0 ✓

4. *Expectations and responsibilities.* Are the expectations I have for my children realistic . . . or too high or low? Do they help with the dishes, make beds, pick up clothes, and do other home chores of which they are capable? Do I add to their duties gradually? Is my preschool child beginning to understand money and what things cost? 2 1 0 ✓

5. *Praise.* Do I use praise, or just nag? Do I notice and reward (even with a kind word) what my young child does, whether it's something small like taking out the garbage or a big achievement like reading his first word in a book? 2 1 0 ✓

6. *Limitations.* Do our family rules fit the age and abilities of my children? Do I set limits that make sense for each child, like a time for going to bed or the amount of T.V. watching permitted? But do I also realize that there has to be some flexibility in schedules, to help children adjust to change? 2 1 0 ✓

7. *Reading.* Do my young children see me reading, and do I read to them? Is it fun for them and me? Do we choose the books together, and have a good time talking about them? How often do I go to the library with them? 2 1 0 ✓

8. *Strengths and Weaknesses.* Do I make an effort to see my children as they really are, not as I'd like them to be? Do I accept the fact that they may not be as good-looking and clever as I sometimes think they are? Am I aware of their limitations, as in catching a ball, cutting with a scissors, skipping or hopping? If they are lagging behind others, am I doing something about it? 2 1 0 ✓

9. *Discipline.* If we are a two-parent family, do we agree on approaches to discipline? Do we stick together in our ideas so that our children can't play one of us against the other? If I'm the only parent, am I consistent in the discipline I use? Do I try to prevent problems by keeping medicines, candy, and valuable breakable things away from little hands? 2 1 0 ✓

10. *Love.* It's the most important factor of all. Do I try to show it through buying them everything they ask for . . . or in more important ways like hugs, touching, smiles, quiet talk, and saying nice things? 2 1 0 ✓

Well, how did you do? A perfect score would be 20, and if you ended up with 16 to 20 points, that may sound fine—but one item you failed on may be enough to mess up your whole relationship. For example, if you never use praise or use it dishonestly, or think that showing your love is a sign of weakness, it may not matter at all how well you did on the others.

Still, a high score . . . and a low score, too . . . may tell you something about your parental effectiveness. These items can also be a guide toward a better understanding of your youngster, and of yourself. And a lot of checks in the "I don't know" column say something important to you too, like,

"Maybe it's time to think more about the young child in my family."

Willard Abraham
Parent Talk
Volume 1–Number 4
Sunshine Press

The ABC of Child Care
Allan Fromme
Pocket Books
1965   322 pp. $1.95

An encyclopedia geared to providing immediate and concise information on the why and how of children's behavior, this book offers concrete advice for dealing with their problems.

Whatever the seeds of aggression may be in our child, we can help him redirect these impulses into more wholesome avenues of expression. This means an attempt to teach him to take these feelings out on still safer objects than he has unwittingly chosen. We do this best in the area of play, by trying to shunt some of his hostility into group rather than individual competitiveness.

Between Parent and Child: New Solutions to Old Problems
Haim G. Ginott
Avon
1977   223 pp. $8.95

"Childrenese" is taught here —a direct, simple, fresh approach to improved parent/child communication. The suggested conversations are easily translated into practice in relating with children. Advice is supported by illustrative dialogues.

How can we help a child to know his feelings? We can do so by serving as a mirror to his emotions. A child learns about his physical likeness by seeing his image in a mirror. He learns about his emotional likeness by hearing his feelings reflected by us.

The function of an emotional mirror is to reflect feelings as they are, without distortion:

"It looks as though you are very angry."

"It sounds like you hate him very much."

"It seems that you are disgusted with the whole set-up." To a child who has such feelings, these statements are most helpful. They show him clearly what his feelings are. Clarity of image, whether in a looking glass or in an emotional mirror, provides opportunity for self-initiated grooming and change.

Developing Leadership for Parent/Citizen Groups
Crystal Kuykendall
National Committee for Citizens in Education
1976   59 pp. $2.00

This booklet, giving insights and basic tools needed to develop leadership potential in parent organizations that aim to improve schools, includes a leadership quiz to measure abilities and a bibliography of books dealing with leadership and public education.

Poor timing can easily lead to defeat, as you doubtless know if your group usually waits for a situation to reach crisis proportions before taking action. It is almost impossible to develop an action plan while tensions are high. Start looking for the warning signs of such problems as school violence, student dissatisfaction, and school deterioration early. Analyze previous crises: how and why did they develop? Think of potential problems and ways to avoid them. Ask students for their insights on the small problems that may erupt into big ones in the future.

Fund Raising by Parent/Citizen Groups
Douglas Lawson
National Committee for Citizens in Education
1977   52 pp. $1.75

This action brochure outlines techniques to raise money by traditional ways such as bake sales or car washes and by professional ways by foundations or corporations.

. . . If you are to raise substantial funds, it is essential that you bring community leaders into your organization—men and women who give money and who have access to others who give, and who are prepared to be active in your group as volunteer fund raisers or as members of your Board, or both. These people are an absolute necessity, not only because they lend credibility to your cause and may even add expertise of a professional nature, but because without them, it will be much more difficult for you to gain access to sources of substantial funding.

Growing With Your Children
Herbert Kohl
Little, Brown
1978   322 pp. $8.95

The author confronts day-to-day issues of parenting, centering around themes of discipline, strength, violence, respect and problems of self-image, being fair, and the like, drawn from the author's experience as a parent of three children.

One of the most difficult responses for children to try out is expressing anger. To express anger is dangerous—one risks the withdrawal of love, physical or emotional; retaliation, and guilt generated by the sense that one was wrong or overreacted. Children observe with fascination the ways adults show anger. They know how they are treated when their parents or brothers and sisters or

P friends are angry at them. They also know how these people respond when they're angry at each other. TV and the movies also provide a whole range of experience with anger. Children see the unambiguously murderous and violent mode of detective stories, as well as the insulting anger of a lot of comedy, and the seething suppression of anger portrayed on soap operas. From this whole repertoire of responses they have to choose their own mode of responding.

How to Influence Children
Charles Schaefer
Van Nostrand Reinhold
1978   198 pp. $9.95

This overview of child-rearing practices describes sixty ways to influence children, based on theories of problem solving, behavior modification and Freudian practices. Early chapters deal with establishing effective discipline; later chapters discuss formation of close parent-child attachments. An appendix reviews basic principles of child development such as self-esteem and aggression.

A positive approach is one in which your intention is to teach a child more adaptive ways of behaving while you show respect, acceptance, and support. With a positive approach, you view and treat a child as a friend rather than an adversary. As a result, the child feels that you are with him rather than against him. A negative or punitive influence approach, on the other hand, has as one of its goals hurting a child by inflicting physical or psychological pain, e.g. loss of self-esteem, intense fearfulness, anxiety, or guilt. Punitive techniques devalue a child and belittle his importance as a human being. Examples of punitive techniques are insults, sar-

casm, ridicule, threats, shouting at or beating a child, and disapproval of the whole child ("You're a bad child."). While these negative methods are often effective in temporarily stopping misbehavior, their adverse effect on the psychological well-being of the child make them inappropriate for effective discipline.

Learning for Little People
Sandy Jones
Houghton Mifflin
1979   232 pp. $7.95

This parents' sourcebook for years three to eight covers art, nature, fantasy, outdoor play, language and so on as well as difficult subjects such as divorce, sex, birth, death, moving. Every chapter contains an article by an experienced parent or specialist; activities; annotated bibliographies; listings of resources and educational play material. The book is fully illustrated, with photographs by Erika Stone.

Where do you begin readjusting a home to make it more comfortable for a young child? Her bedroom. Adults take walls for granted. But to a child, walls are for kicking when you're mad or tense, for bouncing balls off of, for putting art work on, for watching shadows in the night. Making use of wall space for play shows good planning. Put a blackboard, bulletin board, and an unbreakable mirror at child's eye level. If you use wallpaper, select paper that has many bright and intriguing patterns.

Liberated   Parents,   Liberated Children
Adele Faber and Elaine Mazlish
Avon
1974   237 pp. $1.75

The authors describe a group that was established based on Haim Ginott's techniques. They learned how a "language of compassion" slowly but surely helped generate a more loving atmosphere in their homes—and, at the same time, aided their children in developing insights into their own feelings and responsibility for their own lives. The authors write candidly of their failures and frustrations in applying Haim Ginott's teachings—and the lessons they learned through failure, which helped them succeed later on. Filled with observations, examples, actual dialogues and practical living situations, this down-to-earth child-raising manual has important answers for parents looking for a way to bring the principles of Ginott into the realities and stresses of day-to-day life.

When it was my turn, I announced, "I wish to report a first! I was on my way home from a long series of errands—all for David. It was late and cold and my thoughts were racing ahead as to how I could put together a fast supper. My coat was still on when David asked for soup. I hadn't planned to serve soup, but I automatically started looking for a can in the pantry, thinking, 'Why not? How could a loving mother deny her son hot soup on a cold night?' Then I thought about our discussion last week, and it hit me that I didn't really feel loving—I really felt put upon! At that moment finding the can, opening it and having an extra pot to clean seemed like a big imposition. I said, 'David, no soup! I feel pressured. What I could use is some help. Would you peel the carrots, please?'"

Parenting
Patricia Maloney Markin
Association for Childhood Education International
1973   72 pp. $2.50

This anthology of articles supports the concept of parenting as a philosophy propounding a personalized, individualized approach to total human development. Examples of articles included are "Grandpa In the Nursery," "Mister Rogers and Parenting," "Parenting in a Mexican-American Community."

Why, for example, does one so often hear that providing responsible adequate care for children is a special problem for working mothers? It seems that many men are not so conscious of their child-rearing obligations and responsibilities as women are, and at times take pains to deny them. We accord women, not men, the tribute of having held families together. Have men consistently deferred to women's influence in the home, child rearing, family life? Have they given credit to wives and mothers for their children's successful upbringing because it was the expected response?

Parent's Choice
Post Office Box 185
Waban, Mass. 02168
$10.00 per year

A good source of information on movies, television programs, books, games, and records for children. Short information on reviews plus articles on the educational aspects of different programs or products.

Parents' Newspaper
1060 West Elm
Stockton, CA 95203
6 issues for $5.00 per year

Articles, photographs, parent resources to help them learn of ways to teach their children how to grow productively and effectively. There are also treats for kids such as recipes for baking and exercises for kids to do.

Raising Children in a Difficult Time
Benjamin Spock
W. W. Norton
1974   264 pp. $7.00
Pocket Books
1976   264 pp. $1.95

Spock discusses in his commonsense style how mutual respect between parent and child can be established and maintained in this everchanging world. Chapters deal with everything from the child's understanding of religion to controlling aggression; from sex education to the domineering grandmother.

One of the most delightful aspects of children, I think, is the originality of the things they say, especially during the preschool years. Their remarks, their ways of interpreting things, are usually fresher, more vivid even than those of great philosophers and writers. Yet lots of parents never think of paying attention to these gems of perceptiveness, and even correct their children for using unconventional language. Most children will begin to be more conventional around six to eight years of age, and will soon enough be speaking in the platitudes and clichés of adulthood like the rest of us.

Six Approaches To Child Rearing
D. Eugene Mead
Brigham Young University Press
1977   126 pp. $4.95

A technical guidebook for parents that surveys six approaches to child-rearing, this book presents psychoanalytic, developmental-maturational, socio-theological, cognitive-develop-mental, existential-phenomenological and behavioral approaches. Not for the average reader, but fascinating for the parent with interest and/or a psychological background.

Parents need not attempt to be unconditionally accepting of their children all of the time. The adage so popular among parents that you "can love the child but not condone his behavior" is impossible to put into practice. The child is his behavior. Whenever the parent responds with nonacceptance toward the child's acts, the child perceives this as not accepting him.

What Now? A Handbook for New Parents
Mary Lou Rozdilsky and Barbara Banet
Charles Scribner's Sons
1975   148 pp. $7.95

A positive, realistic handbook for new parents on subjects ranging from why babies cry to "what about your life as a couple after the baby comes?" While there is much information on the baby in this small volume, the main focus is on the physical and emotional facts of life that the parents, especially the mother, face.

Recognizing all your feelings (positive and negative) and finding ways to express them without concluding that you are a failure or that you were not cut out to be a mother can free you to discover what kind of mother you really want to be, and can open up the infinite possibilities for personal growth that parenthood can bring.

Your ability to accept and take pleasure in each other will set the tone of your family. In spite of your excitement about the baby, there will be times when all the attention focused on her keeps you apart. Having children makes mar-

P riage less spontaneous and exciting in some ways, and it often takes more effort than you expect to get back together comfortably. If you can express disappointment or resentment you may have about the baby coming between you, you will be able to put more of your energy into re-establishing closeness as a couple.

World's Newest Profession
Ida M. Brodsky
The Profession of Parenting Institute
1975   159 pp. $4.00

In order to maintain the nuclear family, parenthood should be considered a profession. Chapters deal with extended families, sex education, political power in the family, and the like. Since parenthood requires psychiatric skills, social work, political balancing, nursing and nutritional skills, training helps.

It is important to recognize, in terms of this century and the next, that among the many instabilities of contemporary life, people may turn hopefully to their homes for the security they miss outside. Some theorists go on from this observation to declare that only well prepared families can successfully foster the kind of balanced and competent personality that in turn can weather the strains of urban industrial existence.

. . . You may still feel that you should resist his demands when "he doesn't really need anything, he just wants attention." But your baby is not yet old enough to want anything that is not also a need. Attention from adults is a real need; just as real as his physical needs. Without food or warmth he will die; without social attention from adults he will not be able to become a full human being.

Black Families

The two references on books written for black families are excellent for parents who want their specific concerns met. We searched for similar books written by and for other ethnic groups but were unable to locate any. If any reader knows such books, we would be most appreciative if they would write and tell us.

Black Child Care
James P. Comer and Alvin F. Poussaint
Simon & Schuster
1975   447 pp. $1.95

In this book two black psychiatrists discuss the problems of raising black children from infancy to adolescence, and offer special suggestions on how black parents can teach their children to love blackness without hating whiteness and how to teach adolescents to understand and deal with racism in a positive way.

Q. Shouldn't black children learn the realities of life rather than be indoctrinated by "white" ritual and fairy tales?

A. Let's separate the issue of ritual from that of fantasy and fairy tales. The latter help give your child a sense of security in an often dangerous world. They help a child handle failure and help him dream and plan success. They aid learning. They are fun. If common "fantasy figures" (for example, Santa Claus) are "too white," turn them black, as we discuss later. Fantasy and fairy tales will drop

away or change to adult forms as your child grows. Don't worry about them. Ritual, including saying the pledge of allegiance to the flag, is a more complicated matter.

Black Parents' Handbook
Clara J. McLaughlin
Harcourt Brace Jovanovich
1976   211 pp. $3.95

Genetic, medical and environmental problems are different for black parents. This guidebook focuses on child-rearing problems unique to black families, including sickle cell anemia and hypertension as well as black folk medicine practices and the myth of black inferiority.

A common problem in the young black female between two and ten years of age is this recurring bacterial infection on the temple areas of the scalp (Hair sores or Traction). One reason for this condition is the increased traction put on the hair as the result of tight braiding, a popular way to keep hair well-groomed and manageable. Some hair styles (for example, corn row) have been known to cause keloids in African women. Many older girls and adult females suffer this problem because they roll their hair too tightly. The first signs of this condition are small red pimples around the roots of the hair that become white with pus. The infection also causes hair loss. Treatment consists of an antibiotic rubbed into the infected area, as well as medication taken by mouth. It is best to use preventative measures. Do not braid or roll hair too tightly. Hair should be kept loose.

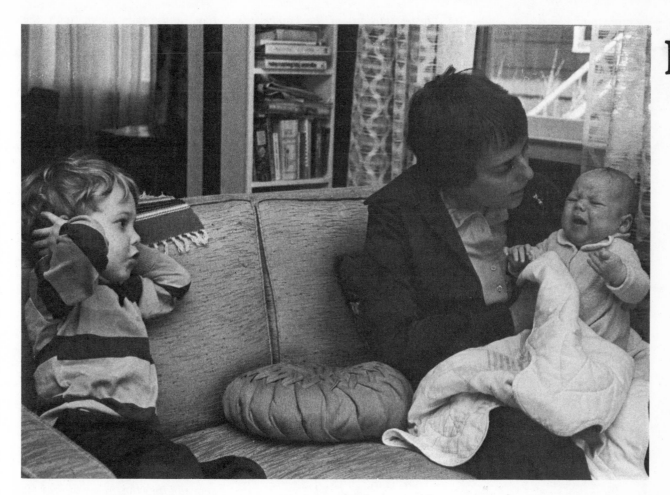

P

Skills and Techniques

Effective Child Rearing
F. William Gosciewski
Human Sciences Press
1976   140 pp. $9.95

This book conveys basic principles of behavioral modification to achieve more effective interaction between parent and child and explains techniques, theories and application of behavioristic psychology. Gosciewski suggests ways parents can maximize a child's potential.

Behavior has a purpose, it is outcome-oriented. This is never more clearly seen than in tantrum and similar crying behaviors. Typically the outburst is designed to gain for the child an outcome which he considers to be otherwise unattainable. Through that behavior or behavioral pattern, the child creates stress for the parent so that the parent is forced to seek a desirable outcome for himself—that is, the cessation of turbulence or crying. Too often under these circumstances the nonbehavioral parent may respond inconsistently, sometimes giving in and other times becoming punitive, thereby unknowingly giving the child sought-after attention. Such unreasonable behavior may begin when the highly frustrated child tries out this technique as a last resort in order to gain some desirable objective. If the parent gives in at that time or in other early attempts, he is ensuring that the child will return to that effective behavior in the future. The more effective that behavior is, the more the child will rely on it.

Family Game
Paul Hersey and Kenneth H. Blanchard
Addison-Wesley
1978   227 pp. $5.95

This book advocates a situational approach to effective parenting, stressing that parents need to know the specifics of each situation, since the child's needs change from one situation to the next. Once specifics are known, the parent can respond with the appropriate style: "telling," "selling," "participating," "delegating," and so on. Numerous strategies for using these styles are offered to help make effective day-to-day decisions.

The concept of a situational approach to child rearing might be stated as follows: Effective parents are those who can adapt their approach to child rearing to meet the unique needs of each of their children and the particular situation or environment in which their family exists. If their children are different, they must be treated differently.

For the Love of Children
Edward E. Ford and Steven Englund
Doubleday
1977   150 pp. $6.95

Methods of rearing children should be based on love, responsibility, discipline, work, play and faith. The authors show how to build a loving parent-child relationship using what they call Reality Therapy. They discuss the effects of television and drugs on the strength of a child and explain how to help children take responsibility for the choices they make.

The role of the parent is not to shield the child from contact with stress—parents couldn't do so if they tried, but in trying they can foster illusions in the youngster's mind. Rather, the role of the parent is to remind the child that stress is inevitable, and that no matter how painful or overwhelming it seems, the child retains the ability to make choices, for better or for worse. Often it will prove difficult to convince an unhappy youngster that he possesses the possibility of autonomy and choice. The child will want to be told, on the contrary, that life has been cruel and mean, and that there is nothing he can do about it. He will want Mom or Dad to intervene and solve the problem. The parents must gently remind the child that there is always something he can do about it, even if the only good choice open to the youngster is to tolerate pain for a while. Fostering a mental attitude of choice-consciousness is thus absolutely essential if the young person is to develop confidence in his ability to live responsibly.

How To Raise Children at Home in Your Spare Time
Marvin J. Gersh
Scarborough Books
Stein & Day
1978   216 pp. $3.95

This child-care book not only offers guidance in baby-proofing your home, handling medical emergencies and toilet training, but also shows mothers how to save countless hours each week for themselves. The author, a pediatrician, uses the most commonly asked questions such as "how come my child won't eat" and "why is he losing weight" to begin his narrative, and attempts to provide practical answers to parents' worries.

Harping on the balanced diet is one way of unbalancing your child. The concept has caused more mother-child dissonance than any other factor with the possible exception of rock 'n' roll. The American child in particular has such a wide choice of foods on which he may thrive that, realistically, there should be no problem. Instead, paradoxically, he suffers from abundance. Since the society can produce, he has to eat.

Mother's Almanac
Marguerite Kelly and Elia Parsons
Doubleday
1974   288 pp. $4.95

With comprehensive, practical suggestions ranging from the mechanics of diapering to meal-time manners, this book, written from a mother's point of view, also contains directions for many crafts and recipes.

A child must learn to be responsible for four things: his toys, his clothes, his pets and himself. Frankly, it's much, much easier to forget about the pets and take care of the rest yourself, but it's quite unfair to your child. The longer he waits to learn the rudiments of responsibility, the more difficult it will be to assume them until one day he'll be looking around for his old mum to make his excuses, pay his bills and baby-sit his children.

Natural Way to Raise a Healthy Child
Hiag Akmakjian
Praeger
1975   285 pp. $4.95

The author expresses his philosophy on child-rearing which is to develop alert, interested, conflict-free children and stresses that the child's key to mental health is dependable emotional availability of parents. Topics include anticipating parenthood, developing learning and speech skills, conscience, and improved eating habits.

Another cause of conflict is to deny a child the food he or she likes until the rest of the meal is eaten. To say to a child, "If you don't eat your squash you can't have pie" would make squash a punishment, not a food. Besides, children don't know what a "meal" is: all they know is that they are hungry and naturally reach for what they like best.

Natural Parenthood
Eda J. LeShan
New American Library
1970   160 pp. $1.25

A positive approach to child-rearing, focusing on how to handle the spoiled child, the child who runs away, the child who has night fears and the child who won't share household duties. Various chapters deal with the deprived child, the teenager and the telephone and even the "care and feeding" of parents.

At the age of three or four, whatever hang-ups you've got are the result of what is happening to you in the bosom of your family; that's where the psychological action is. If you are a pretty sturdy, healthy little kid and if you feel reasonably secure that your parents love you a lot, then you are likely to have the courage it takes to fight whatever you've got to fight about right there, where it's happening. If you can't stand the new baby, you let everybody know about it. If your dumb mother doesn't see that you're getting bigger and should have more automony, you raise all kinds of hell when she tries to boss you around. You work on your problems right where they're happening because you're not afraid to take that chance.

Parenting Skills
Richard R. Abidin
Human Sciences Press
1976   123 pp. $11.95 Manual.
$3.50 Workbook. $13.50 Both.

Exercises are included to reinforce the activities and ideas presented during a parent workshop session, and deal with individual worth, competence, responsibility and behavior-modification principles.

Sharing yourself with your child is a way to build a close relationship with him. It means letting your child know and experience how you feel, your thoughts, and your expectations. Sharing yourself does not involve giving solutions, blaming, criticizing, and judging your children in response to their behavior. You may learn to share yourself when your child has not done anything "good" or "bad," but you want to build the closeness of your relationship.

Parent Power—Child Power
Helen De Rosis
Bobbs-Merrill
1974   230 pp. $6.95

"Problem prevention" is emphasized in this lively, enlightening and supportive guide to child-rearing, which prepares parents by exposing common pitfalls, with special attention to avoiding guilt.

When a child indignantly whines, "But I did sweep it!" you can believe him. Maybe it doesn't look swept, but he did sweep it. Depending on one's goals, one can either let it be, or one can say, "I see that you did sweep it. But it was very dirty and I think it needs some more attention. Will you go over it again?" Even though the youngster cannot bring himself to sweep it again (for that would be acknowledging his ineptitude), he has learned that a floor must be swept differently from the way he did it. But he may very well surprise you if you have not indicated that he is a "slob" or "lazy," by offering to sweep it again. Parents often forget that their children wish to please them.

P

Parents' Guide to Child Raising
Glenn Austin with Julia Stone Oliver and John C. Richards
Prentice-Hall
1978   367 pp. $6.50

The authors emphasize the concept that parents are capable of developing their own decision-making skills while dealing with such questions as how to instill proper eating habits in a child, how to deal with hyperactivity or how to help a child accept a death in the family. Different methods of discipline are discussed to show a parent how to transmit values, self-esteem, sex identity and motivation in their children.

One of the first steps in helping a fearful child is to make him aware that fear is normal. Even the tough ones have fears. So do parents. What counts is how logical the fears are, and, when logical, how you use or control the fear. On a day to day basis, children need to be gradually conditioned to learn to stay alone, and to face challenges such as going shopping alone, joining a group, talking to strangers, and many other essential activities. However, parents must avoid giving the impression that their aim in pushing these activities is to escape the child; rather, play on the fact that parental absence at times is an acceptable and unavoidable necessity. These are teaching tasks that parents should plan for in the day to day care of the child—both short-range and long-term.

P *Parents' Yellow Pages*
Frank Caplan
Doubleday
1978   511 pp. $7.95

This directory for parents provides listings and phone numbers of community organizations and services. Written in a problem-solving manner, it presents a quick overview and alternative solutions to subjects ranging from activities to working mothers. Also includes book reviews, catalogs, evaluation checklists, free or inexpensive pamphlets, and advice for do-it-yourself information gathering. The author includes such information as when to buy your baby's first shoes:

Permit your baby to go barefoot for as long as is practical and safe. Some parents mistakenly rush to the shoe store just as soon as baby can stand. Pediatricians currently recommend tennis shoes or moccasins for beginning walkers and toddlers. Sneakers are inexpensive, will not come off easily, are soft and flexible, and have a non-slippery walking surface—all of which are desirable features.

Positive Parenthood
Paul S. Graubard
New American Library
1977   184 pp. $3.95

The author presents a method to reduce strife in parent-child relationships in three steps, using rewards and praise to deal with problems such as rebelliousness, lying, stealing and the like in a gentle approach to behavior modification.

Children learn very early in life that sex is powerful. They learn that their sexuality affords them pleasure, and that it can provoke a rise from other people. Guiding a child into a healthy and satisfying course with sex is a difficult task, one that sets off conflicting feelings in parents. Most adults would like children to learn that sex is pleasurable and good. On the other hand, they want children to learn to control their impulses and practice sex the "right" way, but children need guidance in this area. They need to avoid social penalties and their own bad feelings about what they do with sex.

Problem Solving Techniques in Childrearing
Myrna B. Shure and George Spivack
Jossey-Bass
1978   242 pp. $12.95

Parents can improve the social adjustments of their children by encouraging the development of interpersonal problem-solving skills. Emphasis is placed on how to approach problems with different types of children—poor and good problem solvers. The authors use scripts to train parents to communicate with their offspring and guide them in their development. Games and sample dialogues are used throughout the book to describe effective solutions.

Whether or not this child is successful right then is not important. What is important is that the child is encouraged to think about the problem, ways to solve it, and the potential consequences of what he might do. In time, this child would likely be able to solve this problem for himself and not have to go to his mother for help.

Proud Parenthood
Joseph L. Felix
Abingdon
1977   158 pp. $6.95

This book encourages parents to draw upon inner intelligence, creativity, love and faith in order to work on personal shortcomings and handle angers, uncertainty, defensiveness and discouragement.

Offering practical suggestions in dealing rationally with discipline and self-control, sixty situations that test parental responses to specific problems of child behavior are included.

Children often appear to be deliberately seeking punishment. Why is this?

One of the most common reasons is the child's own sense of guilt. Punishment relieves the guilt, and this is less painful to the child than his own self-torture. It is common for children to have a bookkeeping sense of justice, which requires that every misdeed incurs a retaliation. Parents often foster this attitude through punishment.

Or the child may be seeking punishment for a lesser crime, hoping to ease his guilt for what he considers a more serious offense.

Raising Happy Healthy Children
Karen Olness
Meadowbrook Press
1977   163 pp. $3.95

Written in diary form, this book deals with rearing children from infancy to the age of seven years, and focuses on problems at each stage.

If parents overreact to pain, their children are likely to do the same. If parents moan over lost possessions, dental appointments, a dent in the fender and other minor stresses, their kids may also become overreactors and poor copers. Children are more likely to be calm in the face of major stresses if they sense calmness in their parents. They will learn how to pick up the pieces and move forward instead of regressing in the face of stress.

Rewarding Parenthood/Rewarding Childhood
V. Thomas Mawhinney
J. P. Tarcher
1978   248 pp. $9.95

Including guidelines on stimulating a child's total emotional and physical development, this book stresses that the parent should consider not only the child's behavior, but her own as well. The author covers how to encourage happiness, emotional strength, coordination, social skills, self-care and independence.

Most babies begin to walk unsupported some time between eleven and fifteen months. Before this occurs, they spend much time walking about while hanging onto tables, chairs, along couches, or perhaps in a walker. To help development of walking, try the following: 1. Stand your baby in front of a couch or padded chair and place a favorite toy about one step out of her reach. 2. While verbally encouraging her to walk to the toy, assist her to take a step. When she steps, praise her and let her play with the toy briefly. As she gains in skill, gradually move her further away from the toy and reduce your assistance slowly.

Toddlers and Parents: Declaration of Independence
T. Berry Brazelton
Delacorte Press
1974   250 pp. $10.00/$6.95

Each chapter is a realistic family profile, recreating the life of one particular small child and the brothers, sisters, parents and other adults shaping his life. Special problems of working parents, single parents, large families, disturbed families and day-care centers are examined. The book concentrates on facets of children and environ-

ments which could cause difficulty and develop into problems.

Susan's quiet period did not last long. . . . As soon as she was up, rattling the bars of her playpen, Mrs. Thompson took her out of it to explore the house. . . . As she tried, she began to explore the floors, the baseboards and lamp cords, the cabinets at her level. Then, her resourcefulness in finding detergents, cleaning fluids, or other toxic substances came to the fore.

. . . The experimentation which is uppermost at this age just cannot be trusted. . . . Far too many infant deaths can be attributed to it. Always have an emetic (such as Ipecac) on hand and a poison booklet to tell you how and when to use it.

What Every Child Needs
Lillian Peairs and Richard H. Peairs
Harper & Row
1974   359 pp. $8.95

A child's formative years pass quickly, and a parent does not get a second chance to shape personality. The authors supply easily understood data to help parents provide an early environment which will allow their children to become creative, self-fulfilling people. The volume is divided into informative sections on anger and hostility, sibling rivalry, untruthfulness and such topics as the importance of friends and developing responsibility.

In our unconscious envy of the freedom children enjoy, we forget their inequality. We forget too that in every generation responsible parents have emerged from the rebellious years of childhood. Kids

the world over rebel against work. What is important to us may not seem important to them. We do not wish to dig holes in the sand. They may not wish to clean house or work in the yard.

P

What Every Child Would Like His Parents to Know
Lee Salk
Warner Books
1972   222 pp. $1.95

Dr. Salk explains what parents can do to protect a child's emotional health, and how to handle specific problems such as undressing in front of a child, stealing, constant disobedience and sex experiences such as "playing doctor."

Many parents feel that it is easier to begin by telling children about the birds and the bees. Sometimes they take them to a farm or read them books about dogs and cats. They hope this approach will purify information about reproduction and decontaminate the facts from any sexual feeling.

Most youngsters couldn't care less about birds and bees. They are interested in the real thing. "Where did I come from?" Children feel suspicious when you sidestep a question or answer it in a roundabout way. Starting with the birds and the bees is simply a gimmick that parents use to get themselves off the hook. We all know the boy who, having been told the facts of life, adopted a facial expression denoting substantial fascination and went off to tell his friends, "Birds and bees do it, too."

P *What to Tell Your Child: About Birth, Illness, Death, Divorce, and Other Family Crises*
Helene S. Arnstein
Condor
1978   302 pp. $2.25

At some time or other, all children's lives are temporarily upset by family events. The author aims through this book to help parents uncover and strengthen their hidden resources for coping with problems such as death, divorce and pressures put on children to experiment with sex and drugs. A listing in the back of the book offers information on organizations that might also offer help to a parent.

Fortunately, most children have a remarkable ability to cope with even the most tragic events, and, though emotional damage may occur, it need not be irreparable. If a parent can offer his child sympathetic understanding, feelings of warmth and closeness, and gentle guidance, a child has an excellent chance of recovering from any cruel experience he has faced. There is in every child a drive and surge toward good health, well-being and a state of equilibrium. And even when life seems darkest, a parent who can help foster this drive in his child will be building up further strengths not only in his child, but in himself.

Your Baby and Child From Birth to Age Five
Penelope Leach
Alfred A. Knopf
1978   512 pp. $15.95

This comprehensive guide to care and development, both physical and psychological, contains photographs, drawings, growth charts, facts and information and a large, handy index. It is designed as a reference for the new mother.

There is no harm in your assuming that these enchanting early smiles are meant for you personally. They soon will be. It is through pleasant social interaction with adults, who find him rewarding and therefore pay him attention, that the baby moves on from being interested in people in general to being able to recognize and attach himself to particular ones. By the time he is around three months old it will be clear that he knows you. He will not smile at you and whimper at strangers. He still smiles at everyone. But he saves his best signs of favor, the smiliest smiles, for you. He becomes both increasingly sociable and increasingly fussy about whom he will socialize with. He is ready to form a passionate and exclusive emotional tie with somebody and you are elected.

A Parent's Guide to Children: The Challenge
Lawrence Zuckerman, Valerie Zuckerman, Rebecca Costa, Michael Yura
Hawthorn Books
1978   81 pp. $2.75

This workbook is structured to give a clear understanding of democratic decision-making to promote consistent, responsible behavior and self-reliance in children. It includes such assignments and learning activities as setting goals, enhancing the family atmosphere, relating to children, and building family togetherness.

Establishing a family council or family meeting on a routine basis is extremely important. Children as well as parents have family and personal concerns that could be resolved through the use of a family council. Participating in a family council allows time for both parents and children to get to know one another better and to experience working in a unit. The entire family works together in a cooperative manner to solve difficult situations, discuss the operations of the household, and work together in the planning of fun activities. The family council is equality in operation.

P.E.T. In Action
Thomas Gordon
Bantam Books
1976   367 pp. $2.50

Gordon outlines the basic Parent Effectiveness Training principles and techniques, emphasizing the right of parent and child to be themselves.

When parents begin to get more effective at using Active Listening in the home, they find it hard to believe it works so well—in many different kinds of situations and with children of all ages. From initial skepticism in many cases, parents come to appreciate the amazing power of this simple way of communicating acceptance and understanding. "I wouldn't have believed it if I hadn't seen it happen with my own eyes," one parent remarked. Her statement represents the attitude that came through in so many of our interviews. Often parents reported incidents involving very brief encounters requiring only one or two Active Listening responses. Other families worked through longer incidents involving complex problems and deep feelings.

P

TA For Families
Adelaide Bry
Harper & Row
1976   167 pp. $1.50

The author uses the techniques of transactional analysis to help family members locate communication problems and learn better ways of feeling and acting toward one another.

Whoever said that family life should be sweet music and soft lights and complete joy every single day is just being plain silly, but the degree and kinds of problems you have all depend upon what you learned when you were a little boy or a little girl. Nobody gets perfect love. But your family can probably be happier than they are, now. But each person in the family has to work at it.

Look At Me
(A production of WTTW/Chicago Public Television)
Viewers' guide to the TV series hosted by Phil Donahue. Prepared by Prime Time School TV
120 South LaSalle St.
Chicago, Ill. 60603

This excellent seven-part series has been created to serve as a resource for parents. Through the narrative of host Phil Donahue, dramatizations and actual film sequences showing parents involved with their children, Look at Me focuses on just how special the relationship is between parent and child and how influential parents are in their children's growth. This viewer guide provides a summary of each episode, including relevant references to various authorities on child development and psychology. The guide also serves as a supplement, suggesting questions and activities that can be pursued on an individual or group basis with spouse, family or friends.

Check with your local PBS station to ask about rerun dates and times in your area, and for more information.

Organizations (See Appendix A)

Administration for Children, Youth and Families

Jewish Board of Family and Children's Services

National Council on Family Relations

National Forum of Catholic Parent Organizations

Parents Without Partners

P.E.E.R.S.

Profession of Parenting Institute

United Synagogue of America

Magazines (See Appendix B)

Family Circle
Marriage and Family Living
Parents' Magazine
Practical Parenting
Redbook

PARTIES. SEE BIRTHDAYS AND PARTIES

PETS
Pleasures and Pitfalls

When you give your child a pet, you don't just add a cat or dog or gerbil to your home, you change the emotional dynamics and psychological currents of your family. You may do your youngster great emotional good, but you also must be cautious of several camouflaged pitfalls.

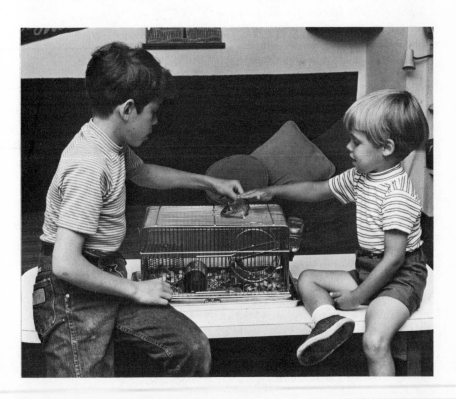

P A pet is too important and plays too great a role in the child's personality development for its choice to be left to mere chance.

What kind of pet is best for your children? Whatever the child has been asking for, get it for him provided it doesn't cause more inconvenience for you than the family can tolerate. Before buying any pet, work through your own feelings about animals, decide how much time you can spare for pet care, and discuss the choice in a family conference. If you can't manage the kind of pet your youngster wants, sit down and reason out with him what kind of animal would fit into your family.

A pet a child can take outdoors and play with around other youngsters has the most value. An animal which is soft and cuddly, responds to a youngster's actions and shows its love and loyalty gives his owner more satisfaction than one which doesn't. Dogs are the first choice of both boys and girls.

What should you do if your youngster fails to care for his pet? Get rid of the pet? Do the work yourself? You, the parent, should realize that caring for an animal is a learned skill acquired gradually by children. Praise your child's enthusiasm when he gives good care to his pet. Get rid of the pet if your child fails to care for it.

What is the best way to handle the death of a pet? Realize that your child will have to go through the work of mourning and learn the agony of losing something he or she loves. Like a vaccination, the loss of a pet can immunize a child against overwhelming emotional shock at the death of a family member. Permit the child to hold a burial service for a dead pet. Let him mourn for a week or two and then replace the pet. If you give him a new pet right away he may get the idea that life has little

value and that he could also be replaced just as quickly.

When a youngster brings home a stray animal you can't keep, what should you do? First, praise the child for his goodness in caring about the animal. Then discuss with him what kind of plan you can make together to find a home for the animal. This helps the youngster learn that his parents aren't arbitrary and that his own innate feelings of caring are good.

Do you need to keep an inventory of your pet's toys? Yes, you should make a list of your pet's toys and check often to be sure none has been chewed or swallowed by the pet or younger children.

How much food and medical attention will the pet require? Choose a pet which will fit into your family budget plans. Large dogs are very nice for pets, but you must realize the high food cost of a very large pet. Pets will get sick, need rabies shots and require a license. Costs vary, depending on the type and health of the animal you obtain.

Suggested Pets for Children

Pets should be given to children only when they are at an age when they can appreciate them, take care of their grooming and other needs, and be willing to feed and water the animal each day.

Common pets:

- gerbils
- hamsters
- white mice
- cats
- dogs
- rabbits

Birds:

- canaries
- cockatiels

- finches
- parakeets
- lovebirds
- doves and pigeons

Fish:

- tetras
- pencil fish
- danios
- rasboras
- barbs
- angelfish
- silver dollar fish
- guppies
- gouramis
- loaches
- swordtail platys

Reptiles:

- harmless snakes
- lizards
- turtles and tortoises (small species)

Amphibians:

- frogs
- toads
- salamanders (most species)
- newts

Insects and other creatures:

- crickets
- grasshoppers
- ants
- harmless spiders
- millipedes
- centipedes (if you are certain yours is a harmless species)
- crayfish
- clams
- mussels
- snails
- butterflies

For Children

Animal Babies
Harry McNaught
Random House
1977   20 pp.   95¢

Beautiful illustrations in warm earth colors accompany a simple description introducing young children to animals they may have an opportunity to see, such as rabbits and deer, and to those they may never see in their environment, such as anteaters and koalas.

Rabbit babies are called kits. They cannot see or hear until they are about ten days old.

A baby deer is called a fawn. The fawn's spotted back helps it hide in the shadowy forest.

Animal Fact/Animal Fable
Seymour Simon
Crown
1979   Unpaged $3.95

In this book, Seymour Simon has collected a fascinating variety of common beliefs about animals and presented them in the form of a guessing game. Each belief appears on the right-hand page with a humorous illustration by Diane de Groat. The answer appears on the following page and is accompanied by an exquisite, scientifically accurate illustration that shows the animal as it really behaves.

Now That You Own a Puppy
Joan Tate
Frederick Fell
1975   64 pp. $2.95

This book for older children is about understanding dogs—why they behave in certain ways; their instincts, habits, sensual perceptions; how to train them through comprehension of animal behavior.

Play for pups is instinctive, but the final outcome of these instinctive actions—hunting, chasing, fighting, killing—does not come about as they would eventually in a wild wolf, for instance. In domestic dogs, games that are played are many and varied, but all have some wild origins. A pup will go and look quite deliberately for something to play with, stick or ball in the garden, for instance. When it sees the ball, or rope, or stick, it knows by instinct what to do with it. When a pup picks up a bit of rag and shakes it, it is using a hunting technique, shaking its prey to stun or kill it.

A Zoo in Your Room
Roger Caras
Harcourt Brace Jovanovich
1975   90 pp. $5.95

The author, a well-known naturalist, explains how any child can actually be a keeper of a zoo in her very own room at home. Sound advice is given on housing and feeding over thirty species of mammals, birds, fish, reptiles, amphibians and insects.

Choosing the kind and number of animals you will care for is important and fun to do, but there are several criteria to use in making your selection.

1. *Size is obviously important. You have to adjust to the actual room you have for your project.*
2. *Food requirements must be another consideration because an animal's diet must be easy to provide and also be inexpensive. . . .*
3. *Safety, then, is a factor that must be taken into account as well. No dangerous animals should be kept in the home zoo.*
4. *A very important consideration is your love for animals. (We can assume that because you want a zoo in the first place.)*

A home zoo is an act of love, and you won't want to keep an animal that would suffer from confinement.

P

PLAYGROUNDS

Manufacturers make a variety of equipment for children, from playground equipment to toys and other paraphernalia. If you are handy, you can make things that are just as much if not more fun for your children to play with. These may be simple toys, a makeshift tent in the backyard, a playground put together by a number of parents. Or as Jeremy Hewes and Jay Beckwith suggest in the book, *Build Your Own Playground*, these projects can be imaginative and creative ways to provide your child and his or her friends with many stimulating and creative hours of outdoor fun. Beckwith, a designer of creative playgrounds, also offers consultation on community-sponsored park playgrounds in *Make Your Backyard More Interesting than T.V.*, McGraw-Hill, 1979, 117 pp., $6.95.

Big Toys, 3113 S. Pine St., Tacoma, WA 98409, (206) 572-7611, offers a full catalog of park-grade, modular components which are especially designed and suitable for backyard use. They are simple to construct and consist of large logs and pipes of park-like quality, in appropriate size and scale for home use.

An alternative to building your own equipment is to order it

P from Child Life Play Specialties, which offers assembled pieces and kits with all the materials pre-cut and pre-drilled. Their play equipment is made from beautiful woods (treated so they won't rot) and is generally expensive. But many parents feel that these high-quality swings, ladders, jungle gyms, sand boxes and play structures are worth the money and the wait for delivery (up to six months). For a free catalogue write to: Child Life Play Specialites, 55 Whitney Street, Holliston, MA 07146, or call (617) 429-4639.

The Children's Design Center also offers quality play equipment. For ordering information and an explanation of their services, see the Toys section.

Create Your Own Playground

MAKING A PLAYGROUND FROM SCROUNGED THINGS

With a little imagination and planning, you can make a play area for your child or for a play group from materials that you can get free for the asking or very inexpensively. Who says playgrounds have to always look the same? It's what the children *do* that counts—running, jumping, swinging—vigorous things that help them to develop their arm and leg muscles.

- *Straw and hay*   From local fields in the fall or from a feed store. For jumping in or using for a thatched roof.
- *Railroad ties*   From railroad companies and crews. For an imbedded balance beam, the sides of a sandbox, or a make-believe car with a mounted steering wheel.
- *Large rocks*   From road construction sites, gravel pits, or the woods. For damming up a stream to make a pool or making stepping stones.
- *Bricks*   Use culled, or seconds from a brickyard or construction company. For building forts or pretend swimming pools. For constructing a climbing wall with concrete.
- *Concrete culverting and clay tile pipes*   From concrete companies, the city sewerage system, the telephone company. For making tunnels and bridges. Be sure they're well embedded in the ground.
- *Tree sections and tree trunks with limbs*   From the city electric company, neighbors, or a lumber mill. For climbing and practicing hammering, sawing, and other woodworking skills.
- *Sand*   From the beach, a construction company, or a sand and gravel pit. For making a sandbox. (Should have drainage bricks underneath and a cover to keep cats and dogs out.)
- *Wooden blocks and pieces of lumber*   Discards from lumber companies and the city utility company. For building structures with hammers and nails, for stacking and other structures.
- *Ropes, rope ladders and cargo nets*   From hardware stores and shipyards. For climbing and swinging.
- *Barrels*   From a hardware store or a distillery. For rolling in, making houses and tunnels. (Be sure to sand away the splinters.)
- *Large, rectangular plastic containers* From textile mills—used for fabric storage. To make play houses and for stacking.
- *Large wooden electric wire spools*   From the electric company. For making tables, stools.
- *Discarded rowboat*   Ask around piers and docks. Use for imaginary voyages, or drill holes for drainage and use as a sandbox.
- *Automobile tires*   From auto junkyards and service stations. Clean them up and paint them bright colors with paint made especially for rubber. Use to roll, to stack, to climb on, as swings.

Sandy Jones
Learning for Little Kids
Houghton Mifflin
1978   232 pp. $7.95

Backyard Vacation: Creative Ideas for Family Fun
Ann Cole, Carolyn Haas, Elizabeth Heller and Betty Weinberger
Parents Are Resources
1974   32 pp. $2.00

This pamphlet offers innovative ways to transform the backyard into a summer vacation spot.
Create Your Own Outdoor Playground from Scrap Materials. You could:

1.   Make a sandbox *from an old tire. Fill it with sand and dump in old pots and pans; unbreakable utensils and toys; empty milk and margarine cartons; cars, dump-trucks, etc.*

2.   *Construct a* balance board *by placing a long piece of wood over some bricks or blocks of wood.*

3.   *Hang a knotted* Climbing Rope *from a tree branch—or make a swing using two pieces of sturdy rope with a tire or board for a seat.*

4.   *Make a tunnel from an old barrel or several large boxes placed end-to-end.*

5.   *Turn a large packing box into a* Playhouse *or a "Pretend Place."*

Build Your Own Playground
Jeremy Joan Hewes and Jay Beckwith
Houghton Mifflin
1975   219 pp. $6.95

A playground need not be a sterile layout of asphalt, slides and swings, and the authors show how to create a play area that encourages children's imagination. The authors discuss such topics as vandalism, building materials, division of labor during construction and planning areas for "special" children.

Scrounging materials can likewise be developed into an art, and a playground has great potential for use of leftovers and castoffs. Some likely sources of interesting and inexpensive materials are government surplus and salvage stores, scrap-metal dealers, state and federal surplus outlets (which often have catalogs), and utility companies. Items that are often available for free include trees (in various forms) from park or highway departments or builders who are clearing sites; tires of all sizes from tire dealers (possibly old inner tubes too); telephone poles or the short end pieces from them from the power and phone companies; and possibly railroad ties from railroad yards.

Child's Play: A Creative Approach to Playspaces for Today's Children
David Aaron and Bonnie P. Winawer
Harper & Row
1965   160 pp. $4.95

Play spaces and playgrounds are stressed as environments for a child's most serious business, since play is a child's work. Examples of creative and developmental play areas are presented.
The cardinal rule about the backyard playspace is that it is not a family activity. Togetherness works well for family outings and some other projects. But the backyard playspace houses a kid's own project. Adults should offer assistance only when asked and such assistance should be limited to the particular request. Parents should volunteer no information other than to tell the children that a new item is on the way. The supervising parent must guard against his natural impulse to take over and make the thing work better. He must not interfere except to ob-

serve how the project is going and to anticipate future requirements.

PLAYING

See also Child Care; Creative Expression; Games and Activities; Nursery and Pre-School Care; Sports; Part I—Learning, Play and First Toys.

In this section we include books which discuss the why of playing as well as how to play with your children.

Play Groups

Play groups are organized by parents to provide systematic play and social activities for children. They can meet as infrequently as once a week for two hours, or five mornings a week. They are usually organized by a group of parents who want to develop ways of assisting each other and who want an opportunity to exchange baby-sitting and free time.

Play groups are a wonderful way for parents to interact and learn with each other.

The Playgroup Handbook
Laura Peabody Broad and Nancy Towner Butterworth
St. Martin's Press
1974   306 pp. $3.95

A guidebook for the mother (or father) planning a playgroup or dealing daily with her own child and his friends. Suggestions are given for: organizing a group, for collecting materials needed for various projects, and for presenting seasonal and non-seasonal activities for preschoolers.

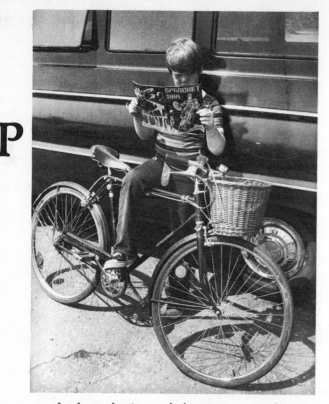

P

In the enthusiasm of planning a group you may find a number of mothers wishing to have their child join. Small numbers are a must. Not only is space a factor to be considered, but the average mother will find herself busy, indeed, with just a small group. For three-year-olds, four in a group is large enough. Remember—four easily distracted people are easier to control than six who have begun to get a little wild in a moment of mother's divided attention. It is amazing the bedlam that can ensue while mother answers the phone or chats with a neighbor who has unexpectedly dropped by. Even with a small group in her care, the playgroup mother must learn to tell a caller, "I have a playgroup here now. I'll call you back later."

Beyond Competition
Sid Sackson
Pantheon Books
1977   100 pp. $2.95

This book provides six games designed to substitute the challenge of cooperation for the concept of competition. Removable sheets are provided for the games. Fun, not winning, is the objective.

In some of the games the cooperation is against an imminent peril, such as being stranded in space or the outbreak of a disastrous war. In others the cooperation is to achieve a worthwhile goal, such as an equitable sharing of resources or the rescue of persons in danger. In all of the games, in order for the group to have a chance of winning, each player must realize how his play affects all the others and, unless the rules specifically prohibit, the options should be discussed in a search for the best play.

Child's Play
Barbara R. Trencher
Humanics Press
1976   157 pp. $9.95

An activities and materials handbook for preschoolers utilizing a humanistic approach, this book aims at establishing positive experiences and sound interpersonal relationships between adults and children. It includes everything from designing creative indoor and outdoor spaces to activities to encourage awareness of the arts.

Body tracings are usually done on large pieces of Kraft brown paper. The child lies on the paper while another child or an adult traces him. Once the outline is made, the child is free to decorate his tracings as he pleases including dressing himself with pieces of scrap material, putting on yarn hair. An adult asks the child to tell a little about himself and his family as the child is working.

Child's Play: A Manual for Parents and Teachers
Lynda Madaras
Peace Press
1977   152 pp. $6.95

This manual is crammed full of toys, games and play projects for young children. It is especially valuable to families seeking workable alternatives in child rearing, with suggestions for setting up a supportive adult community centered around child care. Ideas are included on filmmaking, scrap cities, making books and puppets, and the like. The beginning chapters of the manual provide a step-by-step guide to creating an effective play group, with advice such as:

Methods of discipline often vary widely. For instance, in the playgroup we belong to, two of the families occasionally use spanking to discipline their children. It is not my style, but as long as it doesn't go on within the playgroup, it's not really any of my business. If you are a feminist and one of the parents dresses her little girl in organdy frills or ridicules a little boy who plays with a doll, then you've got a problem. Many of these things can be talked over and do not necessarily mean that you cannot work with such people.

The Complete Book of Children's Play
Ruth E. Hartley and Robert M. Goldenson
Thomas Y. Crowell
1963   484 pp. $4.95

Two outstanding experts give full and authoritative information on every aspect of children's play from birth to adolescence with special chapters on hobbies and pets, television and comics, amusements in car and train, community activities and play that develops minds.

As soon as he enjoys sensations, play begins.

The baby's ears, for example, offer one of our earliest means of reaching him. Most infants are startled by loud, sudden noises, but soft, intimate talking and singing seem to soothe them. They learn to stop crying when they hear footsteps. Even the clink of dishes or the recurrent sound patterns of a clock (especially a chiming one or a cuckoo clock) can be interesting.

How to Play with Your Children (And When Not To)
Brian and Shirley Sutton-Smith
Hawthorn Books
1974   265 pp. $7.95

For centuries, we have believed that playful people were wasting their time and our time, too. But the authors challenge this idea with a staggering discovery—playful people are more versatile. They also say children don't play by instinct—they must be taught to play. The book maps out a way to include play in every family's life-style.

When they have reached five years of age, there are a series of steps you can take in improvisational games with your children. These steps follow the same steps taken by children in their own make-believe play from the age of one year onward. The first step was simply to create make-believe movements. You can begin to do this as early as three years. This is when you and your children or you and a group of children all pretend to walk around heavily like elephants or lightly like pussy cats; or you pretend to jump over the river, walk tall like skyscrapers, or walk small like bugs. This is a movement and music game that you can do with a drum.*

Learning Through Play
Jean Marzollo and Janice Lloyd
Harper & Row
1972   211 pp. $2.95

The authors present activities (such as Curiosity Walks and Silly Sentences) to be played by and with preschool children. These games cover a wide variety of interests and learning areas: the five senses, language development, prereading, measuring, self-esteem, and so on.

The letters of the alphabet are important because we put them together to make words. Many children can recite the alphabet, but have no idea what it means. It's important for you to find ways to help your child understand the purpose of letters. Learning letters is more fun when the letters make up your child's name or when they spell his favorite cereal. Whenever you can, take time to help your child look for letters he knows.

Play Therapy
Virginia M. Axline
Ballantine
1971   373 pp. $1.25

In the days of total direction and orchestration of every move for parents as well as therapists, this book expresses a hands-off, let-the-kid-alone-and-give-him-a-free-space-to-grow approach to therapy. Clinical exchanges between the therapist and kids in play therapy give a clear picture of one of the early child therapists at work in the days when *permissive* meant simply the opportunity to grow and take responsibility for one's self.

A good therapist is in many ways like a favorite teacher. Usually the favorite teacher has earned that distinction because of her basic attitudes toward her pupils—attitudes that usually stress kindliness, patience, understanding, and steadiness, with the added discipline of placing responsibility and confidence in the pupil. The successful teacher or therapist may be young or old, beautiful or homely, smartly or indifferently dressed, but the attitude toward the child is one of respect and acceptance.

Power of Play
Frank and Theresa Caplan
Doubleday
1973   307 pp. $3.95

Play is a child's way of life from infancy on, and is the most natural way for a child to use her capacities to grow and learn. The authors trace the nature of play and look at how adults can be served by play. Humans have prevailed partly because they are more playful and steadfast than other creatures. Being more than a verbal skill, creativity puts the B student ahead of the A student in everyday life, and to create, one must have a sense of adventure and playfulness.

Insight and creativity do not come as a flash of genius; rather they come from a long period of playing, of looking at a problem from unusual perspectives, of holding a situation open for review until several approaches have been found, or from rearranging things in new ways that please one better.

R

RELIGION

See also Moral Development and Values.

Religion, the belief in God and spiritual teaching is practiced in various forms in this country. Many families follow traditional ways to practice religious beliefs by attending churches or temples. Families who do not care to follow the specific practices of a religious group may find alternative ways to express their belief in God. Parents hopefully will choose what is most comfortable for themselves and share their belief system with their children. Children will learn about religion or not by observing their parents and participating if they are given the opportunity.

To Raise a Jewish Child
Rabbi Hayim Halevy Donin
Basic Books
1977   220 pp. $11.95

Written to help parents raise their children to become affirmatively aware of themselves as Jews, this volume focuses on helping children be happy with their Judaism and be prepared to find meaning and purpose in their Jewish identities.

Help is provided in finding and evaluating a Hebrew school, in dealing with secular peer group pressure, and in planning family observances in the home.

So please don't focus in prematurely on his Bar Mitzvah. Tell him the reason he is going to Hebrew school is because he is a Jewish child and must learn about the Jewish people, about the Jewish religion, and about the Jewish way of life. Explain to your child that every Jew must study Torah and the more one knows and studies the better off one is. Let him know that he has to go to a Jewish school until he grows up and that Jewish study is a necessary part of life.

What about Gods
Chris Brockman
Prometheus Books
1978   20 pp. $3.95

People have tried to explain just about everything at one time or another by inventing gods or other imaginary beings. This easy-to-read text for children shares ideas on religion, and cautions readers that gods aren't real and don't help explain anything. Urging children to think about rules, religion and church buildings and gods, the text insists that explanations ought to be scientific, not mythical.

If you've been wondering about gods, you're probably already doing the best thing you can do about something imaginary that many people expect you to believe is real, which is thinking about it. Thinking about gods is not always easy to do though, especially when so many of the people you know probably say they believe in a god. It can also be hard because some people believe it is bad to think about gods and not have faith. They might try to give you a hard time for thinking about gods. But thinking is the only way we have of judging ideas and the information our senses give us.

Thinking is the only way we have of knowing.
   KEEP ON THINKING

When Children Ask About God
Rabbi Harold S. Kushner
Schocken Books
1976   176 pp. $3.95

This book helps parents and teachers present an alternative, nontraditional understanding of what is meant by the word "God," miracles, prayers and so on.

As the child grows older, he begins to outgrow his childish conception of God. He is less likely to be thought of as a Superperson in the sky and more likely to refer to ideas of right and wrong. . . . At about ten, a child will try to sort through the theological baggage that he has accumulated over several years of asking questions and hearing stories. He is aware of contradictions and impossibilities. At this point our answers can do the most good.

Your Child and Religion
Johanna L. Klink
John Knox Press
1972   239 pp. $6.95

Combines quotations from children's letters with statements by specialists to help parents pass their faith on to their children. Klink's book is a kind of "little theology for parents" or a "shorter catechism" to help parents and anyone who deals with children gain a more profound understanding of their faith so it can be explained to their offspring. The book deals with the existence of God, omniscience, human suffer-

ing, prayer, good and evil and the
end of the world.

*It naturally depends upon the
age of the child, how much of this
one can get over to him. But a
child will certainly have a feeling
for human responsibility, that
things happen which are men's
fault, and why should he not accept that God cannot help it when
storms blow?*

Organizations
(See Appendix A)

Jewish Board of Family and Children's Services

National Conference of Christians
and Jews

National Forum of Catholic Parent
Organizations

National Society for Hebrew Day
Schools

United Synagogue of America

R

Please consult with the minis-
ter of your local church for the address of the organization that provides educational information to
the members of the church you
belong to or are interested in.

RIGHTS OF CHILDREN

WHO SPEAKS FOR CHILDREN?

. . . We are all guardians of the children's rights. And if the village conditions which conferred tribal guardians
upon the newborn and his family do not prevail in a complex society, we can reconstitute the mission of the tribal
guardians for a complex society.

The children need spokesmen, advocates, and lobbyists at every level of social and political organization in
which public policy and law affect the development of the child and may impinge upon his human rights. On the
highest levels of government we need powerful spokesmen who can speak with authority and with the strength of
numbers behind them for "the special interests" of children.

Selma Fraiberg
Every Child's Birthright: In Defense of Mothering
Basic Books
1977   188 pp. $10.95
Bantam Books
1979   188 pp. $2.50

Bill of Rights
for Children

The Bill of Rights declares that
every child must be granted:

1. The right to be wanted and
born well.

2. The right to "open systems
that focus on the future."

3. The right to a healthful environment.

4. The right to early childhood
learning experiences which are

suitable to each child's current
needs and which provide a
foundation for future educational experiences.

5. The right to a system of formal
education which provides the
opportunity for accumulating
broad knowledge, helps individuals to achieve their aspira-
tions and promotes humani-
tarian attitudes.

6. The right to become a participating and productive member
of society.

7. The right to receive special attention and support from private and governmental bodies
so that basic needs are met.

8. The right to well-functioning
organizational systems with
sufficient and effective man-
power to provide a broad
spectrum of services.

9. The right to a world and universe free from the threat of
annihilation by war.

—California Council on
Children and Youth

Beyond the Best Interests of the Child
Joseph Goldstein, Anna Freud and
Albert J. Solnit
Free Press
1973   161 pp. $3.95

R Two renowned psychoanalysts and a noted legal authority propose guidelines to prevent needless emotional scars in children who experience divorce-custody battles, stressing that each child should have a chance to be a member of a family where he feels wanted and should have a say in his placement.

We take the view that the law must make the child's needs paramount. This preference reflects more than our professional commitment. It is in society's best interests. Each time the cycle of grossly inadequate parent-child relationships is broken, society stands to gain a person capable of becoming an adequate parent for children of the future.

BirthRights
Richard Farson
Macmillan
1974   240 pp. $6.95
Penguin Books
1974   248 pp. $2.50

Our world is not a good place for children, maintains the author, because every institution in our society discriminates against them. The author reveals the human rights which he believes children should have, such as the right to responsive environmental design, the right to alternative home environments, the right to a single standard for themselves and adults, the right to justice, and the right to political power.

Subjecting children to the prohibitions and deceptions which keep them uninformed and dependent ultimately threatens our democratic process, which requires above all else an informed citizenry. The most potent weapon against tyranny is knowledge that is accessible to all members of society. Whenever one group decides what is and what is not desirable for another to know, whenever a "we-they" condition exists, society becomes vulnerable to totalitarianism.

Childhood for Every Child
Mark Gerzon
Outerbridge & Lazard
1970   250 pp. $7.95

Most Americans wrongly assume that the growth of their children is adequately provided for by the family, school and doctor. The author states that by plying children with synthetic foods, by giving them computers instead of teachers, modern technology has dehumanized the process of growth and children are not allowed to develop naturally.

Young people and other activists have only begun the difficult re-examination of this food fiasco and the possible effects on future generations of kids. Their reaction is incomplete, sometimes inaccurate, and sometimes even faddist. But some reaction is essential if the next generation is to grow at all. Today in our overstuffed nation, we sit entranced at the spectacle of moon exploration while our children wither of malnutrition or gorge themselves on sugary, chemical concoctions. No wonder the post-technological generation, which was bottle-, Gerber-, and Froot Loop-fed, has begun to re-examine their culinary upbringing.

Children Are People Too
Virginia Coigney
William Morrow
1975   228 pp. $6.95

This book shatters the myth that the United States has created a child-centered, child-loving community; stating that we are unintentionally cruel to children and treat them as property. The author provides an ongoing lesson in ways to love children and respect their rights.

Excessive anger can give the parent an unwelcome glimpse of his own childishness, as some of these responses suggest. He stands —driven by rage—on the brink of his own remembered helplessness. Or, he may be made only too well aware of the insecurities of his everyday life. The child's refusal to accept authority is a sharp reminder of the parent's daily helplessness —in work, in marriage, in so many relationships.

The Children's Rights Movement
Beatrice Gross and Ronald Gross
Doubleday
1977   380 pp. $3.95

The authors present changes that need to be made in people's minds and in the patterns of work, education, law and politics to assure that children have healthy options for learning and growing. Including articles by noted physicians, judges and youth workers, the topics range from "Foster Homes that Are Not Too Loving" to "One Kid's Own Bill of Rights."

We define a wanted child as a child who is wanted, in an affectionate and nourishing sense, on a continuing basis by at least one adult—a child who can feel that he is, and will continue to be, valued by those who take care of him.

Conspiracy of Silence—The Trauma of Incest
Sandra Butler
New Glide Publications
1978   208 pp. $10.00

This is an aggressive, empathetic and judgmental book that raises usually unasked and hard-to-answer questions. The most important thing, Butler feels, is not to carry the burden of what someone has done. She feels the first step is to share information, so that the power of two people can become the power of three, four or however many are required to address the phenomena of incest specifically and issues of sexuality generally.

Whatever form the assault takes, the scarring of the child can be deep and lasting. Unlike physical abuse, the damage cannot always be seen, but the scars are there nonetheless. The most devastating result of the imposition of adult sexuality upon a child unable to determine the appropriateness of his or her response is the irretrievable loss of the child's inviolability and trust in the adults in his or her life.

Escape from Childhood—Needs and Rights of Children
John Holt
E. P. Dutton
1974   286 pp. $7.95

Since being subservient and dependent does most young people more harm than good, the rights and privileges of adults should be available to youngsters as well. Such rights include working for money, living away from home, equal treatment under the law and the right to vote.

Work is novel, adventurous, another way of exploring the world. Many defend the boredom and drudgery of the schoolroom by saying that we have to teach children what work is like. Why make the schoolroom dull in order to do that, when most children want to find out what work is like and for a while at least would not find it dull at all? Many children, often the most troublesome and unmanageable, want to be useful, to feel that they make a difference. Real work is a way to do this. Also, work is a part of the mysterious and attractive world of adults, who work much of the time. When a child gets a chance to work with them, he sees a new side of them and feels a part of their world. He also sees a glimpse of his own future. Someday he too will be big and will work most of the time; now he can find out what it will be like.

Weeping in the Playtime of Others
Kenneth Wooden
Mc-Graw Hill
1976   249 pp. $4.95

A moving, dramatic examination of facilities for the incarceration of youth and the wretched treatment inflicted on children by the courts and institutions created to help them. Wooden describes how decisions are made to imprison children and cites economic reasons for the failure to improve their treatment.

Is there a correlation between the inability to read and future delinquency? I am convinced that there is and my conviction is based on a complex of attitudes and platitudes ingrained in our educational system. For the child who falls behind, who . . . hears such words as "dumb," "retarded," "nonreader," and "failure" follow him from kindergarten to high school or whatever grade at which he drops out (the U.S. Office of Education states about one million such children drop out of school yearly), the

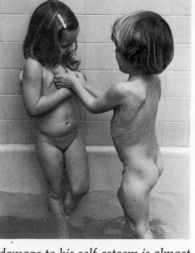

R

damage to his self-esteem is almost certainly irreversible. These years of educational failure shatter the self-confidence of the child. Failure leads to frustration and hopelessness, which in turn can lead to aggressiveness. Acts of aggression, mild or violent, if detected by the schools, police, parents or associated agency, could well mean incarceration for the child.

Organizations (See Appendix A)

National:

Administration for Children, Youth and Families

Appalachian Regional Commission

Child Welfare League of America

Children's Defense Fund

Coalition for Children and Youth

Education Development Center

National Child Labor Committee

National Committee for Prevention of Child Abuse

National Council on Family Relations

U.S. Department of Health and Human Services

Local:

California Children's Lobby

Children's Council of San Francisco—Childcare Switchboard

San Francisco Child Abuse Council

S

SAFETY. SEE FIRST AID AND SAFETY.

SENSORY DEVELOPMENT

See also Developmental Disabilities; Eyesight; Language and Speech.

It might be said that this is where it's all happening! Without the senses, there could be no language as we know it. Senses are critical to our ability to acquire language. If one or more senses are limited, we should determine the extent of the problem as early as possible in the child's life. The other functional senses may have taken over naturally. Or we may have to assist by channeling stimuli through other senses. If we do, our first goal is to determine what senses are functional and to what extent.

Touching-Feeling

Some research indicates that the tactile is one of our most vital senses. Do you know if your child can feel with his body parts the difference between hot and cold, rough and smooth, soft and hard, size, shape?

Smell

The nose protects us by helping us to be more aware of our surroundings.

Taste

Whatever we taste, the spectrum of sensations is infinite but always within the range of sweet, sour, bitter, cold, and hot.

Happiness Is Helping Children Know and Use Their Bodies
Michael K. Grimes
Burgess Publishing Co.
1977   105 pp. $5.95

This manual for parents and teachers helps them teach children how to explore their senses and physical abilities, how to communicate and how to enjoy body movement. Sections cover topics such as spatial relationships, balance, physical activities to develop learning readiness and low-cost equipment.

Movement exploration is a means of problem solving or learning through guided discovery. Motivation is supplied by the teacher's presentation of challenges which first provoke thought, then elicit related action. In responding to a challenge, each child can discover something about how he can move and can experience some measure of success by solving the problem his way. The goal is to help children continue in their efforts to solve problems, their ability to make judgments, and to perform in response to those judgments. As the child adds one small success to another, adds one new skill to another, and grows in his ability to listen, follow cues, and create, he becomes an increasingly alert, confident, thinking, sharing, creating individual—a complete person.

Hearing

Because this is one of our most used senses, it is critical to determine to what extent it is operating. Basically there are two types of hearing:

Acuity (ability to hear sounds of varying intensity). Your own observations as a parent may be very helpful in identifying this limitation.

Speech reception (ability of cochlear nerve to transmit signals to the cortex). More specific observations are needed to determine whether this ability is limited.

Sight

See section on eyes for more information. The eyes are the windows to the world and need protection, care, and attention.

230

Your Child's Sensory World
Lise Liepmann
Penguin Books
1973   315 pp. $2.95

Long before parents must deal with reading, writing and arithmetic problems, they must deal with the real basics—a child's individual sensory patterns. A child's sensory world influences his whole way of life: learning, playing and communicating. Therefore, an awareness of how a child is apt to respond in various situations is vital to a parent. Through a series of games and exercises, this book aids parents in understanding the child's awareness; such things as touch awareness, seeing awareness and communication skills are designed to produce sensitive children.

An idea for expanding hearing sensitivity:

Try a general hearing game with your child while you are both waiting in the dentist's office. He says, "Mommy, what's that bell ringing?" You answer, "You mean the phone next door?" "No, it's a slow, deep bell." "Oh, yes. That must be the church clock on the corner. I never noticed it before." Your child's hearing sensitivity has helped you become more aware of a sound. This should make your child feel proud of himself, and it is fun for both of you besides.

For Children

Anatomy Coloring Book
David Sachs
Aspen Publishing Co.
1972   29 pp. $1.50

This book contains large, easy-to-color pictures of body organs and parts, with health hints below each drawing. For young children.

The ear picks up the sounds you hear. Happy sounds will be yours to hear if dirt, toys and loud noise are kept from your ear.

See Appendix C for Films and Audio-Visual Aids.

SEX EDUCATION
CHILDHOOD SEXUALITY

Children are born with their sexual systems already functioning. Indeed, research photographs by sound waves have shown male infants with erections before birth, and lubrication has been noted in the vaginas of female babies in the twenty-four hours following birth. So one's sexuality (defined as one's sense of self as a male or a female, and how one has been conditioned to behave as a boy or girl, man or woman) continues to develop throughout a long learning process which is subject to many influences. Many parents are unaware of their role in this process—children continuously absorb their parents' feelings about their own selves and others as sexual people. Just as all children learn how to eat, how to talk, how to get along with other people, etc., so do they learn about sexuality.

An example of this learning is a parent's response when seeing his/her child masturbate. Whether the parent is uncomfortable or angry or accepting, a message is communicated to the child about sex which is an important part of that child's earliest sex education. These messages form the foundation of a child's developing values regarding his/her body, its potential for pleasure, and the ways in which that pleasuring is appropriately enjoyed (or perhaps denied). Education for human sexuality is far more complex than merely sharing information and facts.

If parents themselves feel uncomfortable about their own sexual lives, it will be difficult for them to talk to their children about sex. But even with no discussion, a lot of sex education happens anyway, for no message becomes, in itself, a message. Therefore communicating that "this is hard for me to do, but I'm trying" may be more important for a child's learning about sex than long talks or books to read—and infinitely better than total silence. Making it possible for your child to learn about this area of absorbing interest conveys the sense that you care about him/her, a concept intrinsic to its whole well-being. Your child may then feel free to ask questions because you have communicated to him/her that it's okay to do so. You have become, in Dr. Sol Gordon's words, an askable parent!

Children are receptive to and can absorb age-appropriate, accurate information about their sexuality and the sexuality of others. If the communication of caring is maintained, then when the pubertal changes take place and the reproductively "grown-up" children begin facing important decisions about their sexual lives, they will be able to make intelligent decisions, based on a value system developed from clear pictures of their reproductive possibilities and sexual feelings in the light of their responsibilities to themselves and others, rather than from slavish obedience to rules that can crumble under peer pressure or adolescent insecurities. All of this can be done effectively within the philosophical and moral framework intrinsic to each family.

In sum, it is impossible for children not to be sexual, with sexual thoughts, feelings, and responses, for sooner or later, and normally, sexuality must and will make itself manifest in every growing human being. It cannot be totally suppressed, it can only be deflected, distorted—or facilitated. It is the nature of that facilitation that must be our real concern.

Mary S. Calderone
President, Sex Information
and Education Council of the U.S.

Sex Without Shame
Alayne Yates
William Morrow
1978   227 pp. $7.95

S   If they are raised to appreciate sexual pleasures, children will spontaneously expand and enrich their sexuality as part of their own development. The author stresses the crucial role of the parent in encouraging healthy growth in sexual competency. Exercises and games are presented that parents can perform with their offspring to make sexual experiences tangible and less frightening.

The first attempt at really talking about sex may seem earth-shaking to you but can be pleasurable and comforting for your child. Be prepared for some startling misconceptions. My first session with my own children was a revelation. My six-year-old thought that babies resulted from kissing. My five-year-old wondered if boys have to pull on their penis in order to start the stream of urine. My sophisticated ten-year-old had once assumed that girls had a retractable penis they pushed out at will like a bowel movement. At first, the parent learns more than the child.

Organizations (See Appendix A)

American Association of Sex Educators and Counselors

Sex Information and Education Council of the U.S.

SEXUAL EQUALITY

Children should have ample opportunities to be all that they can be; boys and girls should have the chance to explore different roles and experiences, not just "male" or "female" ones. Girls should be allowed to hammer nails and climb if they wish to. Boys should be comfortable cooking and experiencing parenting by playing with dolls.

Children should feel natural about their own skills, abilities and interests, regardless of cultural stereotyping of expected roles. If a young boy is told that "boys don't cry," how is he to handle his need to cry in certain situations? What is he to think about himself and his potential as a man if men and boys aren't supposed to cry?

We all need to be free to express our full range of feelings in ways that are acceptable socially for our age and situation as well as our culture. We need to let children know that it is okay to do this. We as parents and adults need to know that it is all right for us to do this, also.

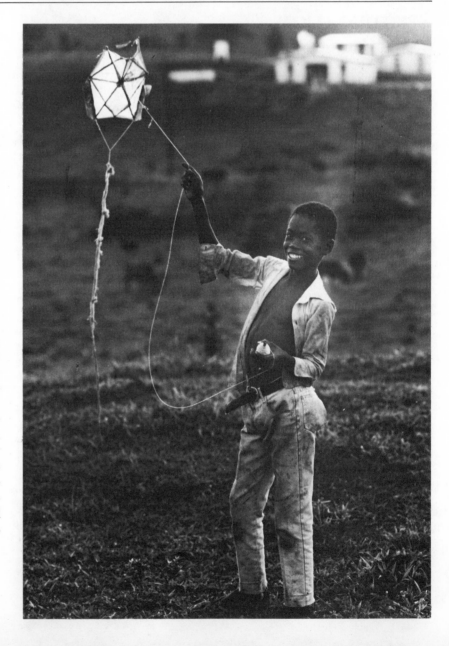

S

SEX ROLES

During this decade the emergence of the women's movement in America has generated a serious re-examination of roles for many women, as well as many men. One area that has been drastically affected by these changes has been child care. Traditionally, the task of child rearing in this society has been left to women. Both nursery and elementary schools have always been dominated by women teachers and men administrators. Women choosing to pursue careers and women forced by economic pressures to support a family, have increased the need for day care. The response to that need has seen many men become active in the education and child-rearing process. To combat sexism in our society, women and men, together, must share the responsibility of raising our children to be free.

Many day care centers are now very sensitive to the stereotyping of children by sex. Boys may play with dolls and girls with blocks. In kindergarten, often an invisible but solid line seems to separate boys' activities from girls'. I can remember my own frustration about not being able to cross over it. Women and men working together, sharing responsibility for all aspects of child care, have eased the burden for many girls and boys, so that stepping across a sex-role-defined line need no longer be as troublesome to the child. Women and men can both change diapers, clean hands, prepare meals, sing songs, tell stories, cuddle and comfort and care for scrapes and bruises as well as manage finances, design curriculum and operate technical aspects of a day care operation.

I can remember my first experience with children. I felt I could only be effective with children 2 years old and over—already verbal and toilet trained. The notion of the baby needing mother (woman) was so ingrained in my mind that I was afraid to deal with infants. As my knowledge increased with experience, the world of the first two years of life was reopened to me. I was able to learn new ways to communicate watching children utter their first words. I learned I could change diapers. I could actually care for a baby. At first, some of the older children seemed confused by a man caring for a baby, but after a short time they grew accustomed to watching me cradling or diapering an infant.

Working with two- to five-year-olds, I can remember incidents where groups of boys would isolate girls trying to enter "their" games. Many girls held back because of this and because of conditioning not to compete with boys. This, however, need not remain a problem very long. Children are quick to accept new ideas and can easily unlearn the sexist conditioning that enters our lives every day. Working together with parents, teaching and practicing equality between women and men in the day care centers, we began teaching children in this new way. Girls began to feel free to run, climb and play ball while boys found they could also pursue interests in cooking and arts and crafts. Activities tended to become more integrated between the sexes. Generally, by eliminating sexist expectations, the results were less defined role playing by children and positive freedom for their growth and development.

Sexism spreads to children very early and quickly in our society through media and advertising. To combat this and to help our children grow up free we must continue to work together (both women and men) in an atmosphere where work is shared equally and without distinction. Children learn more from examples; therefore it is our responsibility to provide the best possible models for them in ourselves and what we do.

Howie Montaug
Teacher Child Care Center

S *Unlearning the Lie*
Barbara Grizzuti Harrison
William Morrow
1973 176 pp. $2.95

An account of one school's encounter with sexism and its attempts to change the curriculum, library and teachers' attitudes to reflect a nonsexist awareness, this is a useful model for teachers and parents who are interested in changing aspects of a school's climate.

Consciousness-raising . . . started to bear fruit: we began to see changes at the school. The staff committed itself to reevaluating its library and its readers and to ordering nonsexist books. The physical setup of nursery and kindergarten classrooms, which had encouraged grouping according to sex, was rearranged to facilitate the movement of children without regard to boy/girl definitions. Several fathers found themselves momentarily at a loss for words when their grade chairperson telephoned to ask if they would contribute a casserole to the school bazaar. Pre-

viously, when a mother telephoned to speak to a parent on a school matter, a father's automatic response had been, "Just a minute, I'll call my wife." We weren't inundated with manmade casseroles, but we felt that by not allowing men to assume automatically that this was their wives' job, we had raised their consciousness.

What is a girl? What is a boy?
Stephanie Waxman
Peace Press
1976 40 pp. $6.95/$3.95

This interesting photographic essay on sex roles and sexual identity gives suggested activities for parent or teacher.

Some people say a girl is someone with a girl's name. Sam is usually a boy's name. But this Sam is a girl. Some people say a boy is someone who is strong. But Lola is lifting a heavy block. And she's a girl. Some people say a boy is someone who doesn't cry. But Eric is crying. And he's a boy.

Organizations
(See Appendix A)

Non-Sexist Child Development Project

Magazines
(See Appendix B)

Ms.
Working Mother

SINGLE PARENTS

See also Divorce.

For a variety of reasons, many parents are separated or divorced. Single parents have a challenging role to play in the lives of their children. Often the responsibility for their children is totally on their shoulders, and they need support and assistance. Single parents can form organizations and groups and exchange baby-sitting, and in many ways provide emotional backup to each other.

SOME DO'S AND DON'TS FOR SINGLE PARENTS

Several years ago I was divorced and had, it seemed, all the typical problems one associates with getting divorced, not least of which was an increasingly difficult time with my son, then 3 years old, now 9. I was working full time teaching elementary school and doing all I could in the evenings for my son, feeling sorry for him and trying to make up to him for what had happened. As a result my life became subject to his every whim and he fast developed into a miniature but extremely powerful tyrant.

I'd like to pass on a few ideas to those of you who are now on your own and may be ready at times to "climb the walls" with your children. Your problems may be the "normal" ones. Those are the ones that are so prevalent we expect them and assume we can do nothing but wait until the next stage and hope they'll outgrow whatever it is. Or perhaps you are having more serious problems which occur less frequently but which are even more devastating at the moment, especially to the single parent who tends to hold himself or herself responsible for all the children's postdivorce emotional problems. Here is a list of some simple do's and don'ts which may help some of you get back on an even keel with your children, feel less defeated by them, and in the process enjoy them more.

Do's

S

- Do spend regularly scheduled time alone with each child at least once a week, doing what that child chooses (as long as it doesn't violate your values), and have a regularly-scheduled family fun time once a week. The activity is determined by consensus of all members, or you may wish to alternate the responsibility for that choice.

- Do reserve talking for pleasant conversation. No matter how powerful your child is, he can't *make* you talk. At a moment of conflict when you're either seething inside, feel a defeat coming, or want to lecture, stop talking and retire from the situation to cool off. The bathroom's a good place if there's reading material available (a very exciting detective story does it for me) and a transistor radio. Or perhaps this is a good time for a bubble bath. Your bedroom may be a better place for you if there's a lock on the door to use when necessary. At any rate, keep out of the warfare. If you stay in it and win, the children are likely to regroup forces for the next attack. However, it's more likely that you'll lose, since children are really much more creative than we parents.

- If you have nobly retained your objectivity and sense of humor in the face of your child's misbehavior, do the unexpected: think about what you would typically do (explain, spank, yell, cry, etc.) and do the opposite. A kiss for example, when a spank is expected, can in some cases work wonders. Once when my son had a tantrum I waited for him to catch his breath and then I lay down on the floor, kicked and screamed, exclaiming, "It's my turn now!" When I began my tantrum he stopped his and after taking turns a few times we both "broke up." Needless to say, your unexpected response has to be changed often and can only be used when you are relatively unshattered by the preceding event.

- Do let your children take responsibility for themselves. They'll learn responsibility when it's given to them. This means you can relax about their schoolwork (it's their business) while retaining your interest in what they're doing. It also means you don't need to rush about reminding, lugging forgotten items to school, or getting dinner three times for those who don't make the first serving. What you do, instead, is to let the children feel the natural consequences of their actions. Going without a meal if arriving for dinner too late is far better for a child's development than learning to be irresponsible. Perhaps more importantly, it is preferable to the usual scolding or lecture given for such transgressions. A key for the successful implementation of natural consequences is kindness and firmness at the same time. Your pleasant attitude takes you out of the punisher role and lets the reality of life be the teacher. Figuring out a natural consequence is sometimes difficult, but it's helpful to ask yourself, "What would happen if I did nothing to intervene in this situation?" There are other times when you can't let the natural consequence occur. At these times with most children, a logical consequence can be agreed on by the family which is not viewed as punishment but which will allow children to feel the natural order necessary for humans to live in cooperation with each other.

- Do respect yourself and your children. Authoritarian methods no longer work well with children, or between husbands and wives for that matter. This means you respect your child's right to make his own choices (how much he eats, what he says, when he goes to sleep, etc.), but you also can choose your own responses, e.g., you can leave the room if he chooses to yell at you, you can choose not to let him accompany you shopping if he's not cleaned up or dressed appropriately, you can ask that he serve himself the amount he wishes to eat and finish that before taking more, etc. Your children will respond more cooperatively when given a choice rather than being told "You must," and you will be helping them learn to respect the rights and feelings of others by insisting on this respect for yourself.

- Do let your children take an active part in running the household as soon as they can toddle about. We all feel more belongingness and happier with ourselves when we are contributing, when we are really needed. Payment for chores done in the home deprives children of the intrinsic satisfaction derived from their contribution to the family, and tends to encourage the attitude of "I'll give only if I get something in return." Your appreciation of their efforts is enough encouragement. My son and I now do all the housework together and I notice a distinct improvement in his attitude toward me. I initiated the idea by saying I wanted to help him feel more important, to feel that this was his house, too, and not just mine.

S
    • Do start listening to your children's ideas and let them help you make decisions which will affect them. They will be much more cooperative if you have all reached a consensus. I have a weekly business meeting with my son and we make plans, decide on rules or consequences, assign jobs for the week, take care of his allowance, and discuss any feelings we might have concerning our relationship.

    • Do encourage your children. It's difficult to feel worthwhile and okay about oneself in this competitive society, and as Dreikurs says, "Children need encouragement like a plant needs water." You can encourage your children most effectively by giving them your time and attention when they are not *demanding* it, by accepting them *as they are* at any time without expectation for change, by frequently demonstrating your affection for them and your appreciation of them, and by giving them your vote of confidence—your absolute belief in their strength and ability to cope with any situation. "I'm sure you can handle that" has become a byword in my household and it's so gratifying to see my son become a more courageous individual.

Don'ts

    • Don't threaten, bribe, or extract promises from your children. These methods, commonly used by parents and teachers, demonstrate your lack of faith and therefore your lack of respect. Furthermore, you'll probably get the misbehavior you expect or fear. Research has convincingly demonstrated that we evoke that which we anticipate.

    • Don't talk too much. This is a particularly difficult rule for me to follow. For some reason males don't usually have as much difficulty with this as females; they act, not talk. When you explain and explain, you are probably satisfying yourself ("I'm teaching my child the right thing to do") but not showing respect for the child. Children are quite intelligent, one explanation is sufficient, and anyway, they usually know when a certain behavior is inappropriate. They learn most from observing the behavior of their parents and other adults, and are quite aware of what is socially acceptable and what is not.

    • Don't do for your children what they are able to do for themselves. They gain confidence and skill through practice, not your help. Although it's far easier to give in and dress a 3- or 4-year-old in the morning, for example, it's more encouraging to him if you can plan a longer time in the morning to allow him to dress himself. To introduce the idea of his dressing himself, you might take some time when there is no pressure and make a game out of his putting his pants on and taking them off, etc., commenting that you believe he is old enough now so that you can let him do this himself. This encourages the attitude "It's a privilege to take on more responsibility!" After he can take care of dressing himself, even though the job may not be perfect, you can remain firm in your resolve not to help him—if necessary you can even take him to nursery school in a state of undress!

    • Lastly, don't pity your child. No person is as unhappy as one who feels unfairly treated and sorry for himself, and this is exactly the feeling that is picked up by children when the surrounding adults feel sorry for "the poor things." Unwittingly, these adults rob children of the capacity to make the best of any situation, and are again demonstrating a lack of faith and respect. As Dr. James Croake pointed out in his article on guilt (*Single Parent*, March, 1974), this insidious pity is very likely to occur during and after a divorce, when parents and relatives feel sorry for the children having to go through such a traumatic situation. In fact, they'll only be traumatized if you expect them to be.

    Perhaps the most satisfying aspect of my professional career has been the knowledge that I can use what I've learned and practice what I preach, in my own family of two. As for you other parents without partners, rest assured that it's really not necessary to drop everything and rush into graduate school to find new and better ways to relate with your children. The guidelines are fairly simple, and as Dr. Pew suggested in a recent *Single Parent* article (April 1974), you can join a group of parents and study the book *Children: The Challenge* together for further elaboration of the concepts presented here as well as other guidelines to follow in relating with your children.

Nancy Catlin,
The Single Parent,
July/August, '74

Bachelor Fatherhood: How to Raise and Enjoy Your Children as a Single Parent
Michael McFadden
Ace Books
1978   158 pp. $1.75

In this book the author covers virtually every aspect of the single father's life. Michael McFadden is a single father—one of the new and increasingly prevalent breed of men who, either by choice or circumstance, are raising their children alone. He offers practical advice on dealing with the divorce and custody hearing, raising small and teen-age children, running a household in the simplest way possible, cooking, and readjusting to life as a bachelor in general.

A group of four single fathers in Manhattan have bought an old brownstone between them and set up a single fathers' commune. A man in Pontiac, Michigan, raising his seven-year-old son, works a night shift and so has a particular problem. What he does is trade with a single mother who works days. He leaves his son at her house on the way to work, then picks up her six-year-old girl and his son on the way home from work. He fixes them breakfast, gets them off to school, then sleeps until they get home. Two hours later the woman picks up her daughter and he has the time alone with his son until he's off to work again.

Getting It Together
Lynn Forman
Berkley Medallion Books
1974   173 pp. $1.50

A guide for divorced mothers to ease the confusion of pulling life together, this book contains advice on reentering the job market; devising a feasible schedule around a job, the child's school and the baby-sitter's hours; dealing with a budget; coping with friends who are either "his" or "yours"; handling the child's reaction when you meet someone new.

Although it may sometimes seem that you have the worst of both worlds—the responsibilities of the married mother without her security, and the aloneness of the single woman, without her freedom—when it comes to those evening hours, in some ways you're better off than either of them.

It's true that the married woman does have someone to share the family burden with. But it's also true that she has that someone's wishes to compromise with, and even her most personal decisions must often be arrived at by mutual consent.

Guide For Single Parents
Kathryn Hallett
Celestial Arts
1974   121 pp. $3.95

Hallett demonstrates how the techniques of transactional analysis can transform the personal loss of divorce, separation or death into an experience of growth rather than paralysis and despair.

A child who is disappointed by his parents' divorce, or who has lost a parent through death, may well decide never to get close to another person again. A child whose feelings are ignored or shut off may decide never to tell or show how she/he feels again. A child who is overprotected or kept "the baby" may continue to seek people who care for and protect him/her. Another child who is left by parents to handle his younger brothers and sisters long before he's able might feel he can only be loved if he takes care of others.

How To Parent Alone
Joan Bel Geddes
Seabury Press
1974   293 pp. $8.95

S

This book is about parent care: how to increase self-confidence, handle financial problems, conquer boredom, overcome loneliness and comfort yourself.

It is advisable for a single parent to read what different experts have to say on subjects like these, but I think it is equally important to read general advice applicable to all children. Even if married parents think they can raise children without consulting books (which I think is doing it the hard way, the hazardous trial-and-error way), no single parent should try, because there is no full-time partner to assist and advise and argue with you. You need to hear someone else's views to balance your own prejudices, both conscious and unconscious, and to supplement your own limitations.

In this sense a good child-care book is a good husband-or-wife substitute. A very incomplete one, no doubt, but a helpful one.

Sex and the Single Parent
Jane Adams
Coward, McCann & Geoghegan
1978   342 pp. $8.95

How does the sexual behavior of single parents help or harm their children? The author deals with the sexual activities and attitudes of single parents. The book discusses feelings of guilt, dependence and self-doubt that plague single parents and the rewards and challenges single-parent families are discovering in their new roles.

Coming to terms with one's sexual identity is a difficult process; when it is further complicated (or enhanced) by single parenthood, it is even harder. Lovers are traditionally "alone in their own universe"—but not lovers who are single parents. There is a part of us that is never truly shared, the part that represents our lifelong commitment to and investment in the children over which we have custody. And no one understands that except another single parent.

Single Parent Experience
Carole Klein
Walker
1973   241 pp. $7.95
Avon
1978   300 pp. $2.50

This serious, level-headed appraisal of the growing social phenomenon of single parenting includes discussions of the reasons for choosing to raise children alone, homosexual parenting, the effects of single parents on the adoption market and the psychological effects of having a single parent.

All the angry writing from advocates of women's liberation, all the strident talk of motherhood myths and baby traps fade in impact at the simple picture of a man cuddling his child with no wife having to smile benign encouragement at his side, ready to grab the baby before he gets hurt by awkward male attempts at affection. And no stronger argument for eliminating biologic and cultural roles and replacing them with human roles exists than in such a picture. For if that hallowed or disputed maternal instinct can be defined at all, it would imply a deep instinct for wanting children, a desire to love them, and cherish, and nurture, and support, and protect them in deeply emotional and not just physical ways. If this is what it means, then the single father is saying, in as clear a voice as we shall ever hear, that if not all women have such feelings, many men do.

For Children

The Boys & Girls Book About
One-Parent Families
Richard A. Gardner
Bantam Books
1981   236 pp. $2.95

This is a book for children living in a one-parent home and designed to be read by children who have a third- to fourth-grade level of reading comprehension. It deals with the feelings that arise as a result of the divorce or death of a parent.

When one parent leaves, however, the children may fear that the other parent may leave as well. They may think, "If my father can leave the house so easily, why can't my mother leave also?" They may then fear that they will be all alone. They may imagine that there will be no one to take care of them, to feed them, to buy them clothes, and to do all the other things that parents do for children.

Organizations
(See Appendix A)

Parents Without Partners

SPORTS.
SEE EXERCISE AND
SPORTS.

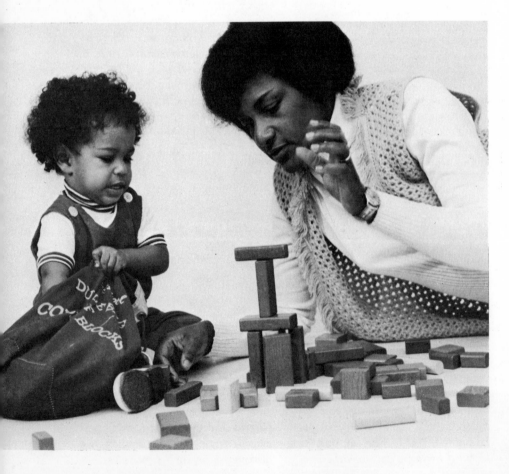

STEPPARENTING

FROM STEPPARENT TO REAL PARENT

S

Less than a generation ago families with stepparents were in a very small minority. Those were the days when the myth of the wicked stepparent could still prevail because the situation was far enough removed from most people's experience for little to be known about the actual family life shared by stepparents and their children.

Today, with divorce and remarriage increasingly common, we see that most stepparents are deeply committed men and women, working with all their hearts and minds to create a sound and happy life for their children, their mates and themselves.

In 1974 alone, two million adults with one million children became available for remarriage. The 1970 Census indicated that 12.4 million children under eighteen live with remarried parents, and it is estimated that fifteen million children are now living in stepfamilies. More than 80 percent of stepfamilies are the result of divorce, and many more fathers than ever before now obtain custody of their children and live with them.

The first step toward successful stepparenthood is to be willing to be flexible and tolerant in order to handle the demands and stresses of a new kind of family life. Even so, of course, there is no guarantee that every day will run smoothly and without conflict. But you will have the opportunity to share yourself, your ideas and skills, and to take part in a full life of challenges and often unexpected satisfactions. As Helen Thomson points out in her book, *The Successful Stepparent:* "A child can profit from a good marriage. He can also profit from a good remarriage. In some ways he can profit more. To be loved by the parents to whom you belong biologically and legally is one thing. To be loved by a person who reaches out to you only because he wants to reach out to you is something different."

Not surprisingly, the kind of parenting that works successfully with one's natural children—treating the child with courtesy, respect and affection, while maintaining consistent expectations and reasonable discipline—works with stepchildren, too. But more patience is needed for the results of that steady reassuring style to take effect. For stepchildren have inevitably suffered a disruption in their lives. They may have had to cope with the stress and sorrow of a fairly recent divorce between their parents, or even with the tragedy of the death of a parent. If the child has been living with only one parent for a long time, then his possessive feeling toward that parent is all too likely to explode into jealousy when the parent remarries. It is only natural for the child to be afraid that the intruding new father or mother will oust him from first place in his parent's heart.

Stepchildren at first are bound to have doubts and anxieties about the future. They need to learn they can count on you to provide them with stability and support before they feel free enough to trust you. After you have gained their trust then the true flowering of their love for you can take place. One stepfather I know told me, "I tried to treat the children as if they were really my own, not worrying about whether or not they would like me. It's not always easy, but I did make an effort to say and do what I thought was best for my two stepdaughters (which wasn't necessarily what they wanted to hear). I think it's important not to try to buy a stepchild's affection by acceding to his or her desires when these go against your better judgment. I tried not to worry from day to day whether or not my stepdaughters accepted me, but to be as real a father to them as I could."

The stepparents' responsibility is often easier to meet when very young children are involved; then the changes may be made more smoothly. With older children, the potential for problems increases, but differences can be resolved if everyone is willing to cooperate. Children need many, varied opportunities for self-expression. In our family, we found that one way to provide this was to create a family circle—a time to sit down together to listen and express ourselves, and to find out what the others felt, needed and wanted. The time this takes is very well spent as the children discover that what they feel is important to their parents and to the other children.

Another opportunity for good and constructive discussion is dinner time. While every dinner can't have the special quality of a family picnic, the very sharing of good things to eat can contribute to the kind of relaxed atmosphere that helps build family solidarity—particularly if the parents make a point of using this time for good talk and not for complaints or recriminations. At first, our dinner was so noisy it was difficult to hear each other. But then we asked the children to listen to each other, assuring them each would be heard. Soon, this "sharing" aspect of our dinner conversation came to be taken for granted.

S It's also important for stepparents, as it is for natural parents, to spend time regularly with each child separately, to learn about his or her needs, feelings and problems. Each child needs to know that he is as important as the others. Parents need time for each other, too—quiet time to talk over plans, problems and solutions, so they can come to an agreement about a given course of action before talking to the children.

The more agreement on everyday family life you and your mate come to beforehand, the better for you and for the children. If they know that both of you have made the important decisions and will be fair and firm, they will be likely to accept—and eventually respect—even those decisions they may initially complain about.

Children need to learn that love is not a scarce commodity—that there is enough for everyone. Not only do they need to realize that the new (mother or) father, say, doesn't threaten their relationship with their mother (or father), but they also need to be reassured that they can feel free to love their stepfather (or stepmother) without feeling guilty or disloyal to their natural father (or mother).

The life you live together now will contribute richly to each of you in the years ahead. A child learns how to be a parent by the examples of the parents who live with him or her each day. Don't expect to be perfect, but do be a real person to that real child. Relax and be yourself, and you will find that time usually solves what at the moment may seem to be insurmountable problems. If, however, frustrations seem overwhelming, undermining your love toward your partner and your confidence in your ability to be a good stepparent, do be willing to seek outside assistance from a counselor.

Finally, remember when you step up to stepparenthood you are bound to face problems and some setbacks. But the rewards and satisfactions are many, and these can only deepen with the passage of time.

Stevanne Auerbach
Parents' Magazine
June 1976

Half-Parent
Brenda Maddox
New American Library
1975   183 pp. $1.75

This guide to more satisfying stepparent-stepchild relationships deals with such issues as why the myth of the cruel stepparent is harsher on stepmothers than stepfathers, financial obligations and inheritance and the best method to handle discipline.

There are a few plain truths about stepparenthood. Stepfamilies can be happy, even happier than families in which there has never been more than one mother or father but it takes more work. The tensions of the stepfamily are special and real. A stepparent cannot be the same as a real parent. There are no new Mommies and new Daddies. Yet there are compensations for the strains. My own particular reward has been to help two young people who are nothing like me to be more like themselves

and to watch the bond grow between the two sets of children.

How to Live With Other People's Children
June and William Noble
Dutton
1979   197 pp. $5.95

This book gives guidance for everyone who might be part of a step relationship (live-in grandparents, temporary guardians) and also presents children's views of their stepparents. The authors stress that anyone who lives with other people's children must create an honest relationship. The Nobles advise the reader on how to prepare for stepchildren, how to deal with bitterness from the prior marriage, how to discipline and how to deal with discrimination by in-laws. Sound advice is given on legal and financial responsibilities, as well as on how to handle a

strongly possessive child and how to handle moodiness and erotic behavior. The authors also deal with the children of people who are not married but are living together.

What children do care about, we learned, is the security that comes form knowing that things are going to continue on an even keel, that faces are not going to change with the seasons. . . . Very few professionals, regardless of how permissively the community views pad crashing and casual split-ups, give much chance to a child's stability in revolving-door households. The situation is not even arguable. And the outcome for the child who is caught up in the adults' maneuvering is predictable: just as a welfare-receiving child becomes a welfare-receiving adult, just as an abused child becomes an abuser, a revolving-door child becomes a revolving-door adult.

Living in Step
Ruth Roosevelt and Jeannette Lofas
Stein & Day
1976   190 pp. $7.95

This is a good book for anyone who wonders what a remarriage with children will be like. The authors discuss the resentments and hostilities, as well as the opportunities for new love and understanding, that accompany the combining of two families. They include interviews with step families and advice on how to adjust, how to establish authority, and how to deal with frustration and loneliness if the stepchildren reject you. An important chapter deals with the lack of laws protecting stepparents.

We have seen couples who have worked out their step problems, each of them sharing with the other concerns for the other's children, each offering what they can and feeling grateful for the help of the other.

There seems to be a common secret to their success. The couple has put themselves first. This means that, when there's a question of priorities, each spouse understands their obligations toward the children and can meet them more successfully because of their commitment to each other. Husband and wife have put their ex-spouses behind them. They're a team, and they gear up together to cope. They're open with each other; they trust each other. Two people who have that sort of relationship can handle a lot of problems.

Stepfamily Bulletin
Human Sciences Press
72 Fifth Ave.
New York, N.Y. 10011
Individual Subscriptions $12.00;
Institutional Subscriptions $24.00

The Stepfamily Bulletin (Fall 1980 first issue) is the newsletter of the Stepfamily Association of America, Inc. It is a unique publication of interest to professionals and non-professionals involved in family study. It includes a children's section, book reviews, a professional activities section and association news.

Stepparenting
Jean and Veryl Rosenbaum
Chandler and Sharp
1977   142 pp. $7.95
E. P. Dutton
1978   145 pp. $3.50

In this book of sound advice and guidelines for developing relationships as stepparent, the authors, who are both stepparents and stepchildren, warn that no matter how kind and loving a stepparent is, he or she is still thought of as an intruder in a child's life. Chapters deal with the right to employ discipline, guilts and jealousies, constant comparing and guidelines for establishing effective communication.

When young children idealize a lost parent, the best way to handle their fantasies is to ignore the grandiose statements. It is dangerous to put down a previous parent. The children will learn the truth themselves later on.

The Successful Stepparent
Helen Thomson
Funk & Wagnalls
1966   237 pp. $1.50

The purpose of this book is to help stepparents with the problems they may encounter in their stepfamily situations. This book presents a way of looking at human feelings and human behavior that many adults have found helpful in their attempts to understand children.

The stepparent, in turn, may spend some uncomfortable moments wondering what he (or she) can think up to say to the kids, for as a rule conversations of this kind don't come easily to grownups not accustomed to children.

Organizations (See Appendix A)

Stepfamily Association of America, Inc.

Stepfamily Foundation of California

For Children

A New Mother for Martha
Phyllis Green
Human Sciences Press
1978   30 pp. $8.95

Written for school age children, this book renders a girl's experience of her mother's death, her father's subsequent remarriage and her struggle to accept both.

Martha looked at the rug. Then she looked at June. "I feel sorry for you, June," she said, softly, "because my father loves my mother most in the world. He could never love you half as much."

Martha watched June, who looked like she was about to cry. Martha thought, I didn't know I could make a grown-up cry. How alone June looks. How alone and lonely.

She couldn't stand the look on June's face. She couldn't stand the silence in the room. She jumped off her father's lap and ran to the guest room and threw herself on the bed.

TELEVISION

WATCH OUT FOR TV

TV. The family pacifier can be educational, entertaining and also boring and violent. Children are spending too much time in front of the set, considering the average figure of 15,000 hours of their childhood growth years spent in front of it. This is more time than is spent in school or in other active leisure time activities. Controversy in recent years has revolved around the amount of time spent not doing other activities, effects on learning and mental and social development, the extent of violence and the advertising bombardment. Parents need to check out what the children are watching and help them make good decisions about what they watch. The suggestions made here will assist in making TV time well spent.

All television is educational television. The question is: what is it teaching?

> Nicholas Johnson
> *How to Talk Back to Your Television Set*
> Atlantic
> 1970 $6.95

TV AND CHILDREN

Much of the programming and commercial message content of television programs being watched by children and youth is potentially, and often demonstrably, a mental and physical health hazard to the young. This is particularly true for those viewers who are at high risk because of ongoing conditions, such as developmental disabilities, mental retardation, psychoses and impulse disorders.

In recognition of this situation, the American Academy of Child Psychiatry and the American Academy of Pediatrics have both issued Position Statements on the effects of television viewing on children and youth. Both groups have recommended to their membership the inclusion, during their work with children and their families, of questions concerning the television viewing habits of the child and his or her family. Child psychiatrists and pediatricians have also been urged to make attempts to assess the impact of television viewing on children and youth and, where appropriate, make specific recommendations concerning viewing habits. Pediatricians and child psychiatrists have been asked to familiarize themselves with current programs provided both by the commercial networks and the public broadcasting system which are deemed to have positive influences on the psychosocial growth and development of their child and adolescent viewers, so that this information can be passed on to children and their families. (This information can be obtained from the national office of Action for Children's Television or from local affiliates of that national organization, or the local P.T.A.) Because most children under the age of eight are unable, on the basis of their cognitive developmental state, clearly to distinguish between program content and commercial messages when viewing television, both the Academy of Pediatrics and the Academy of Child Psychiatry have urged that commercial messages not be broadcast during television programs directed at this audience.

> Michael B. Rothenberg
> Psychiatrist

T

Guide to Assist Parents

TREAT TV WITH T.L.C.*

Talk about TV with Your Child!

- Talk about programs that delight your child.
- Talk about programs that upset your child.
- Talk about the differences between make-believe and real life.
- Talk about ways TV characters could solve problems without violence.
- Talk about violence and how it hurts.
- Talk about TV foods that cause cavities.
- Talk about TV toys that may break too soon.

Choose TV Programs with Your Child!

- Choose the number of programs your child can watch.
- Choose to turn the set off when the program is over.
- Choose to turn on public television.
- Choose to improve children's TV by writing a letter to a local station . . . to a television network . . . to an advertiser . . . to Action for Children's Television.

Look at TV with Your Child!

- Look out for TV behavior your child might imitate.
- Look for TV characters who care about others.
- Look for women who are competent in a variety of jobs.
- Look for people from a variety of cultural and ethnic groups.
- Look for healthy snacks in the kitchen instead of on TV.
- Look for ideas for what to do when you switch off the set . . . .
- Read a book . . . draw a picture . . . play a game.

Evelyn Kaye
The Act Guide to Children's Television
Beacon Press
1979   226 pp. $5.95

---

*Tender, Loving Care

T

The Plug-In Drug
Marie Winn
Bantam Books
1978   258 pp. $2.75

This book concerns itself with the effects of television on children—not the contents of the programs children watch but the effects upon the vulnerable and developing human organism of spending such a significant proportion of each day engaging in this particular experience.

Preschool children are the single largest television audience in America, spending a greater number of total hours and a greater proportion of their waking day watching television than any other age group. According to one survey made in 1970, children in the 2–5 age group spend an average of 30.4 hours each week watching television, while children in the 6–11 group spend 25.5 hours watching. . . . Even the most conservative estimates indicate that preschool children in America are spending more than a third of their waking hours watching television.

Family Guide To Children's Television
Evelyn Kay
Pantheon Books
1974 $8.95/$2.95

This book is out of stock, and probably going out of print. Contact your library to obtain a copy.

Guess who Owns the Airwaves?
Committee on Childhood Television
1511 Masonic Ave.
San Francisco, CA 94117

This pamphlet explains the work that the Committee on Childhood Television is doing to alert people to TV's effect on the lives of children and includes a list of their publications.

TV: The Family School
Edward Morris and Gregory Freida
Avatar Press
1976   63 pp. $3.00

This short, easy-to-read, well-thought-out book takes a fresh, positive look at the living room as a classroom, with television and parents working together as team teachers. It does not editorialize or condone present network programming, but rather offers helpful, specific teaching techniques using TV as an aid to improve language skills and encourage inquisitive thinking in children between the ages of two and twelve.

Point out numbers when they appear on TV screen. Ask child to name them.
Tell child what time favorite programs will come on. Show child where the hands on the clock will be.
Suggest that the child pretend to be a favorite TV character. Suggest or provide a special prop, such as a hat, that would help imitate the character. . . .
Ask child to tell you what happened on a favorite show you did not see. Write the story on paper for your child, in correct lettering, and then read it back. You can type the story instead of printing it. . . .

The Parent Participation TV Workshop Project
Educational Technology Unit
State Department of Education
3rd Floor, 721 Capitol Mall
Sacramento, CA 95814
(916) 445-5065

This project which is run nationally by Teachers Guides to Television and funded in full by a grant from NBC has as its goal to make TV a positive influence on our children and families. Through facilitators at the workshops, parents will learn skills to help them have parent-child dialogues after viewing TV programs for children and will strive to better communication and understanding for parents in regard to their children. The second thrust of this project is to be used in schools in teacher-student curriculums. Students can learn to take a critical look at commercial TV and then discuss programs with their teachers.

Organizations (See Appendix A)

Action for Children's Television
Committee on Childhood Television

T

TOILET TRAINING

Each child has a time when toilet training is most comfortable and will indicate his or her readiness for it. By having a potty seat and no pressure, the child will learn easily and comfortably.

Toilet Learning
Alison Mack
Little, Brown
1978   109 pp. $7.95

In this review of the history of toilet training coupled with a step-by-step guide to accomplishing the task with a minimum of aggravation, one section presents a picture story to be read to children, illustrating what it expected of them.

If the child is able to sit comfortably on the adult toilet after a few tries, it's a good idea to teach her to use it from the beginning. If the child has difficulty climbing on or off, build or buy a low, sturdy step with a wide, deep tread and show the child how to put it in position. If the child finds it hard to balance on the toilet seat, a learning seat that fits over the toilet can be used. If the child feels more comfortable on a learning seat, take it with you when you and the child are away from home, or keep a second one in the trunk of the car.

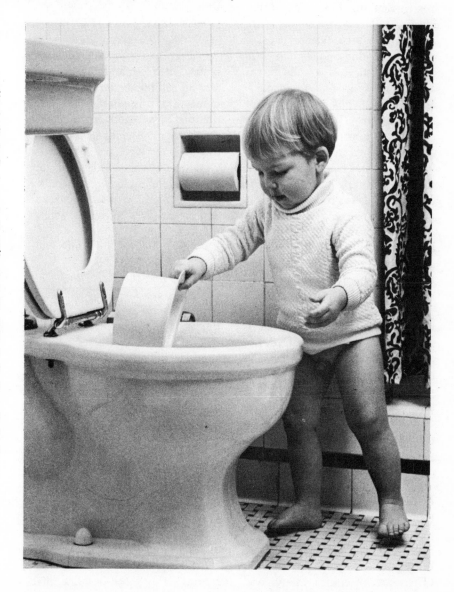

TOYS AND PLAY

See also Creative Expression; Games and Activities; Playing.

T A useful guide on play for young children, Martha Piers and Genevieve M. Landau's *The Wonderful World of Play* is a free booklet available from Hasbro Industries, Inc., 1027 Newport Avenue, Pawtucket, Rhode Island 02861.

All discoveries made through play with ordinary household objects and toys are part of the hidden curriculum of infancy and toddlerhood. These experiences teach optimism, self-confidence, trust—and also caution and fear. In early play experiences, the child learns about time, space and distance. He learns how far it is in terms of energy and traveling time from the crib to the door. He learns about cause and effect in play, how he affects things and what things can do to him. Learning through play is never lost. Lessons are often forgotten, but the enjoyable softness of the favorite doll, the painful bump on the head when we tried to crawl under the table and the magic and fun of games are always remembered.

Your child will need different kinds of toys and different kinds of stimulation at each stage of development. Toys are tools to help children grow. Let boys and girls play with all the same kinds of toys. Choose toys of different textures—wood, plastic, cloth and rubber. You can make many toys yourself.

Choose toys carefully. Toys made by Community Playthings, Child Guidance, Child Craft, Fisher Price and Playskool are highly recommended. They are well conceived, designed for durability and simple and flexible. (There are, of course, many good large and small toy manufacturers.) Be careful what toys you choose. Toys should be chosen for safety and the appropriate age and skill level as well as potential continuous success with the child's use.

Some basic toys are important in the early years: ball (soft, plush or rubber), musical toys (to listen to), noise-making toys (to shake, bang or pound), building toys (to take apart), shape sorter (to help differentiate colors and shapes), cars, push-alongs, carriages, imitative grown-up toys (dishes, pots and pans), wheels and ride-on toys (walkers), cuddly companions (bear, animals, dolls), books and records. Use your imagination and create new toys.

There are countless numbers of toys being manufactured, and not all of them can be in your home. It is important to select durable toys based on your children's interests and age. Later in this section, we have provided a checklist of toys and ideas for your child at different ages. (Appendix E lists toy manufacturers' names and addresses.) We hope this will be useful to you.

Though there are many mail-order houses for children's toys, clothing, and furniture, The Children's Design Center is unique in its philosophy and service. Colleen Burke, the Center's founder, is committed to excellence: "Every product we offer meets our high standards for safety, design excellence, functional integrity, developmental appropriateness and conscientious craftsmanship." While the Design Center has no plans to manufacture its own lines, it has already influenced the juvenile products market by suggesting design changes and improvements prior to choosing a product for inclusion in the catalogue.

To insure rapid delivery of orders, The Children's Design Center has set up a toll-free line (800/833-4755 in the continental U.S., 800/342-4774 in New York State). The staff, young parents themselves, answer questions about products carried by the Design Center, about the tests they have done for the catalogue items, and about baby and child care in general. For a free catalog write to The Children's Design Center, Inc., Geyser Road, Saratoga Springs, New York 12866.

Toy Safety
Pointers on Toys*

- Avoid toys that have sharp edges and protrusions, such as a bird with a pointed beak that can be jabbed in your child's eyes.
- Remove any splinters or projecting nails from boxes or other equipment before giving them to your child. Select toys with rounded edges and smooth surfaces.
- Make sure that plastic is used and not plate glass in toy car, truck, or airplane windows.
- Avoid toys that are poorly constructed, like a rattle that could break apart and free little balls for the child to swallow, and noise makers and squeaker toys with metal mouth pieces or squeakers that fall out.
- Avoid toys that have detachable parts, such as button eyes that your child can put in his ears, nose, or mouth. Dolls with embroidered or firmly glued eyes are safer.
- Check to see that stuffed toys are filled with hygienic material that is washable and can be changed.
- Avoid dolls with fluffy trimmings that the child can pull off and put in his mouth.
- Look for the UL (Underwriters Laboratories) seal on electrical toys. It shows that the toy has been tested for safety of its electrical parts.

---

*Excerpt from *Safe Toys for Your Child*, Administration for Children, Youth and Families, US Government Printing Office

Safe Toys and Equipment

Painting: When painting a child's crib or toys, use only paints that are labelled "lead-free," or "non-toxic." These paints will not contain antimony, arsenic, cadmium, mercury, selenium, or soluble barium, which could be harmful to your child. Since not all paints are so labelled, look for and use only those that are marked: "Conforms to American standard Z66.1-9: For use on surfaces that might be chewed by children."

Outdoor Equipment: Although there is no specific age when a child starts using playground equipment, skates, bikes, or other outdoor toys, he should be old enough to know the dangers of such equipment and be taught to follow certain rules:

- Bicycles, tricycles, or sleds should not be used where there is traffic, and should be used carefully in areas where other children are at play.
- Roller skates should be taken off before crossing the street.

You, as a parent, should see to it that swings and other playground equipment are firmly placed in the ground, away from walls and fences, and out of the direct line of automobile or pedestrian traffic. The equipment should be the right size for the child and assembled according to the directions of the manufacturer.

Dollhouse Magic
P. K. Roche
Dial Press
1980   58 pp. $2.95

This book with photographs and drawings tells how to make and find simple dollhouse furniture: starting with things to save, basic tools and materials and planning each individual room.

A sponge becomes a sofa and a broken watch a clock. A pretty stamp becomes a picture for the wall and a playing card a rug for the floor. All this is a kind of magic, magic that you do yourself —dollhouse magic.

The Woman's Day Book of Soft Toys & Dolls
Joan Russell
Simon & Schuster
1980   255 pp. $7.95

80 excellent creations with step-by-step instructions, full-size patterns, and easy-to-read diagrams allow you to make these toys easily and quickly—with lots of suggestions to encourage your own creativity. Helpful guidelines are given for choosing materials and adapting projects for all ages —from infants to adults.

Your doll will be a treasure if you use very small stitches in machine and hand sewing, pay loving attention to small details and make the clothes from lightweight fabrics with design or texture to fit the size of the doll.

The following list will serve as an age guide for introducing various toys to your children. Many of these items you have at home already. Those toys that are especially recommended are listed with their manufacturer and/or supplier. Refer to Appendix E—Toys and Toy Manufacturers, for addresses and other recommended toys suitable for varied ages.

Toys for Different Ages

T

Babies

- cribmobile
- music boxes mobile
- bells
- colors
- cradle chimes
- stuffed animals

3 to 6 Months

- rattles
- teether
- playpen toys
- crib and play gyms
- baby bouncer
  or
- jolly jumper
- playpen
- feeding chair or table
- unbreakable mirror
- soft dolls

6 to 9 Months

- nested measuring cups, measuring spoons, wooden spoons, clothespins, hard plastic freezer container, cupcake pans and small baking pans, empty Band-Aid boxes or cans, lightweight plastic block, squeaky squeeze toys
- musical rattles
- empty coffee cans with plastic lids
- drum
- blocks
- balls
- floating toys
- busy box
- clutch ball
- texture balls

T

9 to 12 Months

- Baby's First Toys (Platt and Munk)
- Peg Learner (Whitney Brothers)
- Rolly Polly Wooden Ball (Child Guidance)
- Click and Clatter Car (Child Guidance)
- Nesting Blocks (Playskool)
- Nesting Drums (Child Craft)
- Push Wheels (Child Guidance)
- Jack-in-the Box (F. A. O. Schwarz)
- Squeak-a-Boo (Fisher-Price)
- Discover Me Mirror Box (Child Craft)
- Hide and Seek (Child Craft)

12 to 15 Months

- Creative Coaster (Fisher-Price)
- Walker Chair (Playskool)
- First Wagon (Child Craft)
- pull toys
- Indoor Gym (Child Guidance)
- Pound-a-Ball (Child Guidance)

15 to 18 Months

- cardboard boxes
- phone books
- large rubber balls
- sand, mud, and water
- pull toys
- You can make your own toy by attaching beads, milk cartons, bracelets, rattles, or other kitchen utensils to shoelaces
- Rainbow Wagon-O-Blocks (Sife)
- Tike Wagon (Child Craft)
- Toddler Truck (Playskool)

18 Months to 3 Years

- Rocking Horse (Fisher-Price)

- blocks and boards (make bench, bridge, tunnel, walking platform)
- Giant Nesting Cubes (Child Craft)
- kiddie cars
- tricycle
- stick horse
- crayons, newsprint, large sheets of paper
- Shape Sorting Boxes (Child Craft)
- Nesting and Stacking Boxes (Child Guidance)
- Tinker Toys (Tinker Toys)
- Activity Board (Child Guidance)
- Bath Toys (Gabriel)
- puzzles
- records
- books (washable, soft)
- swing set for outdoors
- Kiddie Car (Child Craft)
- rocking horse
- big punching figure
- bean bags
- corrugated cardboard boxes
- Community Playthings (Child Craft)
- Transportation Toys (Mattel)
- Mini-Kitchen (Child Guidance)
- plastic dishes, pots, pans
- Postal Station (Playskool)
- threading toys
- beads
- wheels
- manipulative toys
- popping beads
- Number Sorter (Child Guidance)
- Peg Sorting Board (Child Craft)
- Workbench (Playskool)
- scissors with rounded tips

- Shape Discs (Lauri)
- clay
- paints
- musical horns
- whistles
- cans with plastic lids
- wooden spoons
- pie tins
- metal spoons
- cymbals
- xylophone
- music boxes

3 to 4 Years

- balance board
- tricycle
- wagon
- inflatable rubber ball
- dollhouse
- stuffed animals
- rocking horse
- simple climbing equipment
- dolls and doll clothes
- punching bag
- broom handle
- props for dramatic play
- play telephone
- dress-up clothes
- play money
- locks
- Townsfolk set (Community Playthings)
- housekeeping equipment
- puppets
- Sand Cones (Child Craft)
- Sand Kit (Child Craft)
- art materials
- easels
- play dough
- plasticene
- thread spools

- potato mashers
- felt-tip markers
- squeeze paints
- collage box (paste, assorted pieces of paper, greeting cards and seals, spoons, ribbons, wrappings)
- chalkboard
- construction set
- Snap and Play Blocks (Child Craft)
- Leggo blocks
- lumber scraps
- hammer
- nails (flat head)
- Hexagon Floor Mosaics (ABC)
- sewing cards
- Shape Dominoes (Child Guidance)
- Match Ups (Playskool)
- Fit a Square (Lauri)
- Colors and Things (Playskool)
- Fit a Circle (Playskool)
- Fit a Circle (Lauri)
- mirrors
- plastic pedals
- stethoscope

5 to 10 Years

- ice skates
- roller skates
- snowshoes
- balls, bats, mitts
- puppets
- dress-up mirror
- tape recorder
- bean bags
- target games
- ring toss
- flashlight
- play houses
- blocks

- Derrick (Community Playthings)
- Brio Play Mat (Child Craft)
- dollhouses
- clay
- bulletin board
- coloring supplies
- sewing and embroidering supplies
- design construction kits
- burlap
- yarn
- tapestry needles
- Lego blocks
- locks

- toolbox
- dominoes
- cards and card games
- playing cards (Old Maid, Go Fish)
- Candy Land (Milton Bradley)
- Winnie the Pooh (Parker Brothers)
- Go Together Lotto
- Ed-Ucards
- Alpha Number (Lauri)
- word games
- nature and science activities
- kaleidoscope
- play clocks

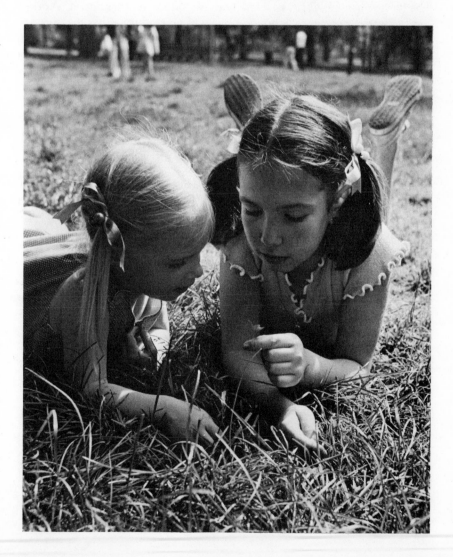

WORKING AND FAMILY LIFE

See also Part I—Sharing Working and Parenting Roles; Single Parenting.

HELPING OURSELVES

Many jobs are so physically distant from our homes that the world of work is an entirely separate realm from the world of family life. If our places of work are near our homes we can, when we wish, go home for lunch; drop by during the day to help resolve a quarrel or comfort a hurt child or just chat; tend to shopping chores, let in an electrician or carpenter, or measure a window for new shades. Children and other family members can stop by at the job with messages or to do errands with us.

The great physical separations of most workers from their homes and neighborhoods reinforce the principle that *our greatest devotion is owed to those who pay our salaries.* Workers are "saved" from the distractions of family matters during work hours. I know of no study that has measured time lost from work, or incompetent or careless work done, because workers were preoccupied with worrying about a sick child left at home, or about the cat who could not be found to be let in before everyone left the house, or about unresolved differences with family members. The unremitting sameness of staying for the entire day in one building—even a new and modern building designed for the worker's comfort—and the sense of having one's life broken into pieces that do not connect with each other may cause a falloff in worker performance significantly greater than any that might come from flexible options of trading work time and family time.

The effect of this separation, this distance between home and job, is unquestionably one of great hardship for families.

> Mary C. Howell
> *Helping Ourselves: Families and the Human Network*
> Beacon Press
> 1975   231 pp. $4.95

The Two-Paycheck Marriage
Caroline Bird
Pocket Books
1980   305 pp. $2.75

Caroline Bird brings us her definitive report on the most important social revolution of our times: the march of wives into the workplace, which is changing the family, marriage, childbearing traditions, life at work and everywhere in our society. This book documents how this massive shift of power from men to women is amending the marital contract of sex for support, and what it is doing to jobs, politics, markets, schooling, and most of all to the family as we always have known it.

Life and health are the most fundamental measures of well-being, and classic studies have shown that working women live longer and feel better all along the way.

According to the Public Health Service, working women and men are ill less often than full-time housewives, and this isn't just because housewives tend to be older than working wives. Among young women 17 to 24 years old, ill health restricted the activities of working wives 10.9 days a year compared with 13.3 for housewives of the same age, and the gap widens as they grow older. As one husband put it, "Working gives a woman something more to talk about than her aches and pains."

When Mothers Work
Evelyn Shafner
Pacific Press
1972   160 pp. $4.95

To work or not to work is the question this book deals with for women who have children. This book not only questions whether a mother should work, but points out vividly some of the things that may happen when she does and urges that any mother who considers working, especially when her children are young, count the cost —financially as well as physically and emotionally—to her family and to herself. The author also describes the ideal situation in which a woman sets priorities as she plans the stages of her life in caring for her children and then feels free to focus on personal pursuits such as a career.

Young adults need to be aware of the amount of money required to maintain a home as a married couple, and to rear children. They should know that with each child added to the household, there may be a reduction in the standard of living for other members of the family. If it is the first child, it may mean that the mother will have to give up her job. Couples should plan for this reduction of income, so that when the baby is born and the mother quits working, they will not discover to their dismay that they cannot exist comfortably on one income.

The Working Mother's Complete Handbook
Gloria Norris and JoAnn Miller
E. P. Dutton
1979   296 pp. $7.95

Drawing on the shared experiences of women, this book shows how women are finding ways to be good mothers and have successful careers at the same time. It discusses your family, your career, and yourself.

One of the quickest ways to wreck your mental health is to insist on doing it all yourself, and great benefits to family life can result when other members of your family assume more home responsibilities . . . When parenting is shared, children benefit from a larger emotional reservoir that helps them function independently and confidently.

Working Mothers
Jean Curtis
Simon & Schuster
1977   214 pp. $3.95

In this book, working mothers, their husbands and children talk about the difficulties they face, the satisfactions they've found, the ways they cope when women combine motherhood and a career.

The author emphasizes the need for compromise and a sense of humor as couples work out their own way of equalizing the burdens and rewards of being individuals and parents.

Coping problems fall roughly into two categories: the practical everyday logistics of running a household and performing at work, and psychological stress, brought on by the pull of conflicting interests and social expectations. Most working mothers seem quite able, on the whole, to manage logistical problems. Many are

superb managers, capable of coping with complex schedules and the thousand details of family life. When they flounder, it is usually because they are overwhelmed by psychological demands, the competing expectations of teachers, doctors, neighbors, friends, colleagues, and sometimes husbands insisting they are doing things the wrong way. They have their limits.

Working Mother magazine often explores the problems of shared roles and the working mother. Two articles outlining the problems and some of the solutions are "Why Husbands Don't Help" (July, 1979) and "I Didn't Ask You to Go to Work" (November, 1979).

For Children

Women At Work
Betty Medsger
Andrews & McMeel
1975   208 pp. $7.95

Black-and-white photographs show women in a myriad of jobs from railway engineer to coal miner to stockbroker, while the text quotes from interviews with working women and shows women living out a great political and human drama.

For Jenny Cirone, who's been lobstering in South Addison, Maine, since she was nine, it doesn't seem strange to be doing something that's done by only one other woman she knows. I think she's barely thought of it, and probably wondered why this outsider with the camera and questions was so curious. "It's true, though, you won't find many of us," she said.

**Organizations
(See Appendix A)**

W National Organization for Women

Magazines (See Appendix B)

Handbook for Working Women
MOMMA
Women Who Work
Working Mother
Working Woman

WORKING WITH CHILDREN

Many career opportunities in addition to parenting provide adults with jobs working with children. Sometimes we do not realize how many people this involves. Teachers, of course, are the largest of this adult group. In addition, there are teacher's aides and support staff that work in the schools. Child-care centers often employ psychiatrists, psychologists, social workers, art therapists, dance therapists, physical therapists, pediatricians and dentists, parent educators and support staff. Today more men are being encouraged to work in day-care, child services and teaching. In addition, there are toy manufacturers, camp staff, clothing manufacturers and people in organizations that work on behalf of children's services.

Organizations

American Association of Elementary-Kindergarten-Nursery Educators
American Montessori Society
Association for Childhood Education International
National Education Association
National Association for the Education of Young Children

Appendix

APPENDIX RESOURCES

Appendix A
Organizations

ORGANIZATIONS

Hundreds of national and local organizations exist in this country for professionals who are involved with children and their parents and for parents with special interests. We have reviewed more than 500 of these organizations. Many are discussed in detail in the areas where they are relevant in this sourcebook. Nearly a hundred more are given here. Some are professional organizations of specialists working with children as teachers, special educators, psychologists and the like. Almost all of the organizations provide publications, referrals or information that parents may find useful.

We have also included selected special organizations and those on a state or a local level that we feel are exemplary and worthwhile. For further information, write to the executive director or the publication and information office of the organization.

If you do not receive the assistance or answers you need from the sources given, or if you have a special problem or are uncertain where to turn, we will be happy to refer you to the appropriate organization. We would also be pleased to hear of any organizations or resources you could recommend. Write to us at the Institute for Childhood Resources, 1169 Howard St., San Francisco, CA 94103.

National Organizations

Action for Children's Television
46 Austin Street
Newtonville, MA   02160
(617) 527-7870

An organization of parents, teachers and physicians designed to combat the harmful effects of television commercians on children, the primary focus of ACT is on a lobbying effort to promote more stringent regulations by the Federal Trade Commission. Primary goals include prohibiting all television advertising directed to children under the age of eight, prohibiting commercials for highly sugared foods and instituting corrective advertising to balance commercials for other sugared foods (i.e., health and nutrition messages).

Publications include: *Promise and Performance: ACT's Guide to TV Programming for Children, Volume 1: Children with Special Needs; The Family Guide to Children's Television: What to Watch, What to Miss, What to Change and How to Do It;* and *Children's TV: The Economics of Exploitation.*

Administration for Children, Youth and Families
c/o U.S. Department of Health and Human Services
Washington, D.C.   20201
(202) 755-7762

This organization serves as a coordinating agency for federal programs for children and their families and acts as an advocate for children by bringing their needs to the attention of the government and the public. Among the programs operated by ACYF are Project Head Start, the Child and Family Resource Program, the Developmental Continuity Project and the Child Development Associate Program. The ACYF also administers a child-welfare research-and-demonstration-grants program.

Publications include a news bulletin and a number of pamphlets and reports, especially through the Children's Bureau.

American Academy of Pediatrics
1801 Hinman Avenue
Evanston, IL   60204
(312) 869-4255

The services of this Pan-American association of pediatricians dedicated to the promotion of higher standards and greater consistency in child health care include a number of public-information and education programs as well as a number of publications designed to stimulate interest in and foster understanding of proper child health care.

Publications include a variety of manuals and pamphlets on all aspects of child health care. Reprints of committee statements on "Pediatrics" and "News & Comment" are also available.

The American Alliance for Health, Physical Education and Recreation (AAHPER)
1201 16th Street, N.W.
Washington, D.C.   20036
(202) 833-5514

Seeks to improve the quality of life through physical education, recreation, leisure and outdoor education. AAHPER is basically a professional organization, though membership is open to any interested persons. Most members are professionals who promote and educate in the related areas of health education, safety, dance, sports and so on.

Publications include: *Update*, the members' newspaper, and three professional journals: *Journal of Physical Education and Recreation*, *Research Quarterly* and *Health Education*. The Alliance also publishes a variety of pamphlets on a wide range of subjects.

American Association of Elementary-Kindergarten-Nursery Educators
NEA Center
1201 Sixteenth Street, N.W.
Washington, D.C.   20036
(202) 833-4390

A professional organization of educators involved with children from preschool through eighth grade. Parents, students and other interested persons are eligible for nonactive membership. The association promotes higher professional standards, better coordination of educational opportunities and better public understanding of the advantages of wisely organized programs for children.

Publications include: three topical issues of *Educating Children: Early and Middle Years*, and three newsletters, which are published annually and are available free to members. In addition, over a hundred tapes and publications are available upon request.

American Association of Marriage and Family Counselors
924 W. Ninth St.
Uplands, CA   91786
(714) 981-0888

The association carries on a number of educational programs to help the public understand more about marriage and family problems, and about the role of professional counseling in preventing marital and family problems.

Publications include: *The Journal of Marriage and Family Counseling*, a quarterly journal.

American Association of Ophthalmology
1100 17th St., N.W.
Washington, D.C.   20036
(202) 833-3447

This organization provides information and conducts research on eye diseases and eye care. They work both with medical professionals and the public, as well as other organizations in the eye field.

American Association of Sex Educators and Counselors
5010 Wisconsin Ave., N.W., Suite 304
Washington, D.C.   20016
(202) 686-2523

Assists those responsible for counseling on sex-related matters and those responsible for sex-education programs in the schools and elsewhere; its central purpose is in training, education and research. The association holds a number of workshops and seminars for members and offers consultation services for both members and non-members.

Publications include: a quarterly newsletter that deals with AASEC's regional and national programs as well as current issues and trends in sex education and counseling, and a variety of other pamphlets and manuals.

American Automobile Association
8111 Gatehouse Road
Falls Church, VA   22042
(703) 222-6000

Dedicated to traffic safety, this organization provides a number of travel and information services. The AAA provides a variety of classroom aids for elementary, high school and college students and teachers. Included are materials on auto maintenance, driving techniques, traffic emergencies, and school, pedestrian and bicycle safety materials.

Publications include a wide variety of pamphlets and manuals.

American Camping Association
Bradford Woods
Martinsville, IN   46151
(317) 342-8456

An organization composed primarily of owners, directors, staff members, and volunteers, the primary purposes are to provide development opportunities for those in the organized camp field and to interpret to the public the values of the organized camping experience. In the interest of improving the camp experience, the association accredits camps based upon minimum standards and on-site visits, which are carried out at least every three years.

Publications include: *ACA Accredited*, *Parent's Guide to Accredited Camps* and a large selection of other publications on camp craft and camp management.

American Dental Association/
American Society of Dentistry for
Children
211 E. Chicago Ave.
Chicago, IL   60611
(312) 440-2500

An educational and professional organization dedicated to improving dental education for children and parents and promoting information. It provides a wide range of publications for young and older children upon request.

American Dietetic Association
430 North Michigan Avenue
Chicago, IL   60611
(312) 280-5000

An educational and professional organization dedicated to improving nutritional well-being, advancing the science of dietetics and nutrition and promoting education in these and allied areas. Its primary purpose is to parallel the advances in medical science and food technology with improved academic and professional standards for the dietetic profession.

Publications include various professional manuals and pamphlets as well as position papers on such topics as *Nutrition and Aging, Child Nutrition* and *Nutrition Education for the Public.* The *ADA Journal* is a monthly publication concerning issues and trends within the profession.

American Foundation for Maternal and Child Health
30 Beekman Place
New York, NY   10022
(212) 759-5510

A nonprofit foundation for research in maternal and child health whose main focus is on the perinatal period and its effect on infant outcome and child development,

the foundation acts as a clearinghouse for information from various medical and social-science disciplines. The foundation also sponsors various conferences on maternal and child health.

American Foundation for the Blind
15 West 16th Street
New York, NY   10011
(212) 924-0420

A private, nonprofit agency that serves as a national clearinghouse for information about blindness, the foundation also promotes the development of educational, rehabilitation and social-welfare services for the blind and multiple-handicapped children and adults. It also conducts research to determine more effective methods of serving the blind and sells special aids and appliances for the blind.

Free publications include: *Is Your Child Blind?, The Preschool Deaf-Blind Child, When You Have a Visually Handicapped Child in Your Classroom,* and a *Catalog of Aids and Appliances.*

American Home Economics Association
2010 Massachusetts Ave., N.W.
Washington, D.C.   20036
(202) 833-3100

Devoted to improving the quality and standards of individual and family life through education, research and public information, the organization provides support for various workshops, leadership conferences, research and production of educational materials. It also serves as a clearinghouse of information and programs related to family concerns.

Publications include *AHEA Action,* a bimonthly newsletter, *Journal of Home Economics,* the bimonthly official organ, the quarterly *Home Economics Research*

Journal and a variety of professional handbooks.

American Library Association
Children's Services Division
50 East Huron Street
Chicago, IL   60611
(312) 944-6780

The Children's Services Division of the ALA fosters improvement and extension of services to children in all types of libraries. Members' interests include the evaluation and selection of library materials for children, interpretation of library materials for children, methods of using such materials with children and concern for production and effective use of good children's materials to groups outside the profession.

Publications include *Top of the News* (issued jointly with Young Adult Services Division), a quarterly, and the annual "Notable Children's Books" list.

American Medical Association
535 North Dearborn Street
Chicago, IL   60610
(312) 751-6000

The AMA is a professional organization dedicated to maintaining standards and disseminating information to professionals and nonprofessionals on drugs, therapy and research, foods and nutrition, physical medicine, cosmetics and medical quackery.

American Montessori Society
150 Fifth Avenue
New York, NY   10011
(212) 924-3209

This nonprofit organization is dedicated to better education through the promotion of Montessori teaching strategies and the incorporation of the Montessori approach into American education.

The Montessori method is a system of education and a philosophy of learning which is concerned with the importance of children developing self-discipline and learning at their own pace when provided with an autoeducative, multisensory environment. The society serves as a clearinghouse for information about Montessori methods, materials, teachers and schools.

Publications include a variety of books about the learning processes of young children and the Montessori philosophy.

American National Red Cross
National Headquarters
Washington, D.C.   20006
(202) 737-8300

An organization dedicated to helping people prepare for emergencies and cope with them when they occur, the Red Cross provides volunteer blood services to a large segment of the nation, conducts community services and serves as an independent medium of voluntary relief and communication between the American people and their armed forces. Services also include training in first aid, home nursing, family health, preparation for parenthood and a variety of youth-oriented courses.

Publications include a variety of pamphlets and manuals on disaster preparedness, safety and first aid.

American Podiatry Association
20 Chevy Chase Circle, N.W.
Washington, D.C.   20015
(202) 362-2700

A professional society dedicated to creating greater public awareness of the benefits of good foot care and initiating programs to meet the foot-health needs of an

expanding population, its special concerns include public information on foot disorders common to children and proper care to insure the normal development of children's feet.

American Society for Psychoprophylaxis in Obstetrics
1411 K Street, N.W.
Washington, D.C.   20005
(202) 783-7050

A nonprofit organization formed to promote the development and acceptance of psychoprophylactic childbirth preparation, its primary program involves the training and certification of teachers in natural-childbirth procedures.

Publications include *Genesis*, the organizational newsletter, and a number of descriptive brochures and pamphlets.

American Speech and Hearing Association
10801 Rockville Pike
Rockville, MD   20852
(301) 897-5700

A national scientific and professional association for speech-language pathologists, audiologists and speech and hearing scientists concerned with communication behavior and disorders, the major goals are to maintain high professional standards, encourage the development of comprehensive clinical service programs and stimulate exchange of information about human communication through conventions, publications and other professional activities.

Publications include *Journal of Speech and Hearing Disorders*, a quarterly; *Language, Speech, and Hearing Services in Schools*, a quarterly; and a variety of other professional publications.

Appalachian Regional Commission
1666 Connecticut Avenue, N.W.
Washington, D.C.   20235
(202) 673-7893

The Appalachian Regional Commission is composed of the governors of the thirteen states that comprise the region and a federal co-chairman appointed by the President. The commission sponsors various programs including housing, community development, energy, environment, natural resources, education, health and child development. The commission boasts a number of innovative health and child-care programs.

The commission publishes a bimonthly magazine, *Appalachia*, which is free to all interested parties.

Association for Childbirth at Home
Box 1219
Cerritos, CA   90701
(714) 994-5880

An organization providing educational services for parents, physicians, midwives and other people who are interested in or involved in home childbirth, the association sponsors seminars, conferences, training and slide shows, and puts out a catalog of birth supplies and a listing of various other publications.

Association for Childhood Education International
3615 Wisconsin Ave., N.W.
Washington, D.C.   20016
(202) 363-6963

A nonprofit association open to all persons concerned with the education and well-being of children, its general goals include promoting more desirable conditions in programs for children, raising the professional standards of teachers and bringing about active cooperation between all groups concerned with the development of children in the home, the school and the community. The association also informs the public of the needs of children.

Publications include *Childhood Education*, the official journal of the association, *ACEI Branch Exchange*, the membership's newsletter, and other titles.

Association for Children and Adults with Learning Disabilities
4156 Library Road
Pittsburgh, PA   15234
(412) 341-1515

This nonprofit organization of parents and professionals was incorporated in 1964 to serve the needs of individuals with learning disabilities with 780 local chapters in the United States and abroad. Their efforts are to improve services to learning disabled persons in areas of public awareness, advocacy, research, education and employment. They have a resource library with over 400 publications at cost price and they act as an information and referral service center.

Association for Sickle Cell Anemia Research
P.O. Box 708
Administration Building, Howard University
Washington, D.C.   20001
(202) 636-7914

The association informs the public about the existence of sickle cell anemia, an inherited blood disease the majority of whose victims are children. ASCAR also educates people who have sickle cell anemia as to how they can live

a healthy and long life, and provides support for research into combating this disease.

They distribute the following pamphlets: *Sickle Cell Anemia and Your Child* and *What Is Sickle Cell Trait?*

Asthma and Allergy Foundation of America
801 Second Avenue
New York, NY   10017
(212) 867-8875

A nonprofit organization dedicated to increasing the knowledge of the causes of and the best treatment for asthma and allergic diseases, its primary objectives include uniting the public, the medical profession, research scientists and public health workers in this regard. Services include the distribution of educational materials and providing professional speakers and community-service programs.

Publications include a variety of pamphlets on asthma and allergic diseases.

Black Child Development Institute
1028 Connecticut Avenue, N.W., Suite 514
Washington, D.C.   20036
(202) 659-4010

Working at the national level to insure the emotional, physical, cognitive and social developmental needs of black children, the institute works to ensure the participation of black parents in the community policies and decisions that affect their children, and to ensure that black children capitalize on the unique experience of the black family and community.

Publications include: *The Black Child Advocate*, the organization newsletter.

Boys' Clubs of America
771 First Avenue
New York, NY   10017
(212) 557-7755

This organization is located primarily in inner-city areas whose various programs provide comprehensive services in supplemental education, guidance, health, recreation, employment and leadership development. Designed as an alternative to boredom and the pitfalls of street life, Boys' Clubs are multipurpose facilities that provide professional adult guidance and supervision on a daily basis. Day-to-day activities vary but arts and crafts, music, reading, mechanics, carpentry, sports, swimming, cooking, camping and educational field trips are among the types offered.

Publications include *Keynote*, a quarterly professional magazine; *Bulletin*, a free semiannual newsletter; *How-To-Do-It*, a semiannual resource publication.

Boy Scouts of America
National Office
North Brunswick, NJ   08902
(201) 249-6000

This organization provides boys and young men with an effective educational program designed to build desirable qualities of character, to train in the responsibilities of participating citizenship and to develop personal fitness. The scouting program includes practical training in a variety of outdoor, recreational, community service and safety procedures and activities.

Publications include handbooks for young people and leaders, merit badge pamphlets and three magazines, one for boys, one for young men and women and their leaders and one for adults.

Camp Fire Girls
4601 Madison Avenue
Kansas City, MO   64112
(816) 756-1950

The membership of this nonprofit, volunteer organization includes youth of both sexes from birth to twenty-one years. The emphasis is on small-group programs making use of informal education, recreation and group-work principles and techniques. The organization is governed by local councils, which often provide such diverse activities as preschool programs, latch-key programs, drop-in centers, juvenile justice programs, career education projects and family life education classes, as well as the traditional outdoor activities and community services.

Publications include *Camp Fire Leadership*, a quarterly magazine, annual reports, program literature, and various surveys and studies.

Child Welfare League of America
67 Irving Place
New York, NY   10003
(212) 254-7410

Organized to provide better understanding of child welfare problems, to formulate and improve standards of work with children and to make knowledge of changing methods available as they prove successful, the league is a federation of private and public child-care agencies in the United States and Canada.

Publications include *Child Welfare*, the organization journal; *CWLA Newsletter;* and a wide range of books on all aspects of child welfare.

Children in Hospitals
31 Wilshire Park
Needham, MA   20970
(617) 444-3877

This nonprofit organization of parents and health-care professionals seeks to educate those concerned about the needs of children and parents for continued ample contact when either is hospitalized. Principal focus is on encouraging hospitals to adopt flexible visiting policies and to provide living-in accommodations whenever possible.

Children's Bureau—See Administration for Children, Youth and Families

Children's Defense Fund
1520 New Hampshire Avenue, N.W.
Washington, D.C.   20036
(202) 483-1470

A nonprofit organization created to provide long-range and systematic advocacy on behalf of the nation's children, its members include professionals and interested laypersons dedicated to reforming institutions, policies and practices affecting the lives of children. Primary concerns include the right to education of children who have been misclassified, the protection of children's right to privacy regarding records kept by various social agencies and the protection of children from medical experimentation and other harmful research.

Coalition for Children and Youth
815 15th Street, N.W.
Washington, D.C.   20005
(202) 347-9380

An organization designed to monitor and discuss public-policy issues such as the impact of legislation, regulations, court decisions and congressional mandates which concern children and youth as well as to disseminate information on such policies and to advocate the

institution of policies more responsive to the needs of children and youth. The coalition also collects information on special issues such as the needs of the poor, women and minorities.

Publications include *CCY Focus*, the organization newsletter.

Council for Exceptional Children
1920 Association Drive
Reston, VA   22091
(703) 620-3660

An organization dedicated to the advancement of the education of all exceptional children—both gifted and handicapped. Council membership consists of professional personnel and other interested persons. The council plays a leading role in the development of legislation designed to meet the educational and social needs of exceptional children and offers a wide range of publication and information services. Referral to other organizations that respond to special needs.

Publications include: *Exceptional Children*, a general journal for the association; *Teaching Exceptional Children*, a teaching journal; and *Cultural Diversity and the Exceptional Child*.

Day Care Council of America
711 14th St., N.W.
Washington, D.C.   20005
(202) 638-2316

An organization dedicated to increasing the availability of children's services and raising the quality of all child-care programs. The council also provides technical assistance to child-care projects, disseminates information to members regarding all aspects of child care and monitors state and federal legislative and regulatory activities.

Publications include *Voice for Children*, a monthly organization magazine; *Resources for Child Care*, a bimonthly newsletter; *Day Care and Early Education* magazine and a variety of books about child care.

Education Development Center
55 Chapel Street
Newton, MA   02160
(617) 969-7100

A nonprofit corporation engaged in educational research and development, the center produces educational programs and training materials for students, parents, teachers and community groups on a variety of subjects. A special focus is the production of a wide range of multimedia materials on topics such as child development, children and families, child abuse, foster parenting, raising a healthy family and single parenting.

Publications include *Day Care and the Public Schools: Profiles of Five Communities*, and *EDC News*, an organization newsletter.

Epilepsy Foundation of America
1828 1st St., N.W., Suite 406
Washington, D.C.   20036
(202) 293-2930

A nonprofit voluntary health organization devoted solely to the interests and needs of epileptics and their medical, social and economic well-being, the foundation's programs include research, information services, counseling and referrals, employment assistance and public health education. A special concern is low-cost insurance and drugs for epileptics. The foundation also acts as an advocate for the rights of persons with epilepsy, especially in regard to their recognition in the development of national programs.

Publications include a number of pamphlets for physicians and other professionals.

Fight for Sight
National Council to Combat Blindness, Inc.
41 West 57th St.
New York, NY   10019
(212) 751-1118

An organization dedicated to aiding scientific research in eye diseases, the organization also operates a number of children's eye clinics that were established primarily for the examination and treatment of disadvantaged children.

Publications include a number of brochures and press releases.

Friends of the Earth
124 Spear St.
San Francisco, CA   94105
(415) 495-4770

An organization dedicated to protecting the public and the environment from such dangers as air pollution, water pollution, soil pollution, radiation and the destruction of species of animals, Friends of the Earth is also one of the leading information and lobbying groups for solar energy, as well as one of the major groups involved in the fight against nuclear power.

Girls' Clubs of America
205 Lexington Avenue
New York, NY   10016
(212) 689-3700

A resource organization for girls which guards the rights of girls of all backgrounds and abilities. The clubs offer opportunities for girls to develop their full potential through a series of outdoor and community-service activities.

Publications include *Girls' Club News*, the organization newsletter.

Girl Scouts of the United States of America
National Headquarters
830 Third Avenue
New York, NY   10022
(212) 751-6900

A nonprofit, informal youth education organization serving girls ages six through seventeen, its activities encourage the development of personal, social and ethical values and individual skills through a wide variety of projects in social and environmental action, youth leadership and career exploration. The National Board charters councils which organize troops, operate camps and plan a wide range of recreational and community-service activities.

Publications include handbooks, leader guides and instructional booklets on various skills as well as such topics as ecology, food, crafts, games, music, first aid and safety.

Home School Institute
c/o Trinity College
Washington, D.C.   20017
(202) 466-3633

Organization to assist parents with tutoring activities at home and other educational materials. Publications include newsletter, a dial home telephone service and a Home Educational learning program.

International Childbirth Education Association
P.O. Box 70258
Seattle, WA   98107
(206) 789-4444

An interdisciplinary organization representing groups and individuals, both parent and professional, who share a genuine interest in family-centered maternity care. The group's services include a comprehensive book center, which features books and pamphlets on childbirth preparation, family-centered maternity care, breastfeeding and related family and professional subjects.

Publications include *Bookmarks*, a semiannual newsletter that contains news and reviews of new books on all aspects of childbirth.

International Transactional Analysis Association
P.O. Box 3932, Rincon Annex
San Francisco, CA   94119
(415) 885-5992

This organization is dedicated to furthering public knowledge and appreciation for the process and benefits of transactional analysis.

Publications include a wide variety of books on transactional analysis as well as books on management, Gestalt therapy, sexuality, families, children and education.

Jewish Board of Family and Children's Services
120 West 57th Street
New York, NY   10019
(212) 582-9100

Recently formed by the merger of the Jewish Board of Guardians and the Jewish Family Service, which has an extensive library in the field of family and children's mental health, the organization gives special attention to books for parents.

Publications include *As Your Child Grows: The First 18 Months; Television: How to Use It Wisely with Children; You, Your Child and Drugs; What to Tell Your Child About Sex;* and *Learning to*

Love and Let Go: A Guide to Helping Children Become Independent.

La Leche League International
9616 Minneapolis Avenue
Franklin Park, IL   60131
(312) 455-7730

A nonprofit organization dedicated to the advocacy of breastfeeding. Its primary objective is to clear up misconceptions about women who don't have enough milk to nurse, women who are too nervous to breast-feed and women with Rh negative blood. Services include a lending library, regular meetings for interested parents, resources to assist new mothers with breastfeeding their babies.

Publications include *La Leche League News*, a monthly newsletter, and a variety of books on the art of breast-feeding.

March of Dimes Birth Defects Foundation
1275 Mamaroneck Ave.
White Plains, NY   10605
(914) 428-7100

A voluntary health organization dedicated to preventing birth defects, it supports research, medical services and professional and public-health education programs designed to reduce birth defects. It also makes available literature, films, audio cassettes, audiovisual materials and exhibits.

Maternity Center Association
48 East 92 Street
New York, NY   10028
(212) 369-7300

A nonprofit health agency devoted to the improvement of maternity care, the association develops and operates demonstration programs of family-centered maternity care, supports and conducts research to improve the

quality and range of maternity services, lobbies public and government leaders with the aim of achieving a more favorable national policy for the care of mothers and babies and sponsors various seminars and workshops on maternity and child care.

Publications include *Birth Atlas, A Baby Is Born, Preparation for Childbearing,* and *Briefs,* a monthly digest magazine.

Muscular Dystrophy Association
810 Seventh Avenue
New York, NY   10019
(212) 586-0808

Supports research and treatment to the individuals with muscular dystrophy and other related neuro-muscular diseases. Extensive research conducted at hospitals and universities throughout the country. Local services can be located by contacting national office or local directory. Write for "Tips —Special Issue for Parents" (Fall 1979)

National Alternative Schools Program
School of Education
University of Massachusetts
Amherst, MA   01002
(413) 545-0941

Information-gathering and surveying issues in alternative education are the main concerns of this organization.

Publications include *Applesauce,* the organization's monthly newsletter by, for and about public alternative schools, which includes updated reports on the various surveys conducted by NASP, an updated list of clearinghouses and centers for regional networking efforts of those involved in alternative education and a list of publications concerning alternative schools and general issues in school reform.

National Association for Gifted
Children
217 Gregory Dr.
Hot Springs, AR   71901
(501) 767-6933

A nonprofit organization
devoted to advancing interest in
and programs for the gifted, its
primary purpose is to further the
education of the gifted so as to enhance their potential creativity.
The association holds an annual
convention in which the latest information, discoveries, new curriculum methods and other matters
pertaining to the gifted are discussed

Publications include *The
Gifted Child Quarterly*, a journal
with contributions from various
experts on theory, practice, new
curriculum and local and national
news about the gifted.

National Association for Retarded
Citizens
2709 Avenue E East
Arlington, TX   76011
(817) 261-4961

An organization dedicated to
the proper treatment of retarded
citizens and to fostering greater
public awareness of their needs, its
primary concerns also include efforts to create self-respect among
the retarded.

Publications include *Mental
Retardation News*, an organization
newsletter concerning various programs and activities for the retarded.

National Association for the Education of Young Children
1834 Connecticut Ave., N.W.
Washington, D.C.   20009
(202) 232-8777

An organization designed to
serve and act on behalf of young
children, its primary focus is on

the provision of education services
and resources. Programs include
conferences and meetings at the
local, state, regional and national
levels and coordinating efforts
with other organizations concerned
with the education, development
and well-being of young children.

Publications include *Young
Children*, a bimonthly journal for
parents and teachers with reports
on various research projects as
well as a wide range of practical articles, and a variety of other
publications on topics concerning
young children.

National Child Labor Committee
1501 Broadway, Room 1111
New York, NY   10036
(212) 840-1801

Formed to promote the physical and mental well-being of young
people in relation to work, the
committee's current goals include
rectifying the unemployment problem of the country's sixteen- to
twenty-four-year-olds and the
education of the children of
migrant farm workers regarding
the abuse of their rights.

National Commission on Resources for Youth
36 West 44 Street
New York, NY   10036
(212) 682-3339

A not-for-profit educational
organization established to expand
opportunities for young people in
their schools and communities, the
commission acts a philosophy of
providing "hands on" experience
for youth in school and community programs. The commission
serves as a national clearinghouse
of ideas for youth participation
programs. By collecting and cata-
loguing information on programs
around the country, the commission prepares case studies and in-

formational films and literature on
programs that meet the proper
standards. Efforts also include providing resources and information
for the establishment of new programs.

Publications include *Re-
sources for Youth*, a quarterly
newsletter.

National Committee for Prevention of Child Abuse
Suite 510
111 East Wacker Dr.
Chicago, IL   60601
(312) 565-1100

An organization that is involved in various programs to
bring about an awareness of the
problem of child abuse, it sponsors
seminars, public service messages
in different media, training of professionals and nonprofessionals
and puts out various publications.

National Conference of Christians
and Jews
43 West 57 St.
New York, NY   10019
(212) 688-7530

An organization dedicated to
fostering understanding among all
ethnic and religious groups and
educating the public in order to
combat racial and religious prejudice. The NCCJ sponsors a variety
of workshops, seminars and in-service training programs for various
community and governmental
organizations.

Publications include a variety
of materials for schools, churches,
synagogues and civic agencies on
important issues of our time.

National Council on Family Relations
1219 University Ave., S.E.
Minneapolis, MN   55414
(612) 331-2774

An interprofessional organization through which professionals

are able to work and plan together for the strengthening of marriage and family life. Members also include academicians and interested laypersons. Primary goals include establishment of professional standards, promotion and coordination of educational efforts, encouragement of research, extension of community services for families and encouragement of sound government policies pertianing to family life.

Publications include three journals, *The Journal of Marriage and the Family; The Family Coordinator;* and *The Journal of Family History;* as well as a quarterly newsletter.

National Education Association
1201 16th St., N.W.
Washington, D.C.   20036
(202) 833-4000

A professional organization of teachers and school administrators, the association also offers a number of programs for parents. Chief among them is a parent-involvement program which seeks to acquaint parents with modern classroom procedures, and a "Briefing for Parents" series which seeks to clarify school programs and activities by presenting essential background information.

Publications include public-information leaflets on a variety of subjects dealing with the formal and informal educational development of children.

National Forum of Catholic Parent Organizations
Suite 350, One Dupont Circle
Washington, D.C.   20036
(202) 293-5954

This organization seeks to provide leadership at the national level to assist parents in under-

standing their role as primary educators of their children and their relation to Catholic educational policymakers and to educational programs. The organization also serves as a forum for Catholic parents, provides information on ways of maximizing the resources available to Catholic schools and religious education centers and encourages governmental support of nonpublic education.

Publications include *Parentcator,* which appears five times yearly.

National Foundation for Gifted and Creative Children
395 Diamond Hill Rd.
Warwick, RI   02886
(401) 942-2253

An organization devoted to educating the public about the importance of early school days and the recognition of gifted and creative children's special needs and talents. The foundation advocates legislation to ensure the special educational attention gifted children are entitled to. It also counsels parents to help them understand the special requirements of gifted children. The foundation maintains a resource center and a testing service as well.

National Foundation for Sudden Infant Death
1501 Broadway
New York, NY   10036
(212) 563-4630

An organization dedicated to arousing the public conscience in order to combat sudden infant death syndrome (SIDS), the foundation conducts a number of regional seminars to educate physicians, nurses and other professionals about SIDS, operates a fund for various research projects and main-

tains a legal defense fund for families with babies who die of SIDS.

National Institute of Child Health and Human Development
Public Health Service
National Institutes of Health
Bethesda, MD.   20014
(202) 496-4000

A component of the National Institutes of Health, the NICHD supports fundamental and clinical studies on fetal development, the birth process and the well-being of mothers, infants and children. Services include dissemination of research results to the public as well as to health professionals and scientific researchers.

Publications include *Facts About Mongolism for Women Over 35; Facts About Sudden Infant Death Syndrome; Little Babies, Born Too Soon, Born Too Small; Malnutrition, Learning and Behavior.*

National Institute of Mental Health
5600 Fishers Lane
Rockville, MD   20852
(301) 443-4515

The federal agency dedicated to the prevention of mental illness and the promotion of mental health, its services include training activities and research and information programs. Major goals include finding new ways to prevent and treat schizophrenia, depression and all other mental illnesses, as well as more common problems such as stress and fatigue. Programs include coordinating services for prenatal clinics, day-care centers, schools and hospitals.

Publications include a wide variety of educational brochures.

National Organization for Women
5 South Wabash, Suite 1615
Chicago, IL   60603
(312) 332-1954

A lobbying organization dedicated to insuring the passage of the Equal Rights Amendment and favorable legislation on various women's issues such as credit, abortion, employment, rape, sports, education and health; it also conducts a national media campaign to improve women's image in magazines, newspapers, radio and television and to call attention to women's accomplishments and importance to society.

Publications include a variety of newsletters and reports on congressional legislation.

National Society for Autistic Children
Suite 1017
1234 Massachusetts Ave., N.W.
Washington, D.C.   20005
(202) 783-0125

The National Society for Autistic Children is an organization working to create programs of education, legislation and research to benefit all children with severe behavioral disorders. Chapters are located throughout the country and are made up of parents, professionals and other interested citizens.

Publications include: *N.S.A.C. Newsletter* as well as an excellent pamphlet, *Could Your Child Be Autistic?*

National Society for Hebrew Day Schools
229 Park Ave. South
New York, NY   10003
(212) 674-6700

This organization is dedicated to the advancement of the Hebrew day-school movement.

Publications include: *Torah Umesorah Report*, a quarterly; *Tempo*, published semiannually; *Olomeinu—Our World*, a children's magazine; as well as texts, audiovisual aids and workbooks, which are listed in a catalog published annually.

Non-Sexist Child Development Project
370 Lexington Avenue
New York, NY   10017
(212) 532-8374

An organization dedicated to instilling nonsexist attitudes in children at an early age; its programs include in-service teacher training and parent-education programs and the development of nonsexist curriculum, classroom materials and toys. A major goal is to create a national awareness of the importance of dealing with sexism in a child's early years.

Publications include a training manual for teachers and preschool and day-care personnel.

North American Center on Adoption
67 Irving Place
New York, NY   10003
(212) 254-7410

A division of the Child Welfare League, the center is devoted to advocating for every child's right to a permanent family. The center's activites include information services about training and programs and policies for childcare professionals, legislators and those who have adopted or wish to adopt children. Included is information on the vast literature written for and about those involved in adoption—adults and children.

Publications include *Adoption Report*, a quarterly newsletter, and *Tanya*, a booklet

describing one family's experience in adopting an exceptional youngster. *ARENA's Waiting Children*, a memorandum featuring children for whom adoptive families are sought, is issued ten times a year.

P.E.E.R.S. (Parents are Effective Early Education Resources)
8040 Roosevelt Blvd.
Philadelphia, PA   19152
(215) 333-6262

This organization of professionals, parents and volunteers provides early intervention services to infants who are developmentally delayed. The organization operates on the premise that parents are the best teachers during a child's early years. Services include information necessary to implement individual stimulation prescriptions, to create optimum learning environments and to take advantage of all available community resources. Weekly parent lectures, demonstrations and many workshops are provided to further this end.

Parents Without Partners
7910 Woodmont Avenue
Washington, D.C.   20014
(202) 654-8850

A nonprofit education organization devoted exclusively to the welfare and interests of single parents and their children, it seeks to provide a comprehensive program on the special problems they encounter as well as assistance on the various readjustments they must make. Services include various workshops, seminars and research projects.

Publications include *The Single Parent*, a magazine which features articles on child-rearing, income taxes, remarriage, psychological problems and adjustments.

Planned Parenthood Federation of America, Inc., of New York City
810 7th Ave.
New York, NY   10019
(212) 541-7800

Dedicated to advancing public knowledge of responsible practices of birth control and parenthood, the organization also seeks to ensure proper medical and legal practices in regard to birth control, parenthood, venereal diseases, abortion and a variety of other relevant issues. A special concern is a justice fund to provide abortions for women of all economic backgrounds.

Publications include a variety of pamphlets and brochures on the different means of birth control and disease prevention.

Profession of Parenting Institute
1609 Poplar St.
Philadelphia, PA   19130
(215) 336-8008

This organization is dedicated to raising parenting to the level of a profession by conducting workshops, training sessions, seminars and annual convocations and initiating legislative action.

Publications include *The World's Newest Profession* and *The Parent Portfolio*, an organization newsletter.

Sex Information and Education Council of the U.S.
84 Fifth Ave.
New York, NY 10011
(212) 929-2300

A nonprofit health-service agency dedicated to the recognition of human sexuality as a health entity, the organization serves as a clearinghouse for information on valuable resources and materials available for health professionals, teachers, parents and young peo-

ple. A special interest is combatting the traditionally reluctant manner in which parents deal with their children's sexuality.

Publications include a variety of books on topics such as homosexuality, masturbation, teenage pregnancy and sexual encounters between adults and children.

United Nations Children's Fund (UNICEF)
331 East 38 St.
New York, NY   10016
(212) 686-5522

Designed to distribute funds for programs for the needy children of the world through a worldwide organization involved in many activities.

Publications include a variety of pamphlets and brochures.

U.S. Department of Health and Human Services
Washington, D.C.   20201
(202) 245-7204

With the general goal of coordinating a broadly based social policy that is responsive to the needs of the public, the department offers a wide variety of government-financed programs. Of special interest is the Head Start program for preschoolers and day care services of the Administration for Children, Youth and Families

Publications include literature on department programs and all aspects of health, education and welfare.

U.S. Department of Agriculture
Washington, D.C.   20250
(202) 655-4000

Programs of this department include the Food Stamp Program, the Nonfood Assistance Program, the Child Nutrition Programs, the National School Lunch Program,

the Special Milk Program and the School Breakfast Program.

Publications include a wide variety of literature on the department's programs and on food and nutrition.

United Synagogue of America
155 Fifth Ave.
New York, NY   10010
(212) 533-7800

This educationally oriented organization serves the conservative Jewish community throughout the United Synagogue Commission on Jewish Education. The commission provides for parent education, develops programs for the Jewish special child, sponsors family meetings and services a network of religious schools. The primary goal is to provide for a meaningful education within the dual context of Jewishness and American civilization.

Publications include *Your Child*, a monthly newsletter, and a number of textbooks dealing with the Jewish experience.

Special and Local Organizations

The organizations in this section have been selected because of the specific services and support they offer parents. Most of these groups are comprised of concerned professionals and/or parents who saw a need for a specific program—i.e., pregnant high school students, day-care and networks for parents who need support or assistance (single parents, stepparents, parents who are significantly upset with themselves, their children, or others, and those who have health problems and work-related difficulties).

Many of the ideas behind these special and local organizations can be transferred to other locales to provide new support networks. Contact the specific organizations for additional information.

Alternative Schools Network
1105 West Lawrence, Room 210
Chicago, IL 60640
(312) 728-4030

A coalition of locally controlled nonpublic schools in the Chicago area, the network serves the schools through fund raising, information sharing and acting as a resource center for alternative community education. The network also sponsors various workshops and conferences concerning the concept of "alternative schools."

Publications include *ASN-NEWS*, a monthly newsletter concerning community and alternative education; *Alternative Curriculum*, a resource book for Chicago area teachers; and *Literacy in 30 Hours*, a book by Cynthia Brown.

Bananas Child Care Information Service
6501 Telegraph
Oakland, CA 94609
(415) 658-7101

A nonprofit child-care information and referral service for northern Alameda County, California, the service offers referrals for all types of child care, housing information, technical assistance, a family day-care law service, health advice, precrisis counseling and information on services and children with handicaps.

Publications include a bimonthly newsletter and a variety of free educational materials.

Bismarck Early Childhood Education Program
400 Ave. E
Bismarck, ND 58501
(701) 255-3866

This public-school program designed to meet the needs of preschool children and their families serves as a coordinating organization for Head Start, Day Care, Special Needs Program and the Child Family Resource Program. The primary objective is to develop the concept of the parents as the primary educators of their children. The program sponsors a number of seminars and discussions for parents on the various approaches and techniques of fostering the successful early education of their children.

California Children's Lobby
P.O. Box 448
Sacramento, CA 95802
(916) 444-7477

An organization dedicated to insuring favorable public opinion and responsible government action for children's causes, its primary objectives include stimulating constructive reforms on administrative as well as legislative levels and establishing an objective evaluation process in order to maintain high-quality services for children.

Publications include *The Cryer*, the organizational newsletter.

Children's Council of San Francisco—Childcare Switchboard
3896 24th St.
San Francisco, CA 94144
(415) 282-7858

A nonprofit child-care information and referral service for the city and county of San Francisco, California, the service offers referrals for all types of child care, housing information, technical assistance to new and existing providers, a family day-care law service, health advice, precrisis counseling and information on services for children with handicaps.

Publications include a bimonthly newsletter and a variety of free educational materials.

Day Care Council of Nassau County
240 Clinton St.
Hempstead, NY 11550
(516) 538-1362

A coordinating, planning and advocacy organization for a broad range of child-care services, the council provides technical assistance, training and information and referral services to providers and users of day-care. The council also provides information on developing day-care centers, criteria on identification of good child care and material concerning government regulations, reimbursement rates, eligibility levels and other pertinent fiscal information.

Publications include *Directory of Day Care Services, Early Childhood Programs and Programs for Children with Special Needs*, and a program evaluation and self-assessment guide to use in various types of child-care programs.

Devereux Foundation
P.O. Box 1079
Santa Barbara, CA 93102
(805) 968-2525

A not-for-profit, nonsectarian, residential and day treatment organization for children with therapeutic needs, the foundation operates twenty-five separate campuses throughout the United States. Services include psychiatric and psychological evaluations, psychotherapy, family counseling, speech therapy, job skill training, perceptual and motor coordination training and off-campus cultural and recreational activities.

Publications include descriptive brochures.

Erikson Institute for Early Education
1525 East 53 St.
Chicago, IL 60615
(312) 493-0200

A tax-exempt organization dedicated to training preprimary teachers and related supervisory personnel, it serves as a center for training teachers and as a nationwide consultation service. The primary goal is to interpret and consistently apply available research findings to the care and education of the very young. A major concern in meeting this goal is the gap between the public's knowledge of preschool children's needs and the recent research that has demonstrated that a large number of children enter school with emotional problems, social difficulties, cognitive skill deficits and health and nutritional inadequacies.

Publications include *Outrider*, the organizational newsletter.

Maryland Committee for Children
608 Water St.
Baltimore, MD 21202
(301) 752-7588

A private, nonprofit organization concerned with enriching existing child-care services and expanding them to meet the needs of families who seek them, the committee's programs include representing the children's interests in the formation of public policy, a consultation service for day-care centers, information services for the public and a series of workshops and seminars for parents and professional day-care staff members.

Publications include an annual report and a variety of brochures and pamphlets.

Parents as Resources Project
464 Central Ave.

Northfield, IL 60093
(312) 441-5617

An organization of parents attempting to help other parents and nonprofessionals work with young children in an educational way, PAR conducts training workshops for parents and paraprofessional staffs of day-care and Head Start centers, family day-care homes and various other child-care agencies and schools. A special project is the training of inner-city parents to be workshop leaders.

Publications include *Recipes For Fun*, a collection of activities for young children; *Workshop Procedures*, a manual for the planning and conducting of workshops; and *Recipes For Holiday Fun*, a parent's guide for holiday activities for children.

Parent Preschool Resource Center of the National Capitol Region
63 Evelyn Ave.
Ottawa, Canada K1S OC6
(613) 238-7561

This organization serves as a library, an information service, a play center and a counseling service. Its guiding philosophy is to offer a wide range of preventive service in order to provide for the physical, mental and emotional well-being of children. Programs include informal workshops and discussions for parents and an open classroom for preschool children.

Publications include *Somebody Else's Place*, a descriptive brochure of the organization.

Resources for Infant Educarers
P.O. Box 32369
San Jose, CA 95152
(408) 297-5920

This nonprofit organization is dedicated to furthering a unique philosophy for the day-to-day care and education of infants and young children. Central to the RIE philosophy is the importance of respecting even the youngest infant as a unique human being instead of an object. Services include consultations and help in designing day-care centers, assistance in the training of personnel and in developing curriculum.

Publications include a variety of descriptive brochures.

San Francisco Child Abuse Council
1304-A Castro St.
San Francisco, CA 94114
(415) 647-4576

A nonprofit organization established to support and coordinate the efforts of those involved in the prevention, identification and treatment of child abuse, its services include case consultations, a hot line for parents and a variety of educational programs for the public, professional groups and agencies.

Publications include *SFCAC News*, a bimonthly newsletter; and a wide selection of pamphlets and brochures.

Stepfamily Foundation of California
900 Welch Rd., Suite 400
Palo Alto, CA 94304
(415) 328-0723

This nonprofit, educational organization is dedicated to providing information about stepfamilies and issues that affect stepparents and stepchildren. Programs include a referral service for families seeking counselors and therapists, research in areas such as stepfamily law and cultural attitudes toward remarriage with children, and professional training services for therapists and counselors.

Publications include a monthly organizational newsletter.

Appendix B
Magazines and Other Parenting Publications

American Baby
575 Lexington Ave.
New York, NY 10022
Write for free copy.

Featuring fashion, beauty and health tips for expectant mothers, health care during and after delivery and general information on baby care, this magazine includes a "Booklets and Samples" section from which parents can order a wide variety of free or inexpensive pamphlets on parenting.

Baby Care
52 Vanderbilt Ave.
New York, NY 10017
Write for free copy

Published quarterly by *Parents'* magazine, this publication features general information for new parents, with topics ranging from "Will Your Marriage Ever Be The Same?" to "Profiles of Play."

Building Blocks
Box 31
Dundee, IL 60118
$1.50/single

The *Building Blocks Newsletter* is designed to provide any adult who works with young children useful, easy-to-follow ideas on what to do with those children.
The "Pages of Projects" series is designed to offer the user 60–70 ideas to facilitate the development of the child in various subject areas —holiday hints, science beginnings and language enrichment.

Children Today
Children's Bureau Administration for Children, Youth & Families
P.O. Box 1182
Washington, D.C. 20013
$6.10/yr. $7.65/foreign
$1.00/single

Current events, programs and research relating to the life of children from infancy through the high school years are covered here. Published six times a year, the magazine considers such topics as families, their creation, development, and learning; adopted children; medicine and children; children from non-English language backgrounds; violence toward youth; neglected children; a child's image in books; day-care; and psychosocial problems with children.

Day Care and Early Education
Day Care Council
711 14 St., N.W.
Washington, D.C. 20005
$9.95/individuals
$15.00/institutions
$19/foreign

Serving the special needs and interests of the child-growth movements, this is a valuable reference tool including current affairs, nutritional concepts, staffing problems, crafts tips, space and equipment selection, book reviews, learning setups, recipes and innovative products.

Early Learning Book Club
Riverside, NJ 08370

This club's selections include many books for children and adults on math, art, games, as well as professional books on early childhood development.

Early Years
Box 1223
Darien, CT 06820
$9.50/yr. $11.50/foreign
$1.50/single

A monthly magazine geared to the basic skills that children must acquire in the early grades, this concentrates on the needs of both teachers and children.

Family Circle
488 Madison Ave.
New York, NY 10022
49¢/single

This all-purpose family magazine is devoted to such issues as cooking, clothing, psychological counseling, car repair, marriage, exercise, money and budgeting, beauty, health, decorating, jobs, diet, child care, gardening and buyer's guide.

First Teacher and *First Teacher for Parents*
P.O. Box 29
Bridgeport, CT 06602
$15/yr.

First Teacher is an illustrated monthly publication for people who care for young children with ideas, activities, and recipes for children.
First Teacher for Parents also published monthly is for relatives

and adult friends of young children, with the same great ideas, activities and recipes for children to learn and do at home.

Growing Up With Gerber
445 State Street
Fremont, MI 49412
$1.00/single

This magazine, published in several volumes that specialize on babies within a given age range, includes a wide variety of articles to answer the questions of new parents. Includes information on child safety, baby foods, baby-sitters, baby health care and more.

Handbook for Working Women
Mail Order Department
Publishing Data Center
Building 3; Brooklyn Navy Yard
Brooklyn, NY 11205
$1.50/single

This quarterly features helpful information for working women. Articles range from "Carefree Shopping by Mail" to "The ½-Hour Cookbook" to "Single Parents— With Double The Work and Double The Pleasure."

MOMMA
Momma Communications, Inc.
Box 308
Station A
Willowdale, Ontario M2W 5S9
$2.00/yr.

This quarterly newsletter for full-time mothers at home is a forum for women to share their concerns and become aware of the many opportunities in their communities for self-growth.

Marriage and Family Living
St. Meinrad, IN 47577
$9.00/yr. $10.00/foreign

This monthly features information on how to make the experience of parenting and being part of a family more enjoyable and productive. Articles range from "Crisis in the Classroom" to "Learning to Like Yourself." The magazine also includes plays and other activities for the family to do together to increase mutual understanding.

Mothering
P.O. Box 2046
Albuquerque, NM 87103
$8.00/yr. $12.00/foreign
$2.25/single

Features include: "Art of Mothering," "Family Health," "Mother to Mother," "Grandmothering," "Midwifery," "Pregnancy and Birth," "Educational Alternatives," "Early Childhood" and "Family Centered Businesses."

Mother's Manual
Box 243
Franklin Lakes, NJ 07417
9 issues $5.40 $.60/single

This bimonthly magazine focuses on the mother-child relationship and is advertised as "America's Foremost Baby Guide." It includes articles ranging from ways of birthing to tips for tiny skiers. It also includes news notes, book reviews, stories of families in process, medicine and children and a Washington report.

Mothers-To-Be and Infant Care
American Baby, Inc.
10 East 52nd St.
New York, NY 10022
$2.00/yr. $.50/single

A quarterly magazine to answer questions about expectant and new motherhood, the magazine includes special features, such as "Learning to Live with an Infant," "Childbirth by the Lamaze Method," "The Pregnant Cook's Book." It also includes features on fashion and beauty, preparing and caring for your baby, medical news and notes, books for parents and booklets and samples.

Ms.
370 Lexington Ave.
New York, NY 10017
$10.00/yr. $1.00/single

The nation's foremost feminist magazine, *Ms.* features guides for homemakers, women in the trades and business women. Feminist news from all around the world is provided. Features include articles on women athletes and clothing, fiction and poetry by women, the women's viewpoint on the arts.

New Baby Talk
Leam Corporation
66 E. 34 St.
New York, NY 10016
$5.25/yr. $5.50/foreign

This monthly magazine focuses on infants and considers subjects ranging from pregnancy to toys. It features questions and answers from a child psychiatrist, suggestions from mothers, shop talk and articles on siblings, swimming and infants, skin care of infants, advice on traveling and visiting with baby and more.

Notes for Parents
James L. Hymes
Southern California Association for the Education of Young Children c/o Natl Association for the Education of Young Children
1834 Connecticut Ave., N.W.
Washington, D.C. 20009
1977 12 Pamphlets $4.50

Notes for Parents is a set of twelve pamphlets for parents of young children. Topics include "Talking and Listening," "Beginning Days of School" and "Give Your Child Responsibility."

What's the good of early schooling? An under-six group is one of the best devices for fostering independence. The simple fact of going off to school; of saying "Goodbye" to one's parents (knowing you will see them again soon); of having one's own work to do . . . If young children could use the words, the boy or girl who has this kind of independence would say: "This is really living."

Parenting News
Institute for Childhood Resources
Parents & Child Care Resources
1169 Howard Street
San Francisco, CA 94103

This periodic newsletter based on *The Whole Child* references new books, resources and parenting ideas. Available for parents, teachers, students and interested others. Write for sample newsletter. Cost of each issue is $2.00 (plus 50¢ postage and handling). Also available is *Choosing Child Care: A Guide For Parents* ($3.50 per copy).

Parents' Magazine
52 Vanderbilt Ave.
New York, NY   10017
$1.00/single $7.95/yr.

This monthly magazine includes sections for parents with (1) children under five, (2) children between five and ten, and (3) children between eleven and eighteen. The magazine runs special features on child-rearing and family health, family food, family fashion, family home and family fun. Articles are included such as one called "Before the Baby Comes."

Practical Parenting
15235 Minnetonka Blvd.
Minnetonka, MN   55343
$5/yr. $6/foreign

This bimonthly newsletter is a forum for the exchange of reader's parenting ideas, problems and tips. Also includes recipes and advice from experts.

Redbook
230 Park Avenue
New York, NY   10017
$7.95/yr. $10.50/Canada
$.95/single

This monthly family magazine offers general information articles, profiles of famous personalities, psychological counseling articles and sections on needlecrafts, home equipment and furnishings, cooking and food, fashion, beauty, and so on. It also includes a novel condensation and short story section each month.

Stepfamily Bulletin
Editors: Elizabeth Einstein, Emily Visher, and John Visher
Human Sciences Press
72 Fifth Avenue
New York, NY   10011
$12.00

This newsletter for stepfamilies and interested professionals provides a rich source of facts and data about step-relationships and remarriages when there are children from a previous marriage. The Bulletin is the official bulletin of Stepfamily Association of America, Inc. and offers current information on state and national stepfamily meetings, professional training workshops, the location of established chapters, and guidelines for organizing local activities. The newsletter features articles concerned with the special attributes of stepfamilies and also significant research findings, book reviews and lists of references, while providing a format for understanding the unique challenges and rewards that arise from the complex cultural, structural

and emotional characteristics of stepfamilies.

Voice for Children
Day Care Council
711 14th St., N.W.
Washington, D.C.   20005
Rates: (Includes one year membership in DCC) $12/individual $50/agency or center $25/single program agency or center $20/library

This magazine, published six times yearly, is the official magazine of the Day Care Council of America. The articles provide information on issues that have national impact on the field of day care, such as "The Federal Interagency Day Care Requirements Issues." It also includes less specialized information of interest to day-care providers on a variety of topics including "Day Care: Facts and Fallacies" and "Training Trainers."

Woman's Day
1 Fawcett Place
Greenwich, CT   06830
$.55/single

This well-known monthly magazine is a constant source of information on home, family and well-being. It offers many special features and articles ranging from children, and psychology to home and garden.

Women Who Work
Family Circle, Inc.
488 Madison Avenue
New York, NY   10022
$1.75/single

A bimonthly publication devoted to providing helpful information to working women; the magazine includes career information, life-style articles, recipes, parenting articles, diet information and more.

Working Mother
McCall Publishing Co.
230 Park Avenue
New York, NY 10017
$7/yr.

This new quarterly is a clearinghouse for information vital to working mothers all over the country and includes life-style information, career news, articles on child care, resolving marriage/career conflicts and more.

Working Woman
600 Madison Ave.
New York, NY 10022
$1.25/single $10.00/yr.

This monthly magazine focuses on specific trades, discusses the dilemma of working while having children, quizzes you on your get-ahead skills, offers help when you want to quit your job and includes articles on how women face success, money making, living/style, national news about working women and reviews of consciousness-raising books.

Young Children
National Association for the Education of Young Children
1834 Connecticut Avenue, N.W.
Washington, D.C. 20009
Members, $6.50/yr.
Non-members, $12.00/yr.
$15.00/foreign
$2.00/single

This publication includes articles of general interest to both parents and early childhood teachers. Information on issues of national significance in the field.

Young Mother
Redbook Publishing Company
230 Park Avenue
New York, NY 10017
$1.00/single

This magazine focuses on health-care information for the pregnant mother and for the new baby. It includes such articles as "Why Babies Cry," "The New Mother's Health," "Dental Care During Pregnancy" and "How Your Baby Grows." It also includes beauty information for the expectant and new mother, recipes for baby food and other articles with general information on raising a baby.

Young Parents Book Club
40 Guernsey Street
Stamford, CT 06904

A wonderful book club which offers a fascinating list of titles that would tempt any concerned parent. Prices are substantially reduced for members. Recent titles offered: *A Book for Grandmothers*, *Fathering*, *Birth Without Violence*, *Great Pets*, as well as offerings for the children themselves.

Additional Parenting Resources

How To Do It Yourself Advocacy Kit
Marlene Posner, Ken Jaffe
California Family Services Agency
2380 Smith Lane, Concord, CA 94518
$4.95 plus 75¢ postage/handling

This unusual kit is a collection of simply prepared ideas, checkpoints and resources presented in ten easy steps for people interested in advocating for the cause of their choice. Useful for PTA groups, citizens concerned with health care, education, early childhood issues, impacting bureaucratic systems and the legislature, this kit is a must for community organizations and agencies.

For Children

Career World
Curriculum Innovations, Inc.
501 Lake Forest Ave.
Highwood, IL 60040
(Minimum 15 subscriptions to one address)
$3.50/per school year per student

This magazine for both elementary and junior high school children explores the world of work, offering interesting information on various jobs as well as articles on how career choices are made. Although this magazine cannot be ordered by an individual parent, it is so worthwhile that we included it in order that you might encourage your child's teacher to order it.

Children's Digest
80 New Bridge Rd.
Bergenfield, NJ 07621
$8.95/yr. $9.95/Canada
$10.95/foreign

Published by *Parents'* magazine, this magazine for school-age children includes informative articles such as "Kids Rights," stories, craft ideas, children's book reviews and more.

Humpty Dumpty's Magazine for Little Children
80 New Bridge Road
Bergenfield, NJ 07621
$8.95/yr. $9.95/Canada
$10.95/foreign

Published by *Parents'* magazine, this magazine includes a variety of wonderful, easy-reading stories and simple games that help very young children learn about their world. A sample issue focused on ". . . how children perceive the world when the lights are out," including such stories as

"Night Noises" and "The Wishing Star." The magazine also includes nature stories, children's recipes and samples of children's artwork.

Sesame Street Magazine
Children's Television Workshop
1 Lincoln Plaza
New York, NY 10023
$.75/single

This magazine is published ten times during the year, monthly except for August and January. It is a wonderful magazine for children which allows them to use their innate curiosity and leads them to explore themselves and the world around them. Each issue is developed to help sharpen children's skills from reasoning and problem-solving to self-expression. There is a section of each issue that is used to give readers suggestions from the Sesame Street Magazine staff, based on their research. It is a carefully designed and researched book and makes the readers an important part of the process, encouraging them to write in with insights and suggestions on how to make the magazine more worthwhile to children.

Note: Scholastic and My Weekly Reader also produce magazines for children, such as *Co-ed, Dynamite* and *My Weekly Reader* which are widely distributed through schools.

Appendix C
Films and Audiovisual Aids

The films and audiovisual aids that follow are useful for educational purposes at parent meetings and discussion groups. Film showings are also excellent fund-raisers for parent groups and schools. We have listed here film companies that have good films that relate to parent interests. Although limited selections are listed here, most of the companies have more titles available. Write directly for information, rental or sale costs. Film catalogs are also included.

Allen Grant Productions
P.O. Box 49244
Los Angeles, Calif. 90049
213/472-0046

What Color Is The Wind? 16mm/ color/27 min. True story of twins, one sighted and one blind.

Suzanne Arms Productions
151 Lytton Ave.
Palo Alto, Calif. 94301
415/321-3340

Five Women Five Births 16mm/ b&w/29 min.

Benchmark Films
145 Scarborough Road
Briarcliff Manor, N.Y. 10510
914/762-3838

Drugs Are Like That 16mm/color/17 min.
Child Behavior—You 16mm/ color/15 min.
Elsa and Her Cubs 16mm/color/ 25 min.

Bradley Wright Films
1 Oak Hill Drive
San Anselmo, Calif. 94960
415/457-6260

On Their Own/With Our Help 16mm/color/25 min.

Camput Film Distribution Ctr.
2 Overhill Road
Scarsdale, N.Y. 10583
914/472-9590

That The Deaf May Speak 16mm/ 42 min.
Play In the Hospital 16mm/50 min.

Children's Home Society of California
5429 McConnel Avenue
Los Angeles, Calif. 90066
213/391-2814

Four Teen Mothers and Their Babies 16mm/55 min.

Churchill Films
662 North Robertson Blvd.
Los Angeles, Calif. 90069
213/657-5110

The Growing Year in Sight and Sound Cartridge filmstrip series/ color

Communications Group West
6066 Sunset Blvd.
Hollywood, Calif. 90028
213/461-4024

We Have Met the Enemy and He Is Us! 16mm/color/12½ min.
A Child's Orientation to Primary School 16mm/color/12½ min.

Davidson Films, Inc.
850 Neill Ave.
Belmont, Calif 94002

Child's Play and the Real World 16mm/18min.
Teachers, Parents, Children 16mm/17 min.
Nurturing 16mm/17 min.

Education Communications, Inc.
2814 Virginia St.
Houston, Tex. 77098
713/522-0897

A Look At You: On the Bus 16mm/9 min.
He's Mentally Retarded 16mm/ 8 min.
A Look At You: The Body 16mm/8 min.

Education Development Center
15 Mifflin Place
Cambridge, Mass. 02138

At the Doctor's 16mm/b&w/ 10 min.
Teacher, Lester Bit Me! 16mm/ color/10 min.
Little Blocks 16mm/color/8 min.

Film Fair Communications
10900 Ventura Blvd.
P.O. Box 1728
Studio City, Calif. 91604
213/877-3191

Robin . . . A Runaway 16mm/ color/32 min.
What Is A Cat? 16mm/animated color/13½ min.
Sleep 16mm/color/11min.

Great Plains National Instructional Television Library
P.O. Box 80669
Lincoln, Neb. 68501
402/467-2502

Ride the Reading Rocket ¾" video series of forty 30-min. programs to teach reading to first-graders

Hallmark Films
51-53 New Plant Court
Owings Mills, Md.   21117

Today's Children 16mm/color/
28 min.
I'll Promise You a Tomorrow
16mm/color/20 min.

High/Scope Foundation
600 North River Street
Ypsilanti, Mich.   48197
313/485-2000

This Is the Way We Go to School
16mm/color/28 min.
Responding to a Baby's Action
16mm/color/24 min.

International Film Bureau
332 South Michigan Avenue
Chicago, Ill.   60604
312/427-4545

Children In the Hospital 16mm/
b&w/44 min.
Our Clothes 16mm/color/17
min.

Joseph T. Anzalone Foundation
P.O. Box 5206
Santa Cruz, Calif.   95063
408/476-7676

Pregnant Fathers 16mm/color/
28 min.
Becoming . . . 16mm/color/30
min.   On the birth experience

J. B. Lippincott Audio/visual Dept.
Division of Higher Education
East Washington Square
Philadelphia, Pa.   19105

The New World
Finding A Place
The Presence of Self

Long Island Film Studio
Box 49403
Atlanta, Ga.   30359

Lead Poisoning—The Hidden Epidemic 16mm/color/10 min.

I feel . . . angry 16mm/color/
11 min.

CRM/McGraw-Hill Films
McGraw-Hill Book Company
Del Mar, Calif.   92014
714/453-5000

Personality: Adolescence 16mm/
color/21 min.
Child's Play 16mm/color/20
min.
Physical Development 16mm/
color/21 min.

Malibu Films
Box 428
Malibu, Calif.   90265
213/456-2859

Bias—A Four Letter Word
16mm/color/22 min.
Anger and How To Cope 16mm/
color/15min.
When In Pain 16mm/color/15
min.

Mass Media Ministries
2116 North Charles Street
Baltimore, Md.   21218
301/727-3270

A Cry of Pain 16mm/color/15
min.   A view of child abuse in
America

The Media Guild
P.O. Box 881
Solano Beach, Calif.   90215
714/755-9191

Juvie 16mm/color/27 min.
Early Words 16mm/color/22
min.
Play-IsTrying Out 16mm/color/
25 min.

Miller-Brody Productions, Inc.
342 Madison Avenue
New York, N.Y.   10017

Think Metric 4 filmstrips with
records or cassettes
A Woggle of Witches 1 filmstrip
with record or cassette

National Association for the Education of Young Children
1834 Connecticut Avenue, N.W.
Washington, D.C.   20009

Animals Unlimited 16mm/color/
19½ min.
At Your Fingertips: Play Clay
16mm/color/10 min.
Growing Up In a Scary World
16mm/color/15 min.

National Audio Visual Center
National Archives and Records
Service
General Services Administration
Reference Section GA
Washington, D.C.   20409
301/763-1896

Sexual Abuse: The Family
16mm/color/30 min.
Operation Head Start 16mm/
b&w/28 min.
Abusive Parents 16mm/color/
30 min.

National Center on Child Abuse
and Neglect
U.S. Children's Bureau
Administration for Children,
Youth and Families
U.S. Department of Health and
Human Services
P.O. Box 1182
Washington, D.C.   20013

Write for complete catalogue that
is a sourcebook for films to be ordered direct from distributors.

National Film Board of Canada
1251 Avenue of the Americas
New York, N.Y.   10019

Child Behavior—You 16mm/
animated/color

The National Foundation/March
of Dimes
Box 2000
White Plains, N.Y.   10602

Born Hooked 16mm/color

New York University Film Library
26 Washington Place
New York, N.Y. 10003
212/598-2250

Films available to groups, organizations only

The Gifted Ones 16mm/color/
22 min.
Growing Up With Deafness
16mm/color/30 min.
Head Start to Confidence 16mm/
color/17 min.

New Yorker Films
43 West 61 Street
New York, N.Y. 10023
212/247-6110

Loving Hands 16mm/color/23
min. The art of baby massage
Diary of a Yonbogi Boy 16mm/
b&w/24 min. Life of a 10-year-
old Korean orphan

Nguzo Saba Films, Inc.
1002 Clayton Street
San Francisco, Calif. 94117
415/731-7336

Umoja: Tiger and the Big Wind
16mm/animated color/8. min. Illustrates *Umoja*—unity
Imani: Beegie and the Egg
16mm/animated color/7. min. Illustrates *Imani*—faith

Paideia
3107 Santa Monica Blvd.
Santa Monica, Calif 90404
213/829-4871

Nursery School—A Chance To Be
16mm/color

Parents' Magazine Films, Inc.
52 Vanderbilt Avenue
New York, N.Y. 10017
212/661-9080

Children in Crisis 4 filmstrip sets
The Parent as Teacher 5 filmstrips with record or cassette

Peach Enterprizes, Inc.
4649 Gerald
Warren, Mich. 48092

*What Did You Say In School To-
day?* 16mm/color/23 min.
James & John 16mm/color/23
min. Twins with Down's Syndrome

Perennial Education, Inc.
477 Roger Williams
P.O. Box 855 Ravinia
Highland Park, Ill. 60035

A Family Talks About Sex
16mm/color/28½ min.
*Teen Sexuality: What's Right For
You?* 16mm/color/29 min.
*Parenting Concerns the First Two
Years* 16mm/color/21 min.

Phoenix Films
470 Park Avenue South
New York, N.Y. 10016
212/684-5910

Elizabeth & the Marsh Mystery
16mm/color/21 min.
Ira Sleeps Over 16mm/color/17
min.
Linda's Film—Menstruation
16mm/color/18 min.

Pittsburgh Child Guidance Center
210 De Soto Street
Pittsburgh, Pa. 15213

*Playing: Pretending—Spontaneous
Drama with Children* 16mm/
b&w/20 min.
*Children and the Arts—A Film
About Growing* 16mm/color/22
min.

Polymorph Films
331 Newbury Street
Boston, Mass. 02115
617/262-5960

Gentle Birth 16mm/color/15
min.

*Stepparenting: New Families, Old
Ties* 16mm/color/25 min.
Day Care Today 16mm/color/
25 min.

Prentice-Hall Media, Dept. N.J.
150 White Plains Road
Tarrytown, N.Y. 10591

Embryology 2 filmstrips with
records or cassettes
Smoking 2 filmstrips with records or cassettes

Psychological Films, Inc.
110 N. Wheeler Street
Orange, Calif. 92669
714/630-4646

Childhood: The Enchanted Years 2
film series 16mm/color/52 min.

Pyramid Films
P.O. Box 1048
Santa Monica, Calif. 90406
213/828-7577

Prenatal Care 16mm/Super 8/
video/25min.
Who Are the DeBolts? 16mm/
color/72 min.

S & L Film Productions
P.O. Box 41108
Los Angeles, Calif. 90041
213/254-8528

*Help Me! The Story of A Teenage
Suicide* 16mm/color/25 min.
Children of Synanon 16mm/
b&w/16 min.

Science Curriculum Improvement
Studies
Lawrence Hall of Science
University of California
Berkeley, Calif. 94720

Don't tell me, I'll find out 16mm/
color/22 min.
Around the Corner 16mm/col-
or/10 min.
Energy & Models 16mm/color/
20 min.

Stanfield House Films
12381 Wilshire Blvd., Suite 203
Los Angeles, Calif.   90026
213/820-4568

Babydance   16mm/color/15 min.
Prenatal care through medium of
dance

Third Eye Films
12 Arrow Street
Cambridge, Mass.   02138
617/354-1500

Great Expectations   16mm/color/
22 min.   Nutrition information
for pregnant women
First Foods   16mm/color/14 min.

Film Catalogues

More Films Kids Like, $8.95
American Library Association
50 East Huron Street
Chicago, Ill.   60611

This excellent film catalogue
published by the American Library
Association is included here because it is a compliation of information on many high-quality children's films. Extensive research
and screenings have helped provide this listing of only the best,
most effective children's films.

Films for Early Childhood
Early Childhood Education Council
196 Bleecker Street
New York, N.Y.   10012

This is another excellent catalogue containing information on
films for parents, teachers and for
children. Write for price.

Clothing and Equipment Suppliers

Notes on Resources for Clothing and Equipment

For further information on the items listed here, send a postcard to the manufacturers; be sure to request current prices. We have searched for companies that produce useful clothing and equipment. The items included can be useful as a guide to purchasing and/or supplementing what is locally available.

Clothing

Bambini
Warren Street Screen Press
329 Warren St.
Cambridge, MA   02141

Handprinted T-Shirts

Casco Bay Trading Post
Freeport, ME   04032

Leather Booties

Cinderella Clothing Industries
112 W. 34th St.
New York, N.Y.   10001

Dresses

Columbia-Minerva Corp.
295 Fifth Ave.
New York, N.Y.   10016

Noah's Ark Kit—Birth Sampler Kits

Danskin Inc.
1114 Ave. of the Americas, 14th Fl.
New York, N.Y.   10036

Leotards, Tights, Playclothes

Janie Press
262 W. 38th St.
New York, N.Y.   10018

Dresses

Jessica of Gunne Sax Factory
274 Brannan St.
San Francisco, CA   94107

Fancy Dresses

Health Tex Inc.
1411 Broadway
New York, N.Y.   10018

Children's Clothes

Kleinerts Incorp.
112 W. 34th St., Suite 1416
New York, N.Y.   10120

Sleepy drye outer pants for diapers/3-way diaper bag/waterproof nylon pants

Lace Palace
1 Rue de La Violette
Brussels, BELGIUM

Brussels Lace
Christening Gown

Wm. G. Leminger Knitting Co.
Mohnton, PA   19540

Square-Toe Socks

Max and Moritz
3200 Bassett
Santa Clara, CA   95080

Children's Clothes

Millicents of San Francisco
275 9th St.
San Francisco, CA   94103

Coats

Mothercare Ltd.
Cherry Tree Road
Watford WD 2 5 SH ENGLAND

Play Shoes
Cosy Toes

Nanette
c/o Mr. Jerry Rosenau
3800 Frankford Ave.
Philadelphia, PA   19124

Children's Wear

Petite Gamin
226 Potrero Ave.
San Francisco, CA 94103

Dresses/Sportswear

Ruth of Carolina
131 2. 33rd St., Rm. 1208
New York, N.Y.   10001

Dresses

Today's Child
550 De Haro St.
San Francisco, CA 94107

Baby & Children's Clothing

Equipment Suppliers

NOTE: These are suggested manufacturers and some sample products.

American Hospital Supply
General Offices
1450 Waukegan Rd.
McGaw Park, Ill.   60085

Crib Dome

Antelope Camping Equipment
21740 Granada Ave.
Cupertino, Calif.   95014

Carrier

J. J. Avery, Inc.
P.O. Box 6459
Denver, Colo. 80206
Lact-Aid

B.B.S. Enterprises, Ltd.
8401 Connecticut Ave., Suite 1011
Chevy Chase, Md. 20015
Safe Sleep Mattress

A Baby Carriage Hospital
5935 W. Irving Park Rd.
Chicago, Ill. 60634
Carriage Bag

Baby-Tenda Corp.
909 State Line Ave.
Kansas City, Mo. 64101
Feeding Table

Barclay Co.
P.O. Box 37
Teaneck, N.J. 07666
Perego stroller

Log House Sales Room
Berea College Student Craft Industries
P.O. Box 2347
Berea, Ky. 40403
Berea Cradle

Bickiepegs, Ltd.
43–47 Jopp's Lane
John Street
Aberdeen, Scotland
Sloping cup

Bowland-Jacobs Manufacturing
Spring Valley, Ill. 61362
Happy Baby Food Grinder

L. J. Broder Enterprises, Inc.
3192 Darvany Dr.
Dallas, Tex. 75220
Sta-Put Feeding Dish

The Carter Company
186 Alewife Brook Pkwy.
Cambridge, Mass. 02138
Child-sized chair

Central Specialties Co.
6030 Northwest Highway
Chicago, Ill. 60639
Kiddie Kab Stroller

Century Products, Inc.
2150 W. 114th St.
Cleveland, OH 44102
Century Motor-Toter Car Seat

Child Craft
Salem, Ind. 47167
Grow-Up Crib

Childcraft Education Corp.
20 Kilmer Rd.
Edison, N.J. 08817
Inflatable Clear Bumpers, Wall Mirror

The Children's Workbench
470 Park Ave. South
New York, N.Y. 10016
Crib-Settee, Highchair/Youth Chair

Collier-Keyworth Co.
Gardner, Mass. 01440
Bobby-Mac Car Seat

Coleco Industries, Inc.
945 Asylum Ave.
Hartford, Conn. 06105
Sno-Jet Baby Boggan

The Comfy-Babe Co.
P.O. Box 326
Downers Grove, Ill. 60515
Mother's Bath Apron, Comfy-Babe Chair

Cosco Household Products, Inc.
2525 State St.
Columbus, Ind. 47201
Cradle Seat, Potty

Craft Pattern
Elmhurst, Ill. 60126
Double-Action Cradle Pattern, Early American Cradle Pattern

Crib-T-Bed, Inc.
2740 Tremainsville Rd.
Toledo, Ohio 43613
Crib-T-Bed

Cross River Products, Inc.
1 Leighton Ave.
Rochester, N.Y. 14609
Duo-Broller Stroller for Twins

Dalco Products
1016 W. Hillcrest Blvd.
Inglewood, Calif. 90301
Safety door knob, lock, and belt

Davol, Inc.
Box D
Providence, R.I. 02901
Nasal Aspirator, Davol Breast Shields

Dexter Diaper Factory
P.O. Box 7367
Houston, Tex. 77008
Dexter B-29 Diaper

EDCOM Systems, Inc.
306 Alexander St.
Princeton, N.J. 08540
Hexagonal Crib, EDCOM Play Corral

F & H Baby Products Co.
Box 12-Y
Vienna, Va. 22180
Safety-Edge

Fraser's WMF Stainless
Division of WMF of America, Inc.
85 Price Parkway
Farmingdale, N.Y. 11735
Plate, cup, and flatware

Frostline Kits
Dept. GB045
425 Burbank
Broomfield, Colo. 80020
Baby-sized Down Comforter Kit

Furniture Designs
1425 Sherman Ave.
Evanston, Ill.   60201
Crib Pattern, Locking Cradle Pattern

GM Love Seats
P.O. Box 60-1813
Minneapolis, Minn.   55460
General Motors Infant Love Seat

Gallic Enterprises, Inc.
P.O. Box 66373
Los Angeles, Calif.   90066
Feed-Ease Baby Bottle Handle

De Ronde Plastic Corp.
23 Bexlin St.
P.O. Drawer D
Montpelier, Vt.   05602
Dub-L-Lox Diaper Pins

Housewares Division
General Electric Co.
1285 Boston Ave.
Bridgeport, Conn.   06602
Electric Baby Dish

Gerber Products Co.
445 State St.
Fremont, Mich.   49412
Carry Bed/Diaper Bag, Car bottle warmer

Gerrico, Inc.
P.O. Box 998
Boulder, Colo.   80302
Deluxe Cuddler, Carry Free Stroller

Gift Fair
P.O. Box 115
Riverside, Conn.   16878
Baby Food Jar Lifter, Diaper Clip, Nipple Spoon

Gladding Corp.
Wood and Youth Products Division
P.O. Box 250
S. Paris, Me.   04281

Baby Sled

Grattan Warehouse, Ltd.
Anchor House
Ingeby Rd.
Bradford BD99 ZXG ENGLAND
EKCO Newborn Baby Bath

Griffin Shoe Co.
P.O. Box 1258
Oakland, Calif.   94604
Griffin Scuffers

Gus File, Inc.
P.O. Box 3006
Albuquerque, N.M.   87110
Medicine Spoon

H & H, Inc.
1185 Glendale Dr.
Salt Lake City, Utah   84110
Portable Fabric Chair Adapter

Happy Family Products
1252 S. La Cienega Blvd.
Los Angeles, Calif.   90035
Happy Napsack, Comfy-Dry Bra Pads, Baby-Walker, Moccasins Kit

Hedstrom Co.
Bedford, Pa.   15522
Twin Totliner

House of Minnel
Deerpath Rd.
Batavia, Ill.   60510
Portable Chair

Iberian Imports
901 Sherman St., Suite 522
Denver, Colo.   80203
Cuddle Bag

Infa-Feeder, Inc.
P.O. Box 15129
Las Vegas, Nev.   89114
Baby Food Feeder

International Design Corp.
1147 W. Ohio St.
Chicago, Ill.   60622

Silvy Crib

Kantwet
Questor Juvenile Furniture Division
771 N. Freedon St.
Ravenna, Ohio   44266
Wink-N-Wake

Kavanaugh International, Inc.
P.O. Box 991
Peabody, Mass.   01960
New Zealand Lambskin

Miles Kimball
35 Algoma Blvd.
Oshkosh, Wisc.   54901
Oshkosh B'Gosh Play-O-Alls

Kindergard Corp.
3357 Halifax St.
Dallas, Tex.   75247
Child Safety Latch

Kleinert's
350 Fifth Ave.
New York, N.Y.   10001
Sleepy-Drye Outer Pants for Diapers, 3-Way Diaper Bag, Waterproof Nylon Pants

La Leche League International, Inc.
9616 Minneapolis Ave.
Franklin Park, Ill.   60131
Woolwick Breast Shield

Life Manufacturing Co., Inc.
20 Meridian St.
E. Boston, Mass.   02128
Zip-A-Babe Harness

Lopuco
6117 Parkway Dr.
West Laurel, Md.   20810
Loyd-B Pump

Medi, Inc.
27 Maple Ave.
P.O. Box 325
Holbrook, Mass.   02343
Baby Bottle Straw

Mills Products, Inc.
125 Perkins Ave.
Brockton, Mass. 02403

Baby Stand Still

N.K.R. Precision Manufacturing Corp.
Box 333, Route 17M
Harriman, N.Y. 10926

Rock-A-Crib Springs

The Netsy Co.
34 Sunrise Ave.
Mill Valley, Calif. 94941

Netsy Milk Cup

Oak Grove Enterprises
Box 47A
Foustell, Mo. 63348

Chummy Portable Baby Carriage

Pansy Ellen Products, Inc.
3287 Edward Ave.
Santa Clara, Calif. 95050

Pansy-ette Infant Bath Aid

Peterson Baby Products
6904 Tijuna Ave.
N. Hollywood Calif. 91605

Safety Bath Sheet, safety restraints

Plakie Toys, Inc.
P.O. Box 3386
Youngston, Ohio 44512

Baby Safe-Nap

Pride-Trimble Corp.
101 E. Alexander Ave.
Burbank, Calif. 95103

Deluxe Play Yard

Quelle, Inc.
Mail Order House
6050 Kennedy Blvd. E.
W. New York, N.J. 07093

Fussack (German baby bag)

Pushka Kit
P.O. Box 1018
Greeley, Colo. 80631

Do it Yourself Baby Carrier

The Reddy Co., Inc.
RFD #2
Montpelier, Vt. 05602

Diaper Dip

Reliance Products Corp.
108 Mason St.
Woonsocket, R.I. 02895

Nuk nipple, Orthodontic Exerciser

Mrs. Janet Rogers
P.O. Box 933
Dunedin, Fla. 33528

Swim-Aid

Roseal Co.
511 17 Ave.
San Francisco, Calif. 94121

Shampooette

Royal Products, Inc.
P.O. Box 90312
East Point, Ga. 30344

Correct Feeding Bottle
Self-Help Handicrafts

Fred Sammons, Inc.
P.O. Box 32
Brookfield, Ill. 60513

Floating Bath Thermometer, Snorkel Cup, Swivel Spoon, Bent-Handled Spoons

Sears, Roebuck & Co.
Sears Tower
Chicago, Ill. 60684

Rear-Mounted Carrier Bicycle Seat, Stay-Dry Pre-Folded Diapers

Snugli Cottage Industries, Inc.
Route 1, Box 685
Evergreen, Colo. 80439

Snugli, a zipper pack

Stephen Shanan Co.
10107 Westview, 211
Houston, Tex. 77043

Protex-A Mat, Mite-Hite Light Switch Extension

Strolee of California
19067 S. Reyes Ave.
Compton, Calif. 90221

Small Changer

Sweet Petite
Route 4
Harrisville Rd.
Mt. Airy, Md. 21771

Papoose Snap Blanket

The Soap Box at Truc
P.O. Box 167
Woodstock, Conn. 06281

German Baby Soap

U-Bild Enterprises
P.O. Box 2383
Van Nuys, Calif. 91409

Wooden Seat Pattern

United De Soto
3101 S. Kedzie Ave.
Chicago, Ill. 60623

Nursery Wallpaper

Western Associated Manufacturers, Inc.
512 Main St.
Winfield, Kans. 67156

Pedi Bares

Westland Plastics, Inc.
800 N. Mitchell Rd.
Newburry Park, Calif. 91320

Jiffy Biffy, Washable Food Catcher

World Famous Sales Co.
3580 N. Elston Ave.
Chicago, Ill. 60618

Aluminum FrameCarrier

Appendix E
Toys and Toy Manufacturers

This list of toys, art supplies and equipment supplements the information in the text.

Please contact local stores to obtain current availability and price information, or write to the companies directly.

Supplies

abc School Supply
Box 13086
Atlanta, Ga.   30324

Cash Register, Spindle Top, Stubby Paint Brush, Fife and Drum and Balance Board

Aldermaston, Inc.
86 Forest Ave.
Glen Cove, N.Y.   11542

Paddy O'Hair

Antelope Camping and Equipment Manufacturing Co.
21740 Granada Ave.
Cupertino, Calif.   95014

Backpack frame and bag, Child Carrier Attachment

Artwood
P.O. Drawer A
Woodland, Ga.   31836

Barn and animals, solid hardwood

Baker and Taylor Educational Products
2 Allwood Ave.
Central Islip, N.Y.   11722

Climb'n Cubes

The Bank Street Bookstore
610 W. 112 St.
New York, N.Y.   10025

Read and Play, Beginning reader book, Picture board of the story scene and playing pieces for acting out the story

Barday School Supplies
29 Warren St.
New York, N.Y.   10007

Water color crayons

Dick Blick
P.O. Box 1267
Galesburg, Ill.   61401

Number Cubes, Rich Art Tempera Maker, Palette Markers, Art-Tote Kit

Camphill Village Gift Shop
Chrysler Pond Rd.
Copake, N.Y.   12516

Cuddly Doll, "Drag" Doll

Carola Creations
144 N. Clinton Ave.
Elmhurst, Ill.   60126

Doll patterns

Central Scientific Co., Inc.
2600 S. Kostner Ave.
Chicago, Ill.   60623

Telescope, Cosmobile

Child Guidance/CBS Toys (Includes Creative Playthings)
41 Madison Ave.
New York, N.Y.   10010

Childcraft Education Corp.
20 Kilmer Road
Edison, N.J.   08817

Waterpump, Bucket and Mop, Women Workers, Brooms, Touch and Match, Water Play Kit, Dressing-Undressing Puzzle

Child Life Play Specialties, Inc.
55 Whitney St.
Holliston, Mass.   01746

Home Exercise Mat, Doorway gym, Firefighter gym kit

Combex Ltd.
117–123 Great Portland St.
London W/N 6AH, England

Fingered Teething Ball

Community Playthings
Rifton, N.Y.   12471

Wall Easel, Blocks and block cart, Variplay triangle set, Right-angle climber and slide, Swedish Variplay set

Construction Playthings
1040 East 85 St.
Kansas City, Mo.   64131

Child-sized gardening tools

Creative Educational Distributor (CED)
159–163 East Lancaster Ave.
Wayne, Pa.   19087

See-sawhorse

Crusader Wood Products
P.O. Box 85
San Marcos, Calif.   92069

Hardwood toys

Developmental Learning Materials
7440 Natchez Ave.
Niles, Ill.   60648

Animal Puzzles, Cuddly Kitty, Body Puzzles, Job Inset Puzzle, Money Dominoes, Photo Number Cards, Picture Lacing Boards

Dollsandreams
454 Third Ave.
New York, N.Y.   10016

A First Picture Book, Rake, Scoop and Digger

Drago School Equipment and Supply
P.O. Box 4868
Hialeah Lake Station
Hialeah, Fla.   33104

Bolt-Tight

Gabriel/CBS Toys
41 Madison Ave.
New York, N.Y.   10010

Bath Toys

Learning Games, Inc.
34 South Broadway
White Plains, N.Y.   10601

Geoboard Kit, Cuisenaire Home Mathematics Kit

Learning Stuff
P.O. Box 4123
Modesto, Calif.   95352

Playground Equipment Design

Love-Built Toys and Crafts
418 Second St./P.O. Box 769
Antioch, Calif.   94509

Toy Patterns and Wooden Parts, crafts book on woodworking

Lyndon Craft Educational Equipment
P.O. Box 12
Rosemead, Calif.   91770

Hollow blocks

Louis Marx Co.
45 Church St.
Stamford, Conn.   06906

Mini Wheels

Mattel Toys
5150 Rosecrans Ave.
Hawthorne, Calif.   90250

Activity Toys & Games

Milo Products Corp.
Grantham, Pa.   17027

So, Sew Stitch Kit, Dado Blocks

Milton Bradley Co.
Springfield, Mass.   01101

Play scenes lotto

Monkey Business
Rt. 3 Box 153A
Celina, Ky.   38551

Monkey Birthing Doll

Mothercare-by-Mail
P.O. Box 228
Parsippany, N.J.   07054

Fit-a-Block Clock, Art Smock

Don Drumm Studios and Gallery
437 Crouse St.
Akron, Ohio   44311

Soft Sculpture Fantasies

Drybranch, Inc.
60 E. Jericho Tpke.
Mineola, N.Y.   11501

Kadima

Edmund Scientific Co.
300 Edscorp Bldg.
Barrington, N.J.   08007

Compass, Jumbo Dial Thermometer, Plastic Fresnel Lens, Giant Balloons

Educational Design Associates
Box 712
Waldorf, Md.   20601

Wildlife Photopuzzles

Educational Teaching Aids (ETA)
159 W. Kinzie St.
Chicago, Ill.   60610

Steering Truck, Infant Wooden Stacking Cubes, Jumbo Wooden Pounding Bench, Nature Lotto

Eduquip-McAllister Corp.
1085 Commonwealth Ave.
Brighton, Mass.   02215

Investigating Optics Kit, Circuit Kit, One-Stringed Instrument

Fisher-Price Toys
A Division of the Quaker Oats Co.
East Aurora, N.Y.   14052

Medical Kit, Play Family Children's Hospital, Music Box Owl, Fisher-Price Activity Center, Floating Family

Fox Blox
24401 Redwood Highway
Cloverdale, Calif.   95425

Animal blocks, Solid Blocks

Fun-da-Mentals
Box 263
South Pasadena, Calif.   91030

Robot, full-color plastic coated cards depict careers in a nonsexist, multiracial way

The Gift Center
United Nations Headquarters
New York, N.Y.   10017

Danish Wooden Rattles, Wooden teething ring, Sphere Within a Circle with a Handle

Go Fly a Kite, Inc.
1434 Third Ave.
New York. N.Y.   10028

Plastic kites

Grandpa's Wooden Toys
Route 9, Box 453
Florence, Ala.   35630

Grandpa's Chair, Block Wagon

Hammatt and Sons
1441 N. Red Gum, Bldg. E
Anaheim, Calif.   92806

Dancing Doll, Deluxe Playground Ball, Blooper Ball

J. L. Hammet Co.
2393 Vaux Hall Road
Union, N.J.   07083

Rake Knitting Frames, Unifix Cubes, Loom Cage

Handcraft Designs
Div. of Bill Muller Wooden Toys, Inc.
Rockhill Industrial Park
87 Commerce Drive
Telford, Pa.   18969

Wooden Hand Car

Mrs. Virginia P. Harman
8210 Lighthouse Court
Annandale, Va.   22003

Spatter Box

Hasbro Industries, Inc.
P.O. Box 675
Central Falls, R.I.   02863

Gingerbread Teethers

Karen Hewitt
Box 45A
East Corinth, Vt.   05040

Thinamabobbin

Holbrook-Patterson, Inc.
170 S. Monroe St.
Coldwater, Mich.   49036

Dollhouse, Balance Boards, Wooden toys and climbing equipment, Table-top sink and stove, Junior gym-pla trainer

J. R. Holcomb Co.
3000 Quigley Rd.
Cleveland, Ohio   44113

Creative Wood Crafts Bag, Hand Puppet Idea Bag

Irwin Toys
Miner Industries, Inc.
200 Fifth Ave.
New York, N.Y.   10010

Toddler Swing

William G. Johnston Co.
P.O. 6759
Pittsburgh, Pa.   15212

Ladder Exerciser

Jonti-Craft Educational Play Equipment
Div. of Rapids Sash and Millwork, Inc.
Sauk Rapids, Minn.   56379

Wheeled Construction Set

Judy Company
Barelay School Supplies
29 Warren St.
New York, N.Y.   10007

The Doctor, Kindergarten Chalk, Counting Songs, Classification Play Tray, Stringing Beads

Kaplan School Supply Corp.
600 Jonestown Rd.
Winston-Salem, N.C. 27103

Alphabet Bingo, Art Darts, Number Bingo, Jumbo Tiddlywinks

Kinder Products
920 Hemingway Dr.
Raleigh, N.C.   27609

Bi-Plane Desk

Kindercastle
Box 272
Commerce, Tex.   75428

Quality wooden line of early learning equipment and toys

Lakeshore Curriculum Materials
8888 Venice Blvd.
Los Angeles, Calif.   90034

Giant blockbuster set, Fat Man, Timberbloc Building set, Giant numbered dice, Child-sized tools

Larbar Corporation
Box 30024
St. Paul, Minn.   55175

Alpha Bag

Lego Systems
555 Taylor Road
Enfield, Conn.   06082

Lego Blocks

Bill Maller Wooden Toys
Rockhill Industrial Park
87 Commerce Dr.
Telford, Pa.   18969

Wooden Car, Rocking Horse

Nasco
901 Janesville Ave.
Fort Atkinson, Wisc.   53538

Alphamat, Wooden Telephone, Giant Gyroscope

Nienhuis Montessori U.S.A.
320 Pinoeer Ave.
Mountain View, Calif.   94041

Counting Lotto

Novo Educational Toy and Equipment Corp.
11 Park Pl.
New York, N.Y.   10007

Anything Muppet, Big Timer, Rocker Scale, Tiddlywinks, Me Too Backpack, Carpenter's Apron

Pathways of Sound
102 Mt. Auburn St.
Cambridge, Mass.   02138

Story Records

Patterns
Box 57 R.R. #1
Blue Hill, Neb.   68930

Learning Book Patterns

Plank & Pin Toys
801 W. Market St.
Bloomington, Ill.   61701

Toys designed to encourage fine and gross motor abilities

Playskool, Inc.
4501 W. Augusta Blvd.
Chicago, Ill.   60651

Baby Bean Pod, Ringed Stack Toy

Plaything Equipment Co.
808 Howard St.
Omaha, Neb.   68102

Nerf Ball

Practical Drawing Co.
P.O. Box 5388
Dallas, Tex.   75222

"When I Grow Up I Want To Be"—Felt figures of a man and a woman for identifying careers

Poppets
1800 E. Olive Way
Seattle, Wash.   98102

Puppets, Doorway Theater

Pumpkinseed
Coldwater Tavern Rd.
Nassau, N.Y.   12123

Geometric Template

Rotadyne, Inc.
8705 Freeway Dr.
Macedonia, Ohio   44056

Tike Slide

S & S Arts and Crafts
Colchester, Conn.   06415

Wooden Beads

Safety Now Co., Inc.
Box 567/202 York Rd.
Jenkintown, Pa.   19046

Scotchlite Rescue Marker, Swing Set Anchor

Sax Arts and Crafts
P.O. Box 2002
Milwaukee, Wisc.   53201

Lapboard

School Days Equipment Co.
973 N. Main St.
Los Angeles, Calif.   90012

Plastic Scales and Weights. Sorting and Order Kit.

Selective Educational Equipment, Inc.
3 Bridge St.
Newton, Mass.   02195

Inexpensive Stopwatch, Elementary Microscope, Hands Free Magnifier, Capturing Magnifier

Stephen Shanan Co.
10107 Westview, 211
Houston, Tex.   77043

Light Switch Extension, Step-Up Stools

Tennis Resources, Inc., West
2563 Greer Rd.
Palo Alto, Calif.   94303

All Ball Tennis

Tonka Toys
5300 Shoreline Blvd
Mound, Minn.   55364

Construction Toys

Toys That Care
P.O. Box 81
Briarcliff Manor, N.Y.   10510

Child-Sized Doctor's Smock

Tucker's Yarn Shop
950 Hamilton St.
Allentown, Pa.   18101

Bucilla ABC Sampler

Tupperware Home Parties
Orlando, Fla.   32802

Tupperware Shape-O

U-Bild Enterprises
Box 2383
Van Nuys, Calif.   91409

Rocking Horse Pattern

Unitarian Universalist Association
25 Beacon St.
Boston, Mass.   02108

One Big Family Dolls

The Vegimill
Bristol, Vt.   05443

The Vegimals

Wynroth Math Programs
Box 578
Ithaca, N.Y.   14850

Math materials, games

Contact: Toy Manufacturers of
          America
          200 Fifth Ave.
          New York, N.Y.   10010
for more information.

Appendix F
Additional Books, Tapes and Other Resources

AUDIO VISUALS

Cassette Communications, Inc.
Write for catalog to:
175 Fifth Avenue
New York, New York 10010
$10.95 + $1.00 (postage & handling)

This group produces cassette tapes on a wide variety of psychological and life-style issues. The approaches and ideas are contributed by a number of established medical and counseling professionals. Topics include *Adoption: A Guide for Parents and Professionals*, Elizabeth Cole and Kathryn Donley, *Risking Intimacy*, Herbert Freudenberger and Penelope Russianoff and *Divorce*, Richard Gardner. They are useful both for organizations and materials.

Problems Parents Face
Write for information to:
Visual Education Corporation
14 Washington Rd.
Box 2321
Princeton, N.J. 08540
$67/series

Lee Salk presents his views on child raising on a set of six audio cassette tapes. He deals with such issues as handling school problems, organizing your own life and developing responsibility in children. Times vary from 12 minutes to 22 minutes.

Inexpensive Booklets

Public Affairs Committee
381 Park Avenue South
New York, N.Y. 10016

The Public Affairs Committee offers a great many inexpensive, excellent booklets for parents. A partial list is included. Each is $.50. Write, giving numbers of booklets you want, and ask for their catalog. Orders must be prepaid.

Divorce Elizabeth Ogg #528

One Parent Families Elizabeth Ogg #543

Helping Children Face Crisis Alicerose Barman #541

Preparing Tomorrow's Parents Elizabeth Ogg #520

Pregnancy and You Aline B. Auerbach and Helene S. Arnstein #482

Your First Months with Your First Baby Alicerose Barman #478

Help for Your Troubled Child Alicerose Barman and Lisa Cohen #454

Breastfeeding Audrey Palm Riker #353S

You and Your Adopted Child Eda J. Le Shan #274

The following publications are available from the Superintendent of Documents, United States Government Printing Office, Washington, D.C. 20402 (write for their catalog).

Breast Feeding (017-026-00084-4) $2.25

Child Development in the Home (017-091-00193-6) $1.50

Day Care for Your Children (017-091-00194-41) $.35

Infant Care (017-091-00228-2) $2.00

Pocket Guide to Babysitting (017-091-00197-9) $2.25

PreNatal Care (017-091-00187-1) $2.00

Your Child From One to Six (017-091-002191-3) $1.75

Your Child From Six to Twelve (017-091-00070-1) $1.75

Suggested books written for professionals which can be useful for parents interested in reading further about young children.

Sueann Robinson Ambron
Child Development
Holt, Rinehart & Winston
1978 524 pp. $16.95

Joanne Hendrick
The Whole Child: New Trends in Early Education
The C. V. Mosby Co.
1975 362 pp. $11.95

Deborah Lott Holmes and Frederick J. Morrison
The Child: An Introduction to Developmental Psychology
Brooks/Cole Publishing Co.
1979 464 pp. $16.95

Contact your nearby college or university for classes in early childhood or child growth and development. Bookstores and libraries at these schools carry other books on children that may be of interest.

An excellent resource for parents, children and teachers is a published catalog which includes order forms from:

Gryphon House
3706 Otis St.
P.O. Box 217
Mt. Rainier, MD 20822

An indexed, illustrated and annotated guide to many books for children and parents. Also features publications of the Day Care Council of America.

Recommended Books

The books included here came to our attention after our deadline for written reviews. They have been recommended as useful additional titles for ordering at bookstore or library. See Appendixes A or G for addresses of publishers or organizations cited.

For those books which do not include a complete description we have included sufficient information for your use.

- Parents: Please let us know what books you find are really useful.
- Publishers: Please continue to send us new books and we will follow up and update our resources and permanent display.

Rahima Baldwin
Special Delivery—The Complete Guide to Informed Birth
Les Femmes Publishing
1979   62 pp. $9.95

Gloria Blum and Barry Blum
Feeling Good About Yourself—A Resource Guide and Curriculum for Social Learning, Self-Esteem and Human Sexuality for Disabled Persons.
Feeling Good Associates
1977   47 pp. $5.00

Michael Brudenell, Malcolm Chiswick, Barbara Nash, Patricia Gilbert, Janet Smy
The Complete Book of Baby Care
Octopus Books
1978   256 pp. $16.95

Frances Wells Burck
Babysense: A Practical and Supportive Guide to Baby Care
St. Martin's Press
1979   283 pp. $9.95

Carrie Carmichael
Non-Sexist Childraising
Beacon Press
1977   158 pp. $4.95

Kenneth B. Clark
Prejudice and Your Child
Beacon Press
1955   234 pp. $1.95

Joseph Bharat Cornell
Sharing Nature With Children (A Parents' and Teachers' Nature-awareness Guidebook)
Ananda Publications
1979   143 pp. $4.95

Ken Davis & Thomas Taylor
Kids & Cash
Oak Tree Publications
1979   275 pp. $8.95

Fitzhugh Dodson
I wish I had a computer that makes waffles . . .
Oak Tree Publications
1978   80 pp. $7.95

Robert Elmers & Robert Aitchison
Effective Parents—Responsible Children
McGraw-Hill
1977   223 pp. $3.95

Jane Ervin
Your Child Can Read and You Can Help—A Book for Parents
Doubleday
1979   361 pp. $10.95

E. Belle Evans, George Saia, and Elmer A. Evans
Designing a Day Care Center
Beacon Press
1974   176 pp. $3.45

Sandy Fuchs
The Marriage and Family Book
Schocken Books
1978   186 pp. $5.95

Diane Gess
Sunshine Porcupine (for kids)
Oak Tree Publications
1979   64 pp. $6.95

Beth Goff
Where Is Daddy? (for children)
Beacon Press
1969   28 pp. $5.95

Martin Goldstein, Erwin J. Haeberle, and Will McBride
The Sex Book—A Modern Pictorial Encyclopedia (for children)
Bantam Books
1971   206 pp. $6.95

Ronald E. Gots and Barbara A. Gots
Caring for Your Unborn Child
Stein & Day
1977   244 pp. $8.95

Ellin Green and Madalynne Schoenfeld
A Multimedia Approach to Children's Literature
American Library Association
1977   159 pp. $6.00

Earl A. Grollman
Concerning Death: A Practical Guide for the Living
Beacon Press
1974 360 pp. $4.95

Earl A. Grollman
Explaining Death to Children
Beacon Press
1967 271 pp. $4.95

Earl A. Grollman
Explaining Divorce to Children
Beacon Press
1969 245 pp. $4.95

Susan and John Hopkins
The Pregnant Woman's Journal
Universe Books
1978 24 pp. $4.95

"ValueTale" Series of Children's Books—Value Communications, Inc.
Ann Donegan Johnson
The Value of Love, The Story of Johnny Appleseed
1979 63 pp. $5.95
Ann Donegan Johnson
The Value of Learning, The Story of Marie Curie
1978 63 pp. $5.95
Spencer Johnson
The Value of Honesty, The Story of Confucius
1979 63 pp. $5.95
Spencer Johnson
The Value of Understanding, The Story of Margaret Mead
1979 63 pp. $5.95

Lynn Johnson
Do They Ever Grow Up?—The Terrible Twos & Beyond
Meadowbrook Press
1978 107 pp. $2.95

Stuart Kahan
The Expectant Father's Survival Kit (What every man needs to know once the test is positive)

Monarch Press
1978 176 pp. $3.95

Robert Kail
The Development of Memory in Children
W. H. Freeman and Company
1979 168 pp. $6.00

M. G. Kains
Gardening for Young People
Stein & Day Publishers
1978 280 pp. $8.95

La Leche League International
The Womanly Art of Breastfeeding
La Leche League International
1958 155 pp. $3.50

Betty Ewing Land
The Art of Grandparentry
Georgetown Press
1974 120 pp. $2.95

Carole Livingston
"Why Was I Adopted?"
Lyle Stuart Inc.
1978 43 pp. $8.95

Martin Lutterjohann
IQ-Tests for Children (How to Test Your Child's Intelligence)
Stein & Day
1979 179 pp. $4.95

Lyn Marshall
Yoga For Your Children
Schocken Books
1979 64 pp. $4.95

Alan Milberg
Street Games
McGraw Hill
1976 306 pp. $12.95/$7.95

Mary Susan Miller/Samm Sinclair Baker
How You Can Help Your Child Get the Best Out of School
Stein & Day
1976 226 pp. $3.95

Leslie Nicholas
How to Avoid Social Diseases—A Practical Handbook
Stein & Day
1973 152 pp. $5.95

Open University (in association with the Health Education Council)
The First Years of Life
Ward Lock Limited
1979 256 pp. $10.00

Robert H. Pantell, James F. Fries, Donald M. Vickery, M.D.
Taking Care of Your Child: A Parents' Guide to Medical Care
Addison-Wesley
1977 409 pp. $10.95/$6.95

Rebecce Rowe Parfitt
The Birth Primer, A Source Book of Traditional and Alternative Methods in Labor and Delivery
Running Press
1977 259 pp. $5.95

Ralph L. Peterson
A Place For Caring and Celebration (The School Media Center)
American Library Association
1979 33 pp. $3.00

Hank Pizer and Christine Garfink
The Post Partum Book
Grove Press, Inc.
1979 215 pp. $9.95

Planned Parenthood Federation of America
What it Means to Become a Parent
1976 20 pp. $.25

Letty Cottin Pogrebin
Growing up Free: Raising Your Child in the 80's
McGraw-Hill
1980 548 pp. $15.95

Elizabeth Pomada
Places to Go with Children in Northern California
Chronicle Books
1976   173 pp. $3.95

Suzanne Ramos
The Complete Book of Child Custody
G. P. Putnam's Sons
1979   330 pp. $10.95

Mary F. Rice and Charles H. Flatter
Help Me Learn (A Handbook for Teaching Children From Birth to Third Grade)
Prentice-Hall
1979   398 pp. $12.95

Nicholas A. Roes
Helping Children Watch TV
Teacher Update, Inc.
1978   49 pp. $2.95

Pam Palewicz-Rousseau and Lynda Madaras
The Alphabet Connection (A Parent's and Teacher's Guide to Beginning Reading and Writing)
Schocken Books
1979   182 pp. $10.95

Niki Scott
The Balancing Act, A Handbook for Working Mothers
Sheed Andrews and McMeel
1978   142 pp. $4.95

Joae Graham Selzer
When Children Ask About Sex—A Guide for Parents
Beacon Press
1974   147 pp. $3.95

Jack G. Shiller
Childhood Injury, A Common Sense Approach
Stein & Day
1977   245 pp. $8.95

Barbara Brooks Simons
(Adventures in Nature)
A Visit to the Forest
Oak Tree Publications
1978   64 pp. $3.95

Liz Smith
The Mother Book
Bantam Books
1978   536 pp. $2.95

Claude Steiner
The Original Warm Fuzzy Tale
(for kids)
Jalmar Press
1977   41 pp. $2.95

Eric Trimmer
The First Seven Years (A Complete Guide for Parents)
St. Martin's Press
1978   142 pp. $8.95

Emily B. Visher and John S. Visher
Step-Families: A Guide to Working with Stepparents and Stepchildren
Brunner/Mazel, Inc.
1979   259 pp. $15.00

Mort Weisinger
1001 Valuable Things You Can Get Free
Bantam Books
1977   211 pp. $1.95

Hal M. Wells
The Sensuous Child—Your Child's Birthright to Healthy Sexual Development
Stein & Day
1978   188 pp. $3.95

Siv Widerberg
The Kids Own XYZ of Love and Sex
Stein & Day
1971   114 pp. $2.25

Aline D. Wolf
Look at the Child
Montessori Learning Center
1978   64 pp. $4.95

Virginia C. Wood
Only Me
Alphapress
1979   64 pp. $3.95

Lawrence Zuckerman, Valerie Zuckerman, Rebecca Costa and Michael T. Yura
A Parents' Guide to Children: The Challenge
Hawthorn Books
1978   81 pp. $2.75

Appendix G
Publishers

If you are unable to find the books listed in *The Whole Child* in your library or bookstore, the following addresses will enable you to order direct from the publisher. Prices may change from those listed when we went to press, so contact the publisher first for current ordering information.

A and W Publishers
95 Madison Ave.
New York, N.Y.   10016

Abingdon Press
201 Eighth Ave. S.
Nashville, Tenn.   37202

Ablex Publishing Co.
355 Chestnut St.
Norwood, N.J.   07648

Academic Press
111 Fifth Ave.
New York, N.Y.   10003

Academy Chicago Ltd.
360 N. Michigan Ave.
Chicago, Ill.   60601

Addison-Wesley Publishing Co.
Reading, Mass.   01867

Administration for Children, Youth and Families—See Appendix A

Adventures in Rhythm
1844 North Mohawk St.
Chicago, Ill.   60614

Aldine Publishing Co.
c/o Lieber-Atherton
1841 Broadway
New York, N.Y.   10023

Allyn and Bacon
470 Atlantic Ave.
Boston, Mass.   02210

American Automobile Association
8111 Gatehouse Rd.
Falls Church, Va.   22042

American Guidance Service
Publishers Building
Circle Pines, Minn.   55014

American Journal of Nursing
Educational Services Div.
10 Columbus Circle
New York, N.Y.   10019

Ananda Publications
900 Allegheny STAR ROUTE
Nevada City, Calif.   95959

And/Or Press
P.O. Box 2246
Berkeley, Calif.   94702

Andrews & McMeel
6700 Squibb Rd.
Mission, Kans.   66202

Arco Publishing
219 Park Ave. South
New York, N.Y.   10003

Aspen Publishing Co.
Box 1201
Aspen, Colo.   81611

Association for Childhood Education International
3615 Wisconsin Ave., N.W.
Washington, D.C.   20016

Association Press
Box O
Wilton, Conn.   06897

Atheneum Publishers
122 E. 42 St.
New York, N.Y.   10017

Avatar Press
P.O. Box 7727
Atlanta, Ga.   30309

Avon Books
959 Eighth Ave.
New York, N.Y.   10019

Ballantine Books
201 E. 50 St.
New York, N.Y.   10022

Bantam Books
666 Fifth Ave.
New York, N.Y.   10019

Basic Books
10 East 53 St.
New York, N.Y.   10022

Beacon Press
25 Beacon St.
Boston, Mass.   02108

Behaviordelia
P.O. Box 1044
Department B
Kalamazoo, Mich.   49005

W. A. Benjamin
2725 Sand Hill Rd.
Menlo Park, Calif. 94025

Berkley Publishing Corp.
200 Madison Ave.
New York, N.Y.   10016

The Bobbs-Merrill Co.
4 West 58 St.
New York, N.Y.   10019

Bowmar
4563 Colorado Blvd.
Los Angeles, Calif.   90039

Brooks/Cole Publishing
555 Abrego St.
Monterey, CA 93940

William C. Brown Co.
2460 Kerper Blvd.
Dubuque, Iowa   52001

Brunner/Mazel, Inc.
19 Union Square West
New York, NY   10003

Bunting & Lyon
238 No. Main St.
Wallingford, Conn.   06492

Burgess Publishing Co.
7108 Ohms Lane
Minneapolis, Minn.   55435

Capra Press
631 State St.
Santa Barbara, Calif.   93101

Celestial Arts
231 Adrian Road
Millbrae, Calif. 94030

Center for Attitudinal Healing
P.O. Box 1012
Tiburon, Calif.   94920

Chandler & Sharp
11A Commercial Blvd.
Novato, Calif. 94947

Charterhouse Books—See David
McKay

Chatham Square Press, Inc.
401 Broadway
New York, N.Y.   10013

Chelsea Publishing Company, Inc.
432 Park Ave. S.
New York, N.Y.   10016

Child Welfare League of America,
Inc.
67 Irving Pl.
New York, N.Y.   10003

Children's Bureau—See
Appendix A

Children's House
Box 11
Caldwell, N.J.   07006

Children's Press
1224 West Van Buren St.
Chicago, Ill.   60607

Chilton Book Co.
Chilton Way
Radnor, Pa.   19089

Chronicle Books
870 Market St.
San Francisco, Calif.   94102

Citation Press—See Four Winds
Press

Herbert Collier
4227 North 32 St.
Phoenix, Ariz.   55003

Condor Publishing Co., Inc.
29 East Main St.
Westport, Conn.   06888

Consumer Reports Books
256 Washington St.
Mt. Vernon, N.Y.   10550

Contemporary Books, Inc.
180 N. Michigan Ave.
Chicago, Ill.   60601

Cornerstone Library
1230 Ave. of the Americas
New York, N.Y.   10020

Council for Exceptional Children
1920 Association Dr.
Reston, Va.   22091

Council on Interracial Books for
Children
1841 Broadway
New York, N.Y.   10023

Coward, McCann & Geoghegan,
Inc.
200 Madison Ave.
New York, N.Y.   10016

Creative Editorial Service
P.O. Box 2244
Hollywood, Calif.   90028

Creative Publications
3977 East Bayshore Rd.
Palo Alto, Calif.   94303

Thomas Y. Crowell Co.
10 East 53 St.
New York, N.Y.   10022

Crown Publishers
One Park Ave.
New York, N.Y.   10016

Dantree Press
44 West 62 St., Suite 4F
New York, N.Y.   10023

Dawne-Leigh Publications
231 Adrian Road
Millbrae, Calif.   94030

John Day Co.—See Thomas Y.
Crowell

Delacorte Press
1 Dag Hammarskjold Plaza
New York, N.Y.   10017

Dell Publishing
1 Dag Hammarskjold Plaza
New York, N.Y.   10017

Delmar Publishers
50 Wolf Rd.
Albany, N.Y.   12205

Delta Books
1 Dag Hammarskjold Plaza
New York, N.Y.   10017

Department of Education
State of California
State Education Building
721 Capitol Mall
Sacramento, Calif.   95814

Dharma Press
2425 Hillside Ave.
Berkeley, Calif.   94704

The Dial Press
1 Dag Hammarskjold Plaza
New York, N.Y.   10017

Dodd, Mead & Company
79 Madison Ave.
New York, N.Y.   10016

Doubleday & Co., Inc.
245 Park Avenue
New York, N.Y.   10017

E. P. Dutton
2 Park Avenue
New York, N.Y.   10016

Education Development Center
School & Society Programs
55 Chapel St.
Newton, Mass.   02160

Educational Facilities Laboratory
477 Madison Ave.
New York, N.Y.   10022

Enterprising Woman
525 West End Ave.
New York, N.Y.   10024

M. Evans & Co., Inc.
216 East 49 St.
New York, N.Y.   10017

The Farm
156 Drakes Lane
Summerton, Tenn.   38483

Farrar, Straus & Giroux
19 Union Square West
New York, N.Y.   10003

Fawcett Publications
Gold Medal Books
1515 Broadway
New York, N.Y.   10036

Fearon-Pitman Publishers
6 Davis Dr.
Belmont, Calif.   94002

Feeling Good Associates
507 Palma Way
Mill Valley, Calif.   94941

Frederick Fell Publishers
386 Park Ave. South
New York, N.Y.   10016

Follett Publishing Co.
1010 West Washington Blvd.
Chicago, Ill.   60607

The Formative Years
P.O. Box 283
Clinton, Conn.   06413

Fountain Publishing Co.
509 Madison Avenue
New York, N.Y.   10022

Four Winds Press
50 West 44 St.
New York, N.Y.   10036

The Free Press
866 Third Ave.
New York, N.Y.   10022

W. H. Freeman
660 Market St.
San Francisco, Calif.   94104

Funk & Wagnalls, Inc.
53 E. 77 St.
New York, N.Y.   10021

Genesis Press
P.O. Box 11457
Palo Alto, Calif.   94301

Georgetown Press
483 Francisco St.
San Francisco, Calif.   94133

Ginn & Co.
191 Spring St.
Lexington, Mass.   02173

Golden Books
3295 Dias
San Jose, Calif.   95122

Golden Press—See Western Publishing

Goodyear Publishing
1640 Fifth St.
Santa Monica, Calif.   90401

Greylock Publishers
13 Spring St.
Stamford, Conn.   16908

Grosset & Dunlap, Inc.
51 Madison Ave.
New York, N.Y.   10010

Grossman Publishing
625 Madison Ave.
New York, N.Y.

Grove Press, Inc.
196 W. Houston St.
New York, N.Y.   10014

Harcourt Brace Jovanovich
757 Third Ave.
New York, N.Y.   10017

Harper & Row
10 East 53 St.
New York, N.Y.   10022

Hart Publishing Co.
12 E. 12 St.
New York, N.Y.   10003

Harvard University Press
79 Garden St.
Cambridge, Mass.   02138

Hasbro Industries, Inc.
41 Madison Ave.
New York, N.Y.   10010

Hawthorn Books
260 Madison Ave.
New York, N.Y.   10016

The Headlands Press
243 Vallejo
San Francisco, Calif.   94111

D. C. Heath & Co.
125 Spring St.
Lexington, Mass.   02173

John Holt Associates
308 Boylston St.
Boston, Mass.   02116

Holt, Rinehart & Winston
383 Madison Ave.
New York, N.Y.   10017

Home and School Institute
Trinity College
Washington, D.C.   20017

The Johns Hopkins University
Press
Baltimore, Md.   21218

The Horn Book, Inc.
31 St. James Ave.
Boston, Mass.   02116

Houghton Mifflin Co.
1 Beacon St.
Boston, Mass.   02107

Human Sciences Press
72 Fifth Ave.
New York, N.Y.   10011

Humanics Press
881 Peachtree St. N.E.
Atlanta, Ga.   30309

Impact Publishers
P.O. Box 1094
San Luis Obispo, Calif   93406

International Universities Press
315 Fifth Ave.
New York, N.Y.   10016

JAB Press, Inc.
P.O. Box 213
Fair Lawn, N.J. 07410

Jalmar Press, Inc.
6501 Elvas Ave.
Sacramento, Calif.   95819

Linda Jenkins
9 Cabernet Court
Lafayette, Calif.   94549

Jossey-Bass, Inc.
433 Montgomery St.
San Francisco, Calif.   94104

William Kaufmann, Inc.
One First St.
Los Altos, Calif.   94022

Alfred A. Knopf
201 E. 50 St.
New York, N.Y.   10022

John Knox Press
341 Ponce de Leon Ave. N.E.
Atlanta, Ga.   30308

Lane Publishing
Menlo Park, CA 94025

Lexington Books
D. C. Heath and Company
125 Spring St.
Lexington, Mass.   02173

Liberty Publishers
3331 Liberty St.
St. Louis, Mo.   63111

Little, Brown & Company
34 Beacon St.
Boston, Mass   02106

Linnet Books
The Shoe String Press, Inc.
Box 4327
995 Sherman Ave.
Hamden, Conn.   06514

MacFadden-Bartell Corp.
215 Lexington Ave.
New York, N.Y.   10016

Macmillan Publishing Co.
866 Third Ave.
New York, N.Y.   10022

Manor Books, Inc.
432 Park Ave. South
New York, N.Y.   10016

Mayfield Publishing
285 Hamilton Ave.
Palo Alto, Calif.   94301

McCall's
230 Park Ave.
New York, N.Y.   10017

McCutchan Publishing Corp.
2526 Grove St.
Berkeley, Calif.   94704

McGraw-Hill, Inc.
1221 Avenue of the Americas
New York, N.Y.   10020

David McKay
2 Park Ave.
New York, N.Y.   10016

March of Dimes Birth Defects
Foundation
1275 Mamaroneck Ave.
White Plains, N.Y.   10603

Meadowbrook Press
16648 Meadowbrook Lane
Wayzata, Minn.   55391

Mental Health Assoc.
1800 N. Kent St.
Arlington, Va.   22209

Merrill-Palmer Institute
71 East Ferry St.
Detroit, Mich.   48202

Charles E. Merrill Publishing Co.
1300 Alum Creek Dr.
Columbus, Ohio   43216

Julian Messner
1230 Avenue of the Americas
New York, N.Y.   10020

Metropolitan Life Insurance Co.
One Madison Ave.
New York, N.Y.   10010

Monarch Press—See Simon &
Schuster

Montessori Learning Center
P.O. Box 767
Altoona, Pa.   16603

William Morrow & Co.
105 Madison Ave.
New York, N.Y.   10016

C. V. Mosby Co.
11830 Westline Industrial Dr.
St. Louis, Mo.   63141

Mynabird Publishing
20 Shoshone Place
Portola Valley, Calif.   94025

National Association for the Education of Young Children
1834 Connecticut Ave., N.W.
Washington, D.C.   20009

National Committee for Citizens in
Education
Suite 410
Wilde Lake Village Green
Columbia, Md.   21044

National Education Association
1201 Sixteenth St., N.W.
Washington, D.C.   20036

New American Library
1633 Broadway
New York, N.Y.   10019

New Glide Publications
330 Ellis St.
San Francisco, Calif.   94102

New School of Exchange
Pettigrew, Ark.   72752

W. W. Norton
500 Fifth Ave.
New York, N.Y.   10110

Oaklawn Press
283 South Lake Ave.
Pasadena, Calif.   91101

Oak Tree Publications
1175 Flintkote Avenue
San Diego, Calif.   92121

Octopus Books
747 Third Ave.
New York, N.Y.   10017

Oliver Press
1400 Ryan Creek
Willets, Calif.   95490

Olympus Publishing
2 Olympus Plaza
1670 East 13 South
Salt Lake City, Utah   84105

O'Sullivan Woodside & Co.
2218 East Magnolia
Phoenix, Ariz.   85034

Outerbridge & Lazard—See E. P.
Dutton

Pacific Press
P.O. Box 3738
Santa Barbara, Calif.   93105

Paddington Press, Ltd.
c/o Grosset & Dunlap
51 Madison Ave.
New York, N.Y.   10010

Pantheon Books
201 East 50 St.
New York, N.Y.   10022

Parents Are Resources
464 Central Ave.
Northfield, Ill.   60093

Parents & Child Care Resources
1169 Howard St.
San Francisco, Calif.   94103

Parents Without Partners
International Office
7910 Woodmont Ave.
Washington, D.C.   20014

Peace Press Publishers
3828 Willat Ave.
Culver City, Calif.   90230

Peek Publications
164 East Dana St.
Mountain View, Calif.   94040

Penguin Books
625 Madison Ave.
New York, N.Y.   10022

Philomel Books
200 Madison Ave.
New York, N.Y.   10016

Pocket Books
1230 Avenue of the Americas
New York, N.Y.   10020

Porter Sargent Pub.
11 Beacon St.
Boston, Mass.   02108

Praeger Publishers
521 Fifth Ave.
New York, N.Y.   10017

Prentice-Hall, Inc.
Englewood Cliffs, N.J.   07632

Profession of Parenting Institute
1609 Poplar
Philadelphia, Pa.   19130

Prometheus Books
1203 Kensington
Buffalo, N.Y. 14215

Public Affairs Committee, Inc.
381 Park Ave. South
New York, N.Y. 10016

G. P. Putnam's Sons
200 Madison Ave.
New York, N.Y. 10016

Random House, Inc.
201 East 50 St.
New York, N.Y. 10022

Rawson, Wade Publishers
630 Third Ave.
New York, N.Y. 10017

Real People Press
P.O. Box F
Moab, Utah 84532

Henry Regnery Co.—See Contemporary Books

Rodale Press Books
33 East Minor St.
Emmaus, Pa. 18049

Ross Laboratories
625 Cleveland
Columbus, Ohio 43216

Routledge & Kegan Paul, Ltd.
9 Park St.
Boston, Mass. 02108

Running Press
38 S. 19 St.
Philadelphia, Pa. 19103

Sagamore Books
Peregrine Smith
P.O. Box 667
Layton, Utah 84041

St. Martin's Press
175 Fifth Ave.
New York, N.Y. 10010

Schocken Books, Inc.
200 Madison Ave.
New York, N.Y. 10016

Scholastic Book Services
50 West 44 St.
New York, N.Y. 10036

Science & Behavior Books
Box 11457
Palo Alto, Calif. 94306

Science Research Associates, Inc.
155 N. Wacker Dr.
Chicago, Ill. 60606

Charles Scribner's Sons
597 Fifth Ave.
New York, N.Y. 10017

Seabury Press
815 Second Ave.
New York, N.Y. 10017

Sex Information and Education Council of the US (SIECUS)
72 Fifth Ave.
New York, N.Y. 10011

Sheed & Ward—See Andrews & McMeel, Inc.

Sierra Club Books
530 Bush St.
San Francisco, Calif. 94108

Simon & Schuster
1230 Avenue of the Americas
New York, N.Y. 10020

Spiritual Company Dharma Press
—See Dharma Press

Stein & Day Publishers
Scarborough House
Briarcliff Manor, N.Y. 10510

Sterling Publishing Co. Inc.
2 Park Ave.
New York, N.Y. 10016

Lyle Stuart, Inc.
120 Enterprise Ave.
Secaucus, N.J. 07094

Sunshine Press
6402 East Chaparral Rd.
P.O. Box 572
Scottsdale, Ariz. 85252

J. P. Tarcher, Inc.
9110 Sunset Blvd.
Los Angeles, Calif. 90069

Charles C. Thomas, Publisher
301–327 E. Lawrence Ave.
Springfield, Ill. 62717

Times Change Press
62 W. 14 St.
New York, N.Y. 10011

Troubador Press
385 Fremont St.
San Francisco, Calif. 94105

Two Step Books
2490 Channing Way
Berkeley, Calif. 94704

U.S. Government Printing Office
Washington, D.C. 20402

Universe Books
381 Park Ave. S.
New York, N.Y. 10016

Universe Books
381 Park Ave. S.
New York, N.Y. 10016

University of California Press
2223 Fulton St.
Berkeley, Calif. 94720

University of Chicago Press
11030 Langley Ave.
Chicago, Ill. 60628

Value Communications, Inc.—See
Oak Tree Publications

Van Nostrand Reinhold Company
135 W. 50 St.
New York, N.Y.   10020

Vantage Press, Inc.
516 West 34 ST.
New York, N.Y.   10001

The Viking Press
625 Madison Ave.
New York, N.Y.   10022

Vintage Books
201 East 50 St.
New York, N.Y.   10022

Wadsworth Publishing
10 Davis Dr.
Belmont, Calif.   94002

Walker & Company
720 Fifth Ave.
New York, N.Y.   10019

Wallaby Books
Simon & Schuster
1230 Avenue of the Americas
New York, N.Y.   10020

Ward Lock Limited
116 Baker St.
London, W1M 2BB

Warner Books, Inc.
75 Rockefeller Pl.
New York, N.Y.   10019

Franklin Watts, Inc.
730 Fifth Ave.
New York, N.Y.   10019

Western Publishing Co., Inc.
1220 Mound Ave.
Racine, Wis.   53404

Workman Publishing
231 East 51 St.
New York, N.Y.   10022

Yale University Press
92A Yale Station
New Haven, Conn.   06520

Brigham Young University Press
Provo, Utah   84602

Appendix H
Children's Museums Throughout the United States

The idea of the creation of a special museum or facility for children is rapidly expanding. The national list is included to provide you with specific places to visit on your next trip with your child.

For other information about children's museums contact the Capitol Children's Museum of the District of Columbia, Washington, D.C.

Alabama

Children's Museum Committee
1109 South 26th St., #6
Birmingham 35205

Arkansas

Museum of Science & Natural History
MacArthur Park
Little Rock 72202

California

Fresno Museum of Natural History
Junior Museum
1944 North Winery Ave.
Fresno 93703

Sulphur Creek Park Nature Center
Hayward 94541

Junior Arts Center
4814 Hollywood Blvd.
Los Angeles 90021

Oakland Museum
1000 Oak St.
Oakland 94607

Palo Alto Junior Museum
1451 Middlefield Rd.
Palo Alto 94301

Sacramento Science Center
3615 Auburn Blvd.
Sacramento 95821

Youth Science Center
Box 2095
Salinas 93901

California Academy of Sciences
San Francisco 94118

The Exploratorium
3601 Lyon St.
San Francisco 94123

Josephine Randall Junior Museum
199 Museum Way
San Francisco 94114

Youth Science Institute
16260 Alum Rock Ave.
San Jose 95127

Coyote Point Museum
Coyote Point Dr.
San Mateo 94401

Alexander Lindsay Junior Museum
1901 First Ave.
Walnut Creek 94596

Colorado

The Children's Museum
931 Bannock St.
Denver 80204

Children's Museum of Denver Inc.
1100 14th St., Room 704
Denver 80222

Rifle Creek Museum—Children's Museum
R.R.1
Rifle 81650

Connecticut

Museum of Arts, Science & Industry
4450 Park Ave.
Bridgeport 06604

Bicentennial Children's Museum
Teacher's College at Fairfield
1561 North Benson Rd.
Fairfield 06430

Monument House—Children's Museum
Park Ave.
Groton 06430

Youthmobile Museum, Inc.
Old Ponsett Rd.
Haddam 06438

Lutz Junior Museum, Inc.
126 Cedar St.
Manchester 06040

New Britain's Youth Museum
28 High St.
New Britain 06051

Children's Museum of New Haven
567 State St.
New Haven 06510

Thames Science Center, Inc.
New London 06320

Karamuseum of Norwalk
133 Lesington Ave.
South Norwalk 06854

Early Learning Center
12 Gary Rd.
Stamford 06903

Mattatuck Museum of the Mattatuck Historical Society—Junior
Museum
119 W. Main St.
Waterbury 06702

Children's Museum of Hartford
950 Trout Brook Dr.
West Hartford 06119

Delaware

Lewes Historical Society
Children's Museum
Lewes 19958

District of Columbia

Children's Museum of Washington
4954 MacArthur Blvd. N.W.
Washington, D.C.

Capital Children's Museum
800 3rd Street N.E.
Washington, D.C. 20002

National Society of Children of
The American Revolution Museum
1776 D Street, N.W.
Washington, DC 20006

Florida

Metropolitan Museum and Art
Centers, Inc.
Coral Gables 33134

The Discovery Center
231 Southwest 2nd Ave.
Fort Lauderdale 33301

Jacksonville Children's Museum,
Inc.
1025 Gulf Life Dr.
Jacksonville 32207

The Junior Museum of Bay County
Panama City 32405

Safety Harbor Museum of History
& Fine Arts, Inc. & Peninsular Ar-
chaeological Society, Inc.
Safety Harbor 33572

St. Petersburg Historical Museum
Children's Museum
335 Second Ave., NE
St. Petersburg 33701

Tallahassee Junior Museum
3945 Museum Dr.
Tallahassee 32311

Children's Museum Committee
c/o Mrs. A. B. Parker
805 South Willow St.
Tampa 33606

Tampa Junior Museum, Inc.
1908 Dekle Ave.
Tampa 33606

Georgia

International Children's Art Gal-
lery
P.O. Box 2002
Atlanta 30301

Museum of Arts & Sciences
4182 Forsythe Rd.
Macon 31204

Cobb County Youth Museum
649 Cheatham Hill Dr.
Marietta 30064

Savannah Science Museum
4405 Paulsen St.
Savannah 31405

Idaho

Herret Arts & Science Center, Inc.
Children's Museum
1220 Kimberly Rd.
East Five Points
Twin Falls   83301

Washington County Museum &
Fiddler's Hall of Fame Children's
Museum
46 W. Commercial St.
Weiser 83672

Illinois

Chicago Children's Museum
1360 N. Lake Shore Dr.
Chicago 60610

Children's Museum
1807 Lincoln Park West
Chicago 60614

Indiana

The Children's Museum
P.O. Box 88126
3000 North Meridian St.
Indianapolis 46208

Mishawaka Children's Museum
410 Lincoln Way East
Mishawaka 46544

Muncie Children's Museum
519 South Walnut
Muncie 47305

Iowa

Children's Museum
P.O. Box 1201
Iowa City 52240

Community Historical Society
Children's Museum
Maxwell 50161

Kansas

Fellow-Reeve Museum
Wichita 67213

Kentucky

Living Arts & Science Center, Inc.
362 Walnut St.
Lexington 40508

Junior Art Gallery
301 York St.
Louisville 40203

Kentucky Railway Museum, Inc.
Children's & Junior Museum
Upper River Rd.
P.O. Box 295
Louisville 40201

Louisiana

Louisiana Arts & Science Center
100 S. River Rd., P.O. Box 3373
Baton Rouge 70821

Contemporary Arts Center
The Ice Cream Factory
900 Camp Street
New Orleans 70130

Louisiana State Museum
Children's Museum
751 Chartres St.
New Orleans 70116

New Orleans Museum of Art
Lelong Avenue, City Park
P.O. Box 19123
New Orleans 70179

New Orleans Recreation Department Children's Museum
1218 Burgundy St.
New Orleans 70116

Grindstone Bluff Museum and Environmental Education Center
Shreveport 71107

Maryland

Cylburn Museum
Cylburn Mansion
4915 Greenspring Ave.
Baltimore 21209

Cloisters Children's Museum
P.O. Box 66
10440 Falls Rd.
Brooklandville 21022

Rosehill Manor Children's Museum
1611 North Market St.
Fredrick 21701

Olde Princess Anne Days, Inc.
Children's Museum
Mansion St.
Princess Anne 21853

Cabin John Regional Park Noah's Ark
7400 Lux Court
Rockville 20854

Maine

1000 Shore Rd.
Cape Elizabeth 04107

Nature Programs For McClellan
Millbridge 04658

Massachusetts

Children's Museum
Museum Wharf, 300 Congress St.
Boston 02210

Children's Art Center
36 Rutland St.
Boston 02118

Museum of Transportation
316 Congress St.
Boston 02210

Children's Museum & Museum Outdoors
Box 98
Dartmouth 02714

Holyoke Museum—Wistariahurst
238 Cabot St.
Holyoke 01040

Thornton W. Burgess Museum
Sandwich 02537

Berkshire Children's Museum
Box 33
Williamstown 01267

Michigan

Kingman Museum of Natural History
West Michigan Avenue at 20th St.
Battle Creek 49017

Children's Museum
67 East Kirby St.
Detroit 48202

Your Heritage House
110 East Perry St.
Detroit 48202

Hackley Art Museum—Junior Museum
296 West Webster St.
Muskegon 49440

Minnesota

A. M. Chisholm Museum
506 West Michigan St.
Duluth 55802

Minnesota Children's Museum
809 Commerce Building
St. Paul 55101

Minnesota Children's Museum
2289 Lilac Lane
White Bear Lake 55110

Missouri

Historic Hermann Museum
Hermann 65041

W. R. Nelson Gallery & Atkins Museum of Fine Arts—Junior Gallery and Creative Arts Center
4525 Oak St.
Kansas City   64111

Nebraska

Children's Museum
P.O. Box 3393
Omaha 68102

New Hampshire

Thomas Bailey Aldrich Memorial
Portsmouth 03801

New Jersey

Monmouth County Historical Association Museum—Junior Museum
70 Court St.
Freehold 07728

Liberty Village
Flemington 08822

Montville Historical Museum—
Children's Museum
84 Main St.
Montville 07045

Morris Museum of Arts & Sciences
Box 125, Convent St.
Morristown 07961

Newark Museum—Junior Museum
43 Washington St.
Newark 07102

Princeton University Junior Museum
Princeton 08540

Gloucester County Historical Society—Children's Museum
58 N. Broad St.
Woodbury 08096

New York

The Brooklyn Children's Museum
145 Brooklyn Ave.
Brooklyn 11213

Hempstead Junior Museum
18 Catherine St.
Hempstead 11550

North Shore Science Museum
Science Activity Center
1526 North Plandome Rd.
Plandome Manor 11030

Metropolitan Museum of Art
Junior Museum
Fifth Avenue at 82nd St.
Manhattan 10028

Massena Historical Center & Museum
Town Hall
Main St.
Massena 13662

Staten Island Children's Museum
15 Beach St.
Staten Island 10304

Rensselaer County Junior Museum
282 Fifth Ave.
Troy 12182

Junior Museum of Oneida City
1703 Oneida St.
Utica 13501

History Center and Museum Children's Museum
Min and Portage Streets
Center of Village Park
Westfield 14787

North Carolina

Charlotte Natural Museum
1658 Sterling Rd.
Charlotte 28209

Durham Children's Museum
North Carolina Museum of Life &
Science
433 Murray Ave.
Durham 27704

Natural Science Center & Zoo,
Inc.
4301 Lawndale Dr.
Greensboro 27408

Creative Museum For Youth
406 Third Ave., NW
Hickory 28601

Rocky Mount Children's Museum
Sunset Park
Rocky Mount 27801

Historic Bethabara
Winston-Salem 27106

Nature Science Park
Museum Drive
Winston-Salem 27105

Ohio

Lake Erie Junior Nature and
Science Center
28728 Wolf St.
Bay Village 44140

Milan Historical Museum
Children's & Junior Museum
10 Edison Dr.
Milan 44846

Little Red Schoolhouse
80 South Main St.
Oberlin 44074

Oklahoma

Oklahoma Art Center
Oklahoma City 73107

Children's Museum of Tulsa
1015 East 19th St.
Tulsa 74120

Oregon

Portland Children's Museum
3037 SW, 2nd Ave.
Portland 97201

Wonderworks—A Children's Museum
Rt. 4, Box 253
The Dalles 97058

Pennsylvania

Please Touch Museum
120 W. Lancaster Ave.
Ardmore 19003

The Ways & Meaning Place at
Boas School
Green & Forster Sts.
Harrisburg 17102

The Children's Museum of NE
Pennsylvania
Kingston 18704

Parkway Program of Franklin Institute
20th St. & Parkway
Philadelphia 19103

Perelman Antique Toy Museum
207 S. 2nd St.
Philadelphia 19106